THIRD EDITION

EKG

Plain and Simple

Karen M. Ellis, RN

Touro Infirmary, New Orleans

Pearson

Boston   Columbus   Indianapolis   New York   San Francisco   Upper Saddle River
Amsterdam   Cape Town   Dubai   London   Madrid   Milan   Munich   Paris   Montreal   Toronto
Delhi   Mexico City   Sao Paulo   Sydney   Hong Kong   Seoul   Singapore   Taipei   Tokyo

Library of Congress Cataloging-in-Publication Data

Ellis, Karen M., author.
  EKG plain and simple / Karen M. Ellis, RN, Touro Infirmary, New Orleans.—Third edition.
      p. ; cm.
  Includes index.
  ISBN-13: 978-0-13-237729-4
  ISBN-10: 0-13-237729-2
  1. Electrocardiography. I. Title.
  [DNLM: 1. Electrocardiography. WG 140]
  RC683.5.E5E442 2011
  616.1'207547—dc22

                                        2010050980

Publisher: *Julie Levin Alexander*
Executive Assistant & Supervisor: *Regina Bruno*
Editor-in-Chief: *Mark Cohen*
Executive Editor: *Joan Gill*
Associate Editors: *Melissa Kerian and Bronwen Glowacki*
Editorial Assistant: *Mary Ellen Ruitenberg*
Development Editor: *Cathy Wein*
Director of Marketing: *David Gesell*
Executive Marketing Manager: *Katrin Beacom*
Marketing Specialist: *Michael Sirinides*
Senior Media Producer: *Amy Peltier*

Media Project Managers: *Lorena Cerisano and Julita Navarro*
Managing Production Editor: *Patrick Walsh*
Production Liaison: *Patricia Gutierrez*
Composition: *Laserwords Private Limited*
Production Editor: *Erika Jordan/Rebecca Lazure*
Manufacturing Manager: *Alan Fischer*
Creative Director: *Christy Mahon*
Art Director: *Kristine Carney*
Printer/Binder: *Courier/Kendallville*
Cover Printer: *Courier/Kendallville*
Cover/Interior Design: *Ilze Lemesis*

10 9 8 7 6

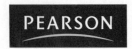

ISBN-10: 0-13-237729-2
ISBN-13: 978-0-13-237729-4

Contents

Introduction

Welcome to the third edition of *EKG Plain and Simple*. We've pulled out all the stops this time. There are lots of changes from the last edition.

More stuff. Better stuff. Not meaning to sound like a TV commercial, but we've got better stuff this edition.

Opening scenarios. Short opening scenarios show the clinical importance of that chapter's information.

Chapter Checkup. This new feature pops in at each chapter's halfway mark and asks a few pertinent questions to assess your understanding of the material. It can help you decide if you're ready to move ahead in the chapter or if you need to stop and review first.

Fewer chapters. Condensed from 19 chapters to 18, this edition simplifies EKG even more by combining information in a logical manner.

Study notes at the end of each chapter. This pulls together all of each chapter's important points in one place and makes studying easier. This is also available for download/printing off the student website.

More practice strips. More strips in each rhythms chapter and 250 in Chapter 12 make learning rhythm interpretation easier.

More tables, new photos, and better art. We've improved the art and added photographs of real-life situations, full color, and more tables so the book is more user-friendly and more visually appealing.

More clinical information on rhythms, heart attack symptoms, and treatment. This helps you see the whole person, not just the EKG.

More clinical anecdotes sprinkled throughout. The material makes more sense when it's shown in the context of a real-life situation. And it helps answer the question, "OK, I know what the rhythm/EKG shows; now what do I do with this information?"

Critical Thinking Exercises. Each chapter has exercises that might include case scenarios, diagrams to label, or other exercises that challenge you to put what you learned into practice.

More scenarios in the final chapter. Chapter 18 is an entire chapter of scenarios that require you to analyze the situation and decide on the rhythm or EKG, the normal treatment, and the expected outcome of that treatment. The added scenarios ensure that modern-day clinical issues are represented (and there are some doozies!).

MyHealthProfessionsKit myhealthprofessionskit This is an exciting addition that includes videos, animations, diagrams, scenarios, games, and practice tests—all certain to help you fine-tune your understanding of the book's material.

Instructor Resources. At MyHealthProfessionsKit, instructors can download chapter synopses, outlines, objectives, frequently asked questions, suggested class activities, and critical thinking questions. Also included is a test bank that allows instructors to generate customized exams and quizzes. There is also an updated comprehensive turn-key lecture package in a clicker-friendly PowerPoint® format.

The book starts, as before, with the basics in Part I. First is a little coronary anatomy and physiology, then EKG waves and complexes, lead morphology, and rhythms. You'll learn what the rhythm is, how to calculate the heart rate, and what the adverse effects and treatments are. There are critical thinking exercises and lots of practice strips to perfect your interpretation skills.

Part II covers 12-lead EKG interpretation. You'll learn what's normal on a 12-lead and what's pathological. Axis, hypertrophy, bundle branch blocks, hemiblocks, myocardial infarction, and pacemakers are just a few topics covered in Part II. Again there are lots of critical thinking exercises and an entire chapter of 12-leads for practice.

This third edition of *EKG Plain and Simple* is written in the same conversational style as the previous editions. Who wants to study some dry, boring textbook?

So turn the page and prepare to learn some good stuff....

Karen Ellis

Acknowledgments

The following people have been instrumental in their contributions to this effort and I'd like to thank them all:

Lehman Ellis, my husband, who bar none has the best smirk I've ever seen, and who always saves the day when my computer—or anything else—messes up. I love you, booboo.

My sons Jason, Mark, and Matthew; my daughter-in-law Lauren; and my soon-to-be daughter-in-law Myshel, for being so wonderful and so funny. They have my sense of humor, I keep telling them. To which their reply is "Wait—you think you're funny?"

ICU staff at Touro Infirmary, who are always on the lookout for good strips and EKGs for me, and who ask my opinion every now and then so I feel like I'm useful. Special shout-out to Terry Lafauci, Kathryn Rives, Holly Gab, Kristen Cannon, Erin Blaum, Becky Rohner, Lacey Sanders, Kimla Bell, Chris Sones, Toni Doyle, Jill Comeaux, Tanya Doucette, Jill Prattini, and Betty Bennet.

Former Emergency Department tech (and new nurse) Patrick Frye, a fellow EKG geek, for asking me disturbingly insightful questions that send me skulking off to do more research. And for being the only one I know who, like me, gets positively giddy at the sight of a really cool EKG.

Emergency Department nurses at Touro Infirmary, for tolerating with good humor my frequent meddling. Special shout-out to Ron Pelas, Paul Overland, Paul Garner, Samantha Santiago, Margaret Pentek, Lisa Mitchell, Lisa Grush, Brian Baudoin, Casey Saavedra, Amy Shepherd, Kelly Krieger, and Christine Troxlair.

Telemetry techs Karen Nix, Roxie Doskey, and Leola Bates, for finding cool strips.

My editors Melissa Kerian and Cathy Wein, whose advice and suggestions were always perfect, and whose respect for an author's autonomy has constantly amazed me. Melissa is my anchor—she's been with me for a while and is always reassuring and helpful. Cathy is a new addition to our team and her contribution has been invaluable. Conference calls with Melissa and Cathy have yielded a bounty of ideas and logistical suggestions. The teamwork has been exceptional.

Mark Cohen, formerly my editor but now a "big cheese," for still being there for me with support and guidance . . . and just a little bit of cheerleading.

Karen

Reviewers

Travis Fox, EMT-P
University of Antelope Valley
Palmdale, California

Scott C. Jones, MBA, EMT-P
Victor Valley College
Victorville, California

Dean C. Meenach, AAS, RN, BSN, CEN, CCRN, EMT-P
Mineral Area College
Park Hills, Missouri

Melyssa Munch, CPI, CMA
Star Career Academy
Brick, New Jersey

Auburne Overton, MHA, RPSGT
Mercy College of Health Sciences
Des Moines, Iowa

Krista T. Rodgers, BS, RMA
Miller-Motte Technical College
Charleston, South Carolina

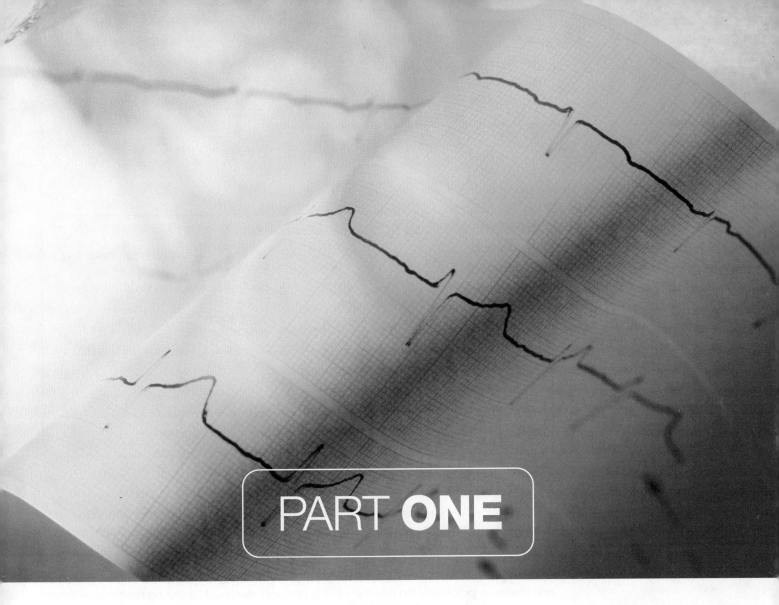

PART ONE

The Basics

1

Coronary Anatomy and Physiology

Upon completion of this chapter, the student will be able to:

- State the location of the heart and its normal size.
- Name the walls and layers of the heart.
- Name all the structures of the heart.
- Track the flow of blood through the heart.
- State the oxygen saturation of the heart's chambers.
- Describe the function and location of the heart valves.
- Describe the relationship of the valves to heart sounds.
- List the great vessels and the chamber into which they empty or from which they arise.
- State what occurs in each phase of the cardiac cycle.
- Name and describe the function of the coronary arteries.
- Differentiate between the two kinds of cardiac cells.
- Describe the sympathetic and parasympathetic nervous systems.
- Describe the *fight-or-flight* and *rest-and-digest* responses.

What It's All About

Mr. Huckabee was very nervous. He was scheduled for heart surgery in the morning. Not only did he have a "bad valve," as his surgeon called it; he also had three blocked coronary arteries, one of which was so bad it could cause a heart attack any minute. All this had been discovered when Mr. Huckabee's heart rhythm became erratic and began causing symptoms. The doctor did a full cardiac workup on him and found the blockages and the valve problems. So now he's in the hospital, nervously awaiting his surgery. When his nurse Jill asked him to tell her what he understood was to happen in surgery the next morning, he replied he really didn't know—the surgeon had told him so much so fast that he really didn't understand any of it. Jill took out a model of the heart and pointed out the heart valves and coronary arteries, explaining what they do and how his symptoms— heart rhythm disturbances, occasional chest pain, shortness of breath, and swelling of the legs—were all related to his heart problems. Jill then explained how the surgery would correct the problems. Mr. Huckabee visibly relaxed afterward, saying he was grateful Jill took the time to teach him about his heart. Mrs. Huckabee, who'd been listening to Jill's explanations, whispered "she's good" to her husband after Jill left the room, adding "I hope she's your nurse tomorrow night after the surgery. She really seems to know a lot."

Introduction

The function of the heart, a muscular organ about the size of a man's closed fist, is to pump enough blood to meet the body's metabolic needs. To accomplish this, the heart beats 60 to 100 times per minute and circulates 4 to 8 liters of blood per minute. Thus, each day the average person's heart beats approximately 90,000 times and pumps out about 6,000 liters of blood. With stress, exertion, or certain pathological conditions, these numbers can quadruple.

The heart is located in the **thoracic (chest) cavity**, between the lungs in a cavity called the **mediastinum**, above the diaphragm, behind the **sternum** (breastbone), and in front of the spine. It is entirely surrounded by bony structures for protection. This bony cage also serves as a means to revive the stricken heart, as the external chest compressions of CPR compress the heart between the sternum and spine and squeeze blood out until the heart's function can be restored.

The top of the heart is the **base**, from which the great vessels emerge. The bottom of the heart is the **apex**, the pointy part that rests on the diaphragm. The heart lies at an angle in the chest, with the bottom pointing to the left. See Figure 1-1.

Layers of the Heart

The heart has three layers:

- **Epicardium**   The outermost layer of the heart. The coronary arteries run along this layer.
- **Myocardium**   The middle and thickest layer. The myocardium is made of pure muscle and does the work of contracting. It's the part that's damaged during a heart attack.
- **Endocardium**   The thin innermost layer that lines the heart's chambers and folds back onto itself to form the heart valves. The endocardium is watertight to prevent leakage of blood into the other layers. The cardiac conduction system is found in this layer.

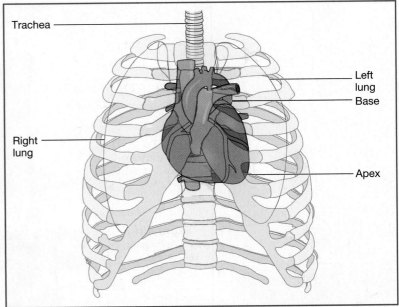

FIGURE 1–1

Heart's location in thoracic cavity.

Surrounding the heart is the **pericardium**, a double-walled sac that encloses the heart. Think of it as the film on a hard-boiled egg. The pericardium serves as support and protection and anchors the heart to the diaphragm and great vessels. A small amount of fluid is found between the layers of the pericardium. This **pericardial fluid** minimizes friction of these layers as they rub against each other with every heartbeat. See Figure 1-2 for an illustration of the heart's anatomy.

Heart Chambers

The heart has four chambers (see website for animations showing the heart layers and heart chambers):

- **Right atrium**   A receiving chamber for deoxygenated blood (blood that's had some oxygen removed by the body's tissues) returning to the heart from the body, the right atrium has an oxygen (O_2) saturation of only 60% to 75%. The blood in this chamber has so little oxygen, its color is dark maroon. Carbon dioxide (CO_2) concentration is high. The right atrium delivers its blood to the right ventricle.
- **Right ventricle**   The right ventricle pumps the blood to the lungs for a fresh supply of oxygen. O_2 saturation is 60% to 75%. Again, the blood is dark maroon in color. CO_2 concentration is high.
- **Left atrium**   This is a receiving chamber for the blood returning to the heart from the lungs. O_2 saturation is now about 100%. The blood is full of oxygen and is now bright red in color. CO_2 concentration is extremely low, as it was removed by the lungs. The left atrium delivers its blood to the left ventricle.
- **Left ventricle**   The left ventricle's job is to pump blood out to the entire body. It is the major pumping chamber of the heart. O_2 saturation is about 100%. Again, the blood is bright red in color. CO_2 concentration is minimal.

The atria's job is to deliver blood to the ventricles that lie directly below them. Since this is a short trip and minimal contraction is needed to transport this blood to the ventricles, the atria are thin-walled, low-pressure chambers.

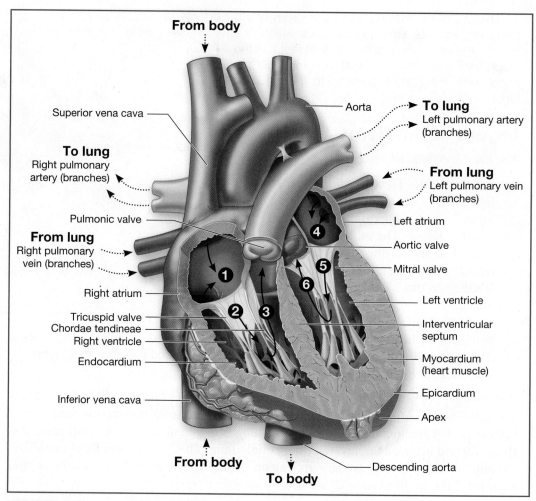

From body

Superior vena cava

Aorta

To lung
Left pulmonary artery
(branches)

To lung
Right pulmonary
artery (branches)

From lung
Left pulmonary vein
(branches)

Pulmonic valve

Left atrium

From lung
Right pulmonary
vein (branches)

Aortic valve

Mitral valve

Right atrium

Left ventricle

Tricuspid valve
Chordae tendineae
Right ventricle

Interventricular
septum

Endocardium

Myocardium
(heart muscle)

Inferior vena cava

Epicardium

Apex

From body

Descending aorta

To body

FIGURE 1–2

The heart: Its layers, chambers, and blood flow.

The ventricles, on the other hand, are higher-pressure chambers because they must contract more forcefully to deliver their blood into the pulmonary system and the systemic circulation. Since the right ventricle must pump its blood only to the nearby lungs, and pulmonary pressures are normally low, the right ventricle's pressure is relatively low and its muscle bulk is relatively thin. The left ventricle generates the highest pressures, as it not only must pump the blood the farthest (throughout the entire body); it also must pump against great resistance—the **blood pressure**. Because of this heavy workload, the left ventricle has three times the muscle bulk of the right ventricle and plays the prominent role in the heart's function.

The heart is divided into right and left sides by the **septum**, a muscular band of tissue. The septum separating the atria is called the **interatrial septum**. The septum separating the ventricles is called the **interventricular septum**.

Heart Valves

The heart has four valves to prevent backflow of blood. Two are semilunar valves and two are AV valves:

Semilunar valves separate a ventricle from an artery and have three half-moon-shaped cusps. The term *semilunar* means half moon. There are two semilunar valves:

- **Pulmonic valve**   This valve is located between the right ventricle and the pulmonary artery.
- **Aortic**   The aortic valve is located between the left ventricle and the aorta.

Atrioventricular (AV) valves are located between an atrium and a ventricle. They are supported by chordae tendineae (tendinous cords), which are attached to papillary muscles (muscles that outpouch from the ventricular wall) and anchor the valve cusps to keep the closed AV valves from flopping backward and allowing backflow of blood. There are two AV valves:

- **Tricuspid**   This valve, located between the right atrium and ventricle, has three cusps.
- **Mitral**   The mitral valve, also called the *bicuspid valve,* is located between the left atrium and ventricle. It has two cusps.

Valves open and close based on changes in pressure. *And they open only in the direction of blood flow.* Blood flows down from atrium to ventricle, and up from ventricle to aorta and pulmonary artery. For example, the tricuspid and mitral valves are located between the right atrium and ventricle and the left atrium and ventricle, respectively. Since blood flows down from atrium to ventricle, these valves open only one way—down. Thus, when the atria's pressure is higher than the ventricles' pressure, the tricuspid and mitral valves open to allow blood to flow into the waiting ventricles. The aortic and pulmonic valves open upward only when the pressure in the ventricles exceeds that in the waiting aorta and pulmonary artery. Blood then flows up into those arteries.

Valve closure is responsible for the sounds made by the beating heart. The normal lub-dub of the heart is made not by blood flowing through the heart, but by the closing of the heart's valves. S_1, the first heart sound, reflects closure of the mitral and tricuspid valves. S_2, the second heart sound, reflects closure of the aortic and pulmonic valves. Between S_1 and S_2, the heart beats and expels its blood (called **systole**). Between S_2 and the next S_1, the heart rests and fills with blood (called **diastole**). Each heartbeat has an S_1 and S_2. Note the valves on Figure 1-2.

Great Vessels

Attached to the heart at its base are the five great vessels (see website for a virtual tour of the heart and an animation of the heart vessels):

- **Superior vena cava (SVC)**   The SVC is the large vein that returns deoxygenated blood to the right atrium from the head, neck, and upper chest and arms.
- **Inferior vena cava (IVC)**   The IVC is the large vein that returns deoxygenated blood to the right atrium from the lower chest, abdomen, and legs.
- **Pulmonary artery**   This is the large artery that takes deoxygenated blood from the right ventricle to the lungs to load up on oxygen and unload carbon dioxide. It is the *only* artery that carries deoxygenated blood.
- **Pulmonary veins**   These are four large veins that return the oxygenated blood from the lungs to the left atrium. They are the *only* veins that carry oxygenated blood.
- **Aorta**   The aorta is the largest artery in the body. It takes oxygenated blood from the left ventricle to the systemic circulation to feed all the organs of the body.

Note the great vessels on Figure 1-2.

SA node starts beat

Blood Flow through the Heart

Now let's track a single blood cell as it travels through the heart:

Superior or inferior vena cava → right atrium → tricuspid valve → right ventricle → pulmonic valve →→ pulmonary artery →→ lungs →→ pulmonary veins →→ left atrium →→ mitral valve →→ left ventricle →→ aortic valve →→ aorta →→ body (systemic circulation)

- The blood cell enters the heart via either the **superior** or **inferior vena cava.**
- It then enters the **right atrium.**
- Next it travels through the **tricuspid valve** into the **right ventricle.**
- Then it passes through the **pulmonic valve** into the **pulmonary artery,** then into the **lungs** for oxygen/carbon dioxide exchange.
- It is then sent through the **pulmonary veins** to the **left atrium.**
- Then it travels through the **mitral valve** into the **left ventricle.**
- It passes through the **aortic valve** into the **aorta** and out to the **body (systemic circulation).**

chapter CHECKUP

We're about halfway through this chapter. To evaluate your understanding of the material thus far, answer the following questions. If you have trouble with them, review the material again before continuing.

1. Name the heart layers, chambers, valves, and great vessels. Describe the function of each.
2. Track the flow of blood through the heart.

Blood flow through the heart is accomplished by way of the cardiac cycle. Let's look at that now.

The Cardiac Cycle

The **cardiac cycle** refers to the mechanical events that occur to pump blood. There are two phases to the cardiac cycle—diastole and systole. During diastole, the ventricles relax and fill. During systole, the ventricles contract and expel their blood. Each of these phases has several phases of its own. See Figures 1-3 and 1-4.

coronary arteries

Diastole

systemic

- **Rapid-filling phase** This is the first phase of diastole. The atria, having received blood from the superior and inferior vena cava, are full of blood and therefore have high pressure. The ventricles, having just expelled their blood into the pulmonary artery and the aorta, are essentially empty and have lower pressure. This difference in pressure causes the AV valves to pop open and the atrial blood to flow down to the ventricles. Imagine the atria as a sponge. When the sponge is saturated with water, the water pours out in a steady stream at first.

- **Diastasis** Diastasis is the second phase of diastole. The pressure in the atria and ventricles starts to equalize as the ventricles fill and the atria empty, so blood flow slows. As the sponge becomes emptier, the flow slows to a trickle.

Quick Tip

Rapid-filling phase = atria dumping blood into ventricles

Diastasis = slowing blood flow

Atrial kick = atria contracting to squeeze remainder of blood into ventricles

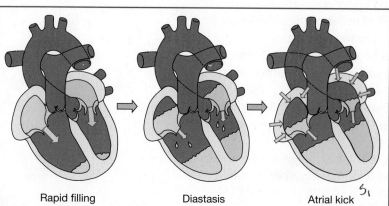

Rapid filling   Diastasis   Atrial kick S_1

FIGURE 1–3

Phases of diastole.

■ **Atrial kick** (See website for animations showing atrial contraction and the atrial cycle.) Atrial kick is the last phase of diastole. The atria are essentially empty, but there is still a little blood to deliver to the ventricle. Since the sponge is almost empty of water, what must be done to get the last little bit of water out of it? The atria therefore contract, squeezing in on themselves and propelling the remainder of the blood into the ventricles. The pressure in the ventricles at the end of this phase is high, as the ventricles are now full. Atrial pressure is low, as the atria are essentially empty. The AV valve leaflets, which have been hanging down in the ventricle in their open position, are pushed upward by the higher ventricular volume and its sharply rising pressure until they slam shut, ending diastole. S_1 is heard at this time. Atrial kick provides 15% to 30% of ventricular filling and is an important phase.

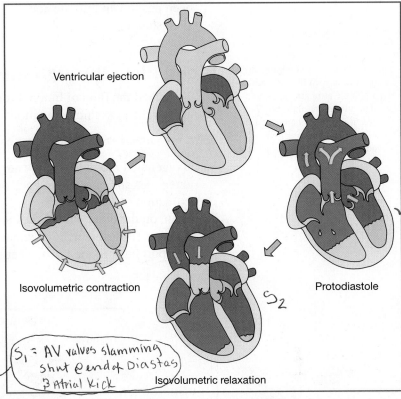

Ventricular ejection

Isovolumetric contraction

Protodiastole

S_2

Isovolumetric relaxation

[handwritten:] S_1 = AV valves slamming shut @ end of Diastas) ß Atrial Kick

FIGURE 1–4

Phases of systole.

Some heart rhythm abnormalities cause a loss of the atrial kick. This causes an immediate decrease in **cardiac output** (amount of blood pumped by the heart every minute). *[handwritten:]* ↓ Atrial Kick = ↓ Cardiac output

[handwritten:] S_2 = Semilunar Pulmonic ß Aortic valves slam shut @ end of Systole ß Isometric relaxation

Systole

① ■ **Isovolumetric contraction** (see website for animations showing ventricular contractions and the cardiac cycle). This is the first phase of systole. The ventricles are full, but the pressure in them is not high enough to exceed the blood pressure and pop the semilunar valves open. Since the ventricles cannot increase their pressure by adding more volume (they're as full as they're going to get), they squeeze down on themselves, forcing their muscular walls inward, putting pressure on the blood inside and causing the ventricular pressure to rise sharply. No blood flow occurs during this phase because all the valves are closed. This phase results in the greatest consumption of myocardial oxygen.

② ■ **Ventricular ejection** This is the second phase of systole. With the ventricular pressures now high enough, the semilunar valves pop open and blood pours out of the ventricles into the pulmonary artery and the aorta. Half the blood empties quickly and the rest a little slower.

③ ■ **Protodiastole** Protodiastole is the third phase of systole. Ventricular contraction continues, but blood flow slows as the ventricular pressure drops (since the ventricle is becoming empty) and the aortic and pulmonary arterial pressures rise (because they are filling with blood from the ventricles). Pressures are equalizing between the ventricles and the aorta and pulmonary artery.

④ ■ **Isovolumetric relaxation** This is the final phase of systole. Ventricular pressure is low because the blood has essentially been pumped out. The ventricles relax, causing the pressure to drop further. The aorta and pulmonary artery have higher pressures now, as they are full of blood. Since there is no longer any forward pressure from the ventricles to propel this blood further into the aorta and pulmonary artery, some of the blood in these arteries starts to flow back toward the aortic and pulmonic valves. This back pressure causes the valve leaflets, which had

Quick Tip

Isovolumetric contraction = ventricles squeezing but not pumping

Ventricular ejection = pumping vigorously

Protodiastole = pumping less

Isovolumetric relaxation = relaxing, valves closing to end systole been pushed up into the aorta and pulmonary arteries in their open position, to slam shut, ending systole. S_2 is heard now.

Blood Flow through the Systemic Circulation

We've tracked the flow of blood through the heart. Now let's track its course as it heads throughout the systemic circulation:

Aorta ➔➔ arteries ➔➔ arterioles ➔➔ capillary bed ➔➔ venules ➔➔ veins ➔➔ vena cava

- Oxygenated blood leaves the aorta and enters arteries, which narrow into arterioles and empty into each organ's capillary bed, where nutrient and oxygen extraction occurs.
- Then, on the other side of the capillary bed, this now-deoxygenated blood enters narrow venules, which widen into veins, and then return to the vena cava for transport back to the heart. Then the cycle repeats.

See Figure 1-5.

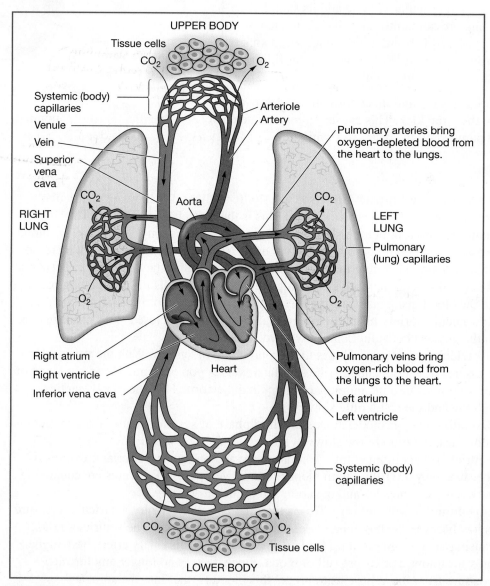

FIGURE 1–5

Systemic circulation.

Coronary Arteries

The heart must not only meet the needs of the body; it has its own needs. With the endocardium being watertight, none of the blood in the chambers can get to the myocardium to nourish it. So it has its own circulation—the coronary arteries—to do that. Coronary arteries arise from the base of the aorta and course along the epicardial surface of the heart and then dive into the myocardium to provide its blood supply. Unlike the rest of the body, however, the myocardium does not receive its blood supply during systole. Only in diastole is the heart able to feed itself. Blood cannot enter the coronary arteries during systole

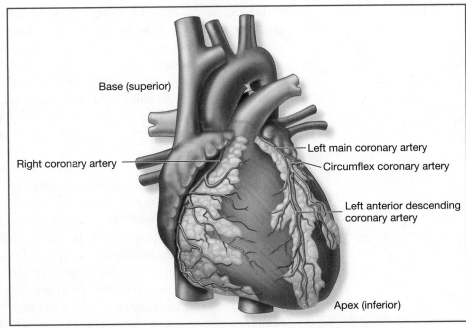

FIGURE 1–6

Coronary arteries.

because the heart muscle is contracting and essentially squeezing the coronary arteries shut. During diastole, the heart muscle stops contracting and the blood can then enter the coronary arteries and feed the myocardium. Let's look at the three main coronary arteries. See Figure 1-6.

- **Left anterior descending (LAD)**   The LAD is a branch off the left main coronary artery. The LAD supplies blood to the anterior wall of the left ventricle.
- **Circumflex**   The circumflex, also a branch of the left main coronary artery, feeds the lateral wall of the left ventricle. Since the LAD and the circumflex coronary arteries are branches off the left main coronary artery, blockage of the left main itself would knock out flow to both these branches. That can produce a huge heart attack sometimes referred to as the *widow-maker.*
- **Right coronary artery (RCA)**   The RCA feeds the right ventricle and the inferior wall of the left ventricle.

Once the myocardium has been fed by the coronary arteries, the deoxygenated blood is returned to the right atrium by **coronary veins.**

Heart Cells

The heart has two kinds of cells:

- **Contractile cells**   The contractile cells cause the heart muscle to contract, resulting in a heartbeat.
- **Conduction system cells**   The conduction system cells create and conduct electrical signals to tell the heart when to beat. Without these electrical signals, the contractile cells would *never* contract.

Nervous Control of the Heart

The heart is influenced by the **autonomic nervous system (ANS)**, which controls involuntary biological functions. The ANS is subdivided into the sympathetic and parasympathetic nervous systems.

The **sympathetic nervous system** is mediated by **norepinephrine**, a chemical released by the adrenal gland (see website for an animation regarding nervous system influence on the heart). Norepinephrine speeds up the heart rate, increases blood pressure, causes pupils to dilate, and slows digestion. This is the fight-or-flight response, and it's triggered by stress, exertion, or fear. Imagine you're walking your dog at night and an assailant puts a gun to your head. Your intense fear triggers the adrenal gland to pour out norepinephrine. Your heart rate and blood pressure shoot up. Your pupils dilate to let in more light so you can see the danger and the escape path better. Digestion slows down as the body shunts blood away from nonvital areas. (Is it essential to be digesting your pizza when your life is at stake? The pizza can wait.) So the body puts digestion on hold and shunts blood to vital organs, such as the brain, to help you think more clearly and to the muscles to help you fight or flee.

The **parasympathetic nervous system** is mediated by **acetylcholine**, a chemical secreted as a result of stimulation of the **vagus nerve**, a nerve that travels from the brain to the heart, stomach, and other areas. It slows the heart rate, decreases blood pressure, and enhances digestion. This is the rest-and-digest response. Parasympathetic stimulation can be caused by any action that closes the **glottis**, the flap over the top of the **trachea** (the windpipe). Breath holding and straining to have a bowel movement are two actions that can cause the heart rate to slow down. It is not uncommon for paramedics to be summoned to the scene of a "person found down" in the bathroom. Straining at stool causes vagal stimulation, which causes the heart rate to slow down. If the heart rate slows enough, **syncope** (fainting) can result. In extreme cases, the heart can stop, requiring **resuscitation**. Although the heart is influenced by the autonomic nervous system, it can also, in certain extreme circumstances, function for a time without any input from this system. For example, a heart that is removed from a donor in preparation for transplant is no longer in communication with the body, yet it continues to beat on its own for a while. This is possible because of the heart's conduction system cells, which create and conduct electrical impulses to tell the heart to beat.

In a nutshell, the sympathetic nervous system hits the accelerator and the parasympathetic nervous system puts on the brakes.

chapter one notes TO SUM IT ALL UP . . .

- **Heart's function**—Pump enough blood to meet the body's metabolic needs.
- **Heart has three layers:**
  - *Epicardium*—Outermost layer—where coronary arteries lie.
  - *Myocardium*—Middle muscular layer—does the work of contracting—damaged during a heart attack.
  - *Endocardium*—Innermost layer—watertight—lines the chambers and forms the heart valves. The conduction system is in this layer.
- **Heart has four chambers:**
  - *Right atrium*—Receiving chamber for deoxygenated blood returning to heart from body. Oxygen saturation is 60% to 75%. Blood is dark maroon.
  - *Right ventricle*—Pumps deoxygenated blood to lungs so it can be oxygenated. Oxygen saturation is 60% to 75%. Blood is dark maroon.
  - *Left atrium*—Receiving chamber for oxygenated blood coming from lungs. Oxygen saturation is 100%. Blood is bright red.
  - *Left ventricle*—Major pumping chamber of heart—pumps oxygenated blood to systemic circulation. Oxygen saturation is 100%. Blood is bright red.

- **Interventricular septum**—Band of tissue that separates right and left ventricles.
- **Interatrial septum**—Separates right and left atria.
- **Four heart valves**—Job is to prevent back flow of blood. Valves open in direction of blood flow—AV valves open downward, semilunar valves open upward.
  - *Pulmonic valve*—Semilunar valve between right ventricle and pulmonary artery.
  - *Aortic valve*—Semilunar valve between left ventricle and aorta.
  - *Tricuspid valve*—AV valve between right atrium and right ventricle.
  - *Mitral valve*—AV valve between left atrium and left ventricle.
- **Five great vessels:**
  - *Superior vena cava (SVC)*—Large vein—returns deoxygenated blood from upper body to the heart.
  - *Inferior vena cava (IVC)*—Large vein—returns deoxygenated blood from lower body to the heart.
  - *Pulmonary artery (PA)*—Takes deoxygenated blood from right ventricle to lungs—only artery in the body that carries deoxygenated blood.

- *Pulmonary veins*—Take oxygenated blood from lungs to left atrium—only veins that carry oxygenated blood.
- *Aorta (Ao)*—Main artery of the body—carries oxygenated blood to the body.

■ **Blood flow through heart:**

Superior/inferior vena cava → right atrium → tricuspid valve → right ventricle → pulmonic valve → pulmonary artery → lungs → pulmonary veins → left atrium → mitral valve → left ventricle → aortic valve → aorta → body

■ **Cardiac cycle**—Mechanical events that occur to pump blood. Two phases—diastole and systole. **Diastole**—ventricles relax and fill with blood. **Systole**—ventricles contract and expel blood.

■ **Diastole**—three phases:
- *Rapid filling*—Atria full of blood, ventricles empty. Pressure differential causes AV valves to pop open—blood rapidly fills ventricles.
- *Diastasis*—Pressures equalize between atria and ventricles—flow into ventricles slows.
- *Atrial kick*—Atria contract to squeeze remainder of blood into the ventricles.

■ **Systole**—four phases:
- *Isovolumetric contraction*—Ventricles contracting, no blood flow occurring because the aortic and pulmonic valves are still closed. Huge expenditure of myocardial oxygen consumption.
- *Ventricular ejection*—Valves open—blood pours out of ventricles into pulmonary artery and aorta.
- *Protodiastole*—Pressures equalize between ventricles and pulmonary artery and aorta—blood flow slows.

- *Isovolumetric relaxation*—Ventricles relax—pulmonic and aortic valves close.

■ **Blood flow through the systemic circulation:**

Aorta → arteries → arterioles → capillaries → venules → veins → vena cava

■ **Coronary arteries**—Supply blood flow to myocardium. Three coronary arteries:
- *Left anterior descending (LAD)*—Branch off left main coronary artery—provides blood flow to anterior wall of left ventricle.
- *Circumflex*—Also a branch off left main coronary artery—provides blood flow to lateral wall of left ventricle.
- *Right coronary artery*—Provides blood flow to right ventricle and inferior wall of left ventricle.

■ **Two kinds of heart cells:**
- *Contractile cells*—Cause the heart to contract, resulting in a heartbeat.
- *Conduction system cells*—Create and conduct electrical impulses to tell the heart when to beat.

■ **Heart influenced by the autonomic nervous system (ANS), which controls involuntary biological functions.** ANS subdivided into sympathetic (SNS) and parasympathetic nervous systems (PNS). Sympathetic nervous system hits the accelerator; parasympathetic puts on the brakes.
- *SNS*—Mediated by hormone norepinephrine—causes fight-or-flight response—speeds up heart rate, increases blood pressure, dilates pupils, and slows digestion.
- *PNS*—Mediated by acetylcholine—causes rest-and-digest response. Slows heart rate, lowers blood pressure, enhances digestion.

Practice Quiz

1. The function of the heart is to _____ _____

2. Name the three layers of the heart. _____ _____ _____ _____

3. Name the four chambers of the heart. _____ _____ _____ _____

4. Name the four heart valves. _____ _____

5. The purpose of the heart valves is to _____ _____

6. Name the five great vessels of the heart. _____ _____

7. List the phases of diastole. _____ _____ _____

8. List the phases of systole. _____ _____ _____

9. Name the two divisions of the autonomic nervous system. _____ _____

10. The three main coronary arteries are _____ _____

Putting It All Together—Critical Thinking Exercises

These exercises may consist of diagrams to label, scenarios to analyze, brain-stumping questions to ponder, or other challenging exercises to boost your understanding of the chapter material.

1. Label the heart diagram.

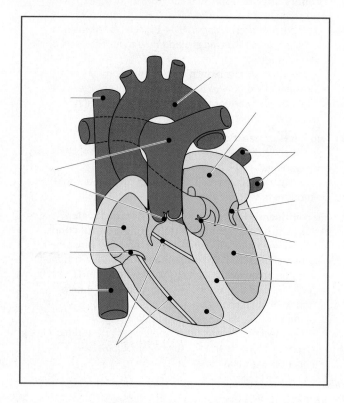

2. Number the following structures 1–14 in order of blood flow through the heart:

_____ superior and inferior vena cava

_____ tricuspid valve

_____ mitral valve

_____ aortic valve

_____ pulmonic valve

_____ body

_____ aorta

_____ pulmonary artery

_____ lungs

_____ pulmonary veins

_____ right atrium

_____ left atrium

_____ right ventricle

_____ left ventricle

3. What would happen to the tricuspid and mitral valves if their chordae tendineae "snapped" loose?

Electrophysiology

2

CHAPTER 2 OBJECTIVES

Upon completion of this chapter, the student will be able to:

- Define the terms *polarized, depolarization,* and *repolarization* and relate them to contraction and relaxation.
- Describe and label the phases of the action potential.
- Define *transmembrane potential.*
- Draw and explain the P wave, QRS complex, T wave, and U wave.
- Explain where the PR and ST segments are located.
- Define the *absolute* and *relative refractory periods* and the implications of each.
- Be able to label, on a rhythm strip, all the waves and complexes.
- Explain the delineations of EKG paper.
- On a rhythm strip, determine if the PR, QRS, and QT intervals are normal or abnormal.

- Name the waves in a variety of QRS complexes.
- Define *pacemaker.*
- List the different pacemakers of the heart and their inherent rates.
- Track the cardiac impulse from the sinus node through the conduction system.
- Define the four characteristics of cardiac cells.
- Describe the difference between *escape* and *usurpation.*
- Define *arrhythmia.*
- Tell what happens:
  When the sinus node fails
  When the sinus node and atria both fail
  When the sinus node, atria, and AV node all fail

What It's All About

Mrs. Mahoney was admitted to the hospital because Dr. Parker wanted to watch her closely while he adjusted her heart rhythm medications. Mrs. Mahoney had an extensive cardiac history—she'd already had two heart attacks and had cardiac arrested with the last one. "I'm lucky to be alive," she joked with her nurse Toni. On admission her PR interval was 0.16 seconds, QRS interval was 0.08 secs, QT interval 0.36 secs, heart rate was 88, sinus rhythm—all normal. Toni checked Mrs. Mahoney's rhythm, intervals, and heart rate every 4 hours per hospital protocol. Sixteen hours after being started on her new medication, Mrs. Maloney's PR interval had increased to 0.24 secs and her QT interval was 0.48 secs—a big change. Her QRS interval was unchanged. Toni notified Dr. Parker, who cut back on the dose of medication. "This is why I wanted her in the hospital for this," the physician told Toni. "With that drastic a change in her intervals, she could easily have developed a lethal arrhythmia. And she's already done that once. Thanks for paying close attention to those numbers."

Introduction

Cardiac cells at rest are electrically negative on the inside compared with the outside. Movement of charged particles (**ions**) of sodium and potassium into and out of the cell causes changes that can be picked up by sensors on the skin and printed out as an EKG.

Depolarization and Repolarization

The negatively charged resting cardiac cell is **polarized**. There are sodium ions primarily outside the cell (extracellular) and potassium ions primarily inside the cell (intracellular). Though both these ions carry a positive electrical charge, the intracellular

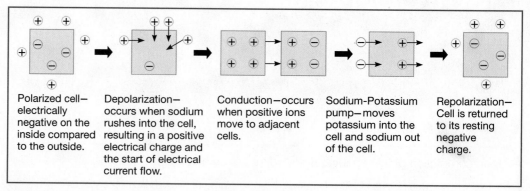

Polarized cell—electrically negative on the inside compared to the outside.

Depolarization—occurs when sodium rushes into the cell, resulting in a positive electrical charge and the start of electrical current flow.

Conduction—occurs when positive ions move to adjacent cells.

Sodium-Potassium pump—moves potassium into the cell and sodium out of the cell.

Repolarization—Cell is returned to its resting negative charge.

FIGURE 2–1

Depolarization and repolarization.

potassium has a much weaker positive charge than the extracellular sodium. Thus, the inside of the cell is electrically negative compared with the outside. The polarized state is a state of readiness—the cardiac cell is ready for electrical action. When the cardiac cell is stimulated by an electrical impulse, a large amount of sodium rushes into the cell and a small amount of potassium leaks out, causing a discharge of electricity. The cell then becomes positively charged. This is called **depolarization**. An electrical wave then courses from cell to cell, spreading this electrical charge throughout the heart. During cell recovery, sodium and potassium ions are shifted back to their original places by way of the **sodium-potassium pump**, an active transport system that returns the cell to its negative charge. This is called **repolarization**. See Figure 2–1.

Depolarization and repolarization are the myocardium's electrical stimuli. Myocardial contraction and relaxation should be the mechanical response. Depolarization should result in muscle contraction; repolarization should result in muscle relaxation. *Electrical stimulus precedes mechanical response. There can be no heartbeat (a mechanical event) without first having had depolarization (the electrical stimulus).* To illustrate this principle, let's look at your vacuum cleaner. Its mechanical function is to suck up dirt, but it can't do its job without being plugged into an electrical source first. So if your power goes out, your vacuum cleaner won't work, will it? Likewise, if the heart's electrical system "goes out," the heart's pumping will stop. *Electrical stimulus precedes mechanical response.*

What happens if you plug in your vacuum and it still doesn't work? There could be a mechanical malfunction that prevents it from working. Likewise with the heart: The electrical stimulus may be there, but if there is a bad enough mechanical problem with the heart itself, it won't be able to respond to that stimulus by pumping.

The heart's electrical and mechanical systems are two separate systems. They can malfunction separately or together. Electrical malfunctions show up on the EKG. Mechanical malfunctions show up clinically.

Imagine this scenario: A man has a massive heart attack that damages a large portion of his myocardium. His heart's electrical system has not been damaged, so it sends out its impulses as usual. The heart muscle cells, however, have been so damaged that they are unable to respond to those impulses by contracting. Consequently, the EKG shows the electrical system is still working, but the patient's heart is not beating. He has no pulse and is not breathing. The vacuum was plugged in, but it was broken and couldn't do its job. *Electrical stimulus precedes—but does not guarantee—mechanical response.*

Quick Tip

Depolarization *should* result in muscle contraction. Repolarization *should* result in muscle relaxation.

The Action Potential

Let's look at what happens to a ventricular muscle cell when it's stimulated. See Figure 2–2. There are four phases to the **action potential:**

- *In phase 4.* The cardiac cell is at rest. It is negatively charged with a resting **transmembrane potential** (the electrical charge at the cell membrane) of −90 millivolts. Electrically, nothing is happening. (Note phase 4 is a flat line. *Flat lines indicate electrical silence.*)
- *In phase 0.* The cardiac cell is stimulated. Sodium rushes into the cell, and potassium leaks out, resulting in a positive charge within the cell. This is called depolarization. You can see that at the top of phase 0, the cell's charge is above the zero mark, and the cell is thus positively charged. Phase 0 corresponds with the QRS complex on the EKG. The QRS complex is a spiked waveform that represents depolarization of the ventricular myocardium.

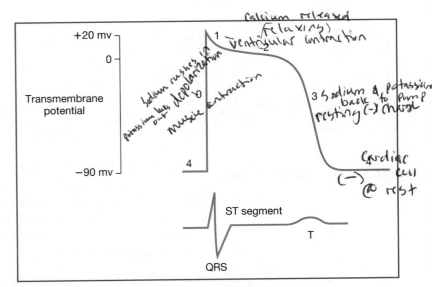

FIGURE 2–2

Action potential.

- *Phases 1 and 2 are* **early repolarization.** Calcium is released in these two phases, resulting in ventricular contraction. Phases 1 and 2 correspond with the ST segment of the EKG. The ST segment is a flat line on the EKG that follows the QRS complex and represents a period of electrical silence. But the heart is not physically at rest—it is contracting. Phase 2 is called the **plateau phase**, because the waveform levels off here.
- *Phase 3 is* **rapid repolarization.** Sodium and potassium return to their normal places via the sodium-potassium pump, thus returning the cell to its resting negative charge. Phase 3 corresponds with the T wave of the EKG. The T wave is a broad rounded wave that follows the ST segment and represents ventricular repolarization. The cardiac cell then relaxes.

Refractory Periods

The word **refractory** means "resistant to." Let's look at the periods when the cardiac cell resists responding to an impulse. See Figure 2–3.

- **Absolute** The cell cannot accept another impulse because it's still dealing with the last one. Absolutely no stimulus, no matter how strong, will result in another depolarization.
- **Relative** A strong stimulus will result in depolarization.
- **Supernormal period** Even a weak stimulus will cause depolarization. The cardiac cell is "hyper." Stimulation at this time can result in very fast, dangerous rhythms.

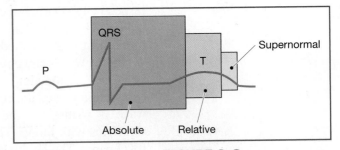

FIGURE 2–3

Refractory periods.

EKG Waves and Complexes

Depolarization and repolarization of the atria and ventricles result in waves and complexes on the EKG paper. Let's examine these waveforms. See Figure 2–4.

- **P wave** Represents atrial depolarization. The normal P is small, rounded, and upright, but many things can alter the P wave shape.
- **T$_a$ wave** Represents atrial repolarization—usually not seen, as it occurs at the same time as the QRS complex.

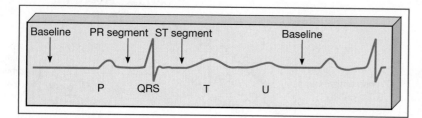

FIGURE 2–4

EKG waves and complexes.

- **QRS complex**   Represents ventricular depolarization. The normal QRS is spiked in appearance, consisting of one or more deflections from the baseline. The QRS complex is the most easily identified structure on the EKG tracing. Its shape can vary.
- **T wave**   Represents ventricular repolarization. The normal T wave is broad and rounded. If the QRS is upright, the T wave usually is also. If there is a QRS complex, there *must* be a T wave after it. *Any tissue that depolarizes must repolarize.* Many things can alter the T wave shape.
- **U wave**   Represents late ventricular repolarization and is not normally seen. If present, the U wave follows the T wave. It should be shallow and rounded, the same deflection as the T wave (i.e., if the T wave is upright, the U wave should be also).

See Table 2–1 for a summary of the waves and complexes.

TABLE 2–1   Waves and Complexes Summary

Kind of Wave	Represents	Normal Shape
P wave	Atrial depolarization	Small, rounded, upright in most leads
T_a wave	Atrial repolarization	Usually not seen as it's inside QRS
QRS complex	Ventricular depolarization	Spiked upward and/or downward deflections
T wave	Ventricular repolarization	Broad, rounded, upright if the QRS is upright
U wave	Late ventricular repolarization	Shallow, broad, rounded, same deflection as T wave

Each P-QRS-T sequence is one heartbeat. The flat lines between the P wave and the QRS and between the QRS and T wave are called the **PR segment** and the **ST segment**, respectively. During these segments, no electrical activity is occurring. (Flat lines indicate electrical silence.) The flat line between the T wave of one beat and the P wave of the next beat is called the **baseline** or **isoelectric line**. The baseline is the line from which the waves and complexes take off.

Atrial contraction occurs during the P wave and the PR segment. Ventricular contraction occurs during the QRS and the ST segment. When the atria depolarize, a P wave is written on the EKG paper. Following this, the atria contract, filling the ventricles with blood. Then the ventricles depolarize, causing a QRS complex on the EKG paper. The ventricles then contract.

Waves and Complexes Identification Practice

Following are strips on which to practice identifying P waves, QRS complexes, and T waves. You'll recall that P waves are normally upright, but they can also be inverted (upside down) or biphasic (up *and* down). P waves usually precede the QRS complex, so find the QRS and then look for the P wave. Some rhythms have more than one P wave and others have no P at all. Write the letter *P* over each P wave you see.

The QRS complex is the most easily identified structure on the strip because of its spiked appearance. Write *QRS* over each QRS complex.

T waves are normally upright but can also be inverted or biphasic. Wherever there is a QRS complex, there must be a T wave. Write a *T* over each T wave.

1.

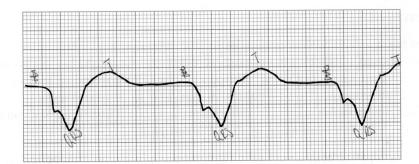

2.

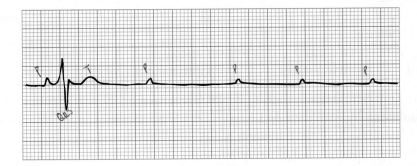

3.

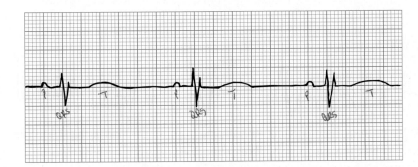

4.

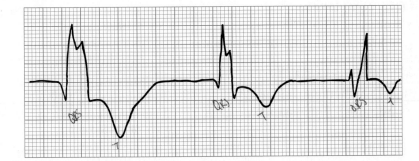

5.

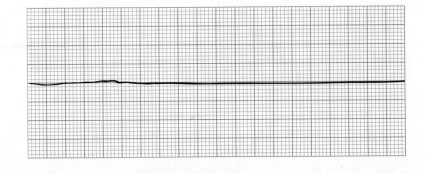

QRS Nomenclature

Now that we know what a QRS complex looks like, let's fine-tune that a bit. The QRS complex is composed of waves that have different names—Q, R, and S—but no matter which waves it's composed of, it's still referred to as the QRS complex. Think of it like this: There are many kinds of dogs—collies, boxers, and so on—but they're still dogs. Likewise, the QRS complex can have different names, but it's still a QRS complex. Let's look at the waves that can make up the QRS complex.

- **Q wave**   A negative deflection (wave) that occurs before a positive deflection. There can be only one Q wave. If present, it must always be the first wave of the QRS complex.
- **R wave**   Any positive deflection. There can be more than one R wave. A second R wave is called **R prime**, written **R′**.
- **S wave**   A negative deflection that follows an R wave.
- **QS wave**   A negative deflection with no positive deflection at all.

As in the alphabet, Q comes before R and S comes after R. See Figure 2–5. The dotted line indicates the baseline. Any wave in the QRS complex that goes above the baseline is an R wave; any wave going below the baseline is either a Q or an S wave.

See Table 2–2 for a summary of the QRS waves.

Quick Tip

When you name the QRS waves, you're naming the upward and downward spikes that comprise the QRS complex.

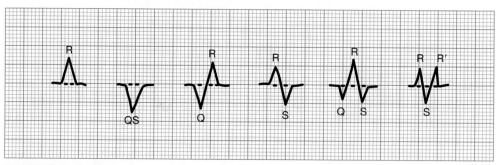

FIGURE 2–5

Examples of QRS complexes.

TABLE 2–2   Summary of QRS Waves

QRS Wave	Deflection	Location	Comments
Q wave	Negative	Precedes R wave	If present, Q wave is *always* first wave of QRS complex
R wave	Positive	Can stand alone or be preceded or followed by Q and/or S	Can have more than one; second R wave is called R prime, written R′
S wave	Negative	Follows R wave	
QS wave	Negative	Stands alone	

QRS Nomenclature Practice

Name the waves in the following QRS complexes:

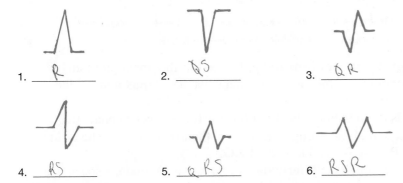

1. _R_   2. _QS_   3. _QR_

4. _RS_   5. _QRS_   6. _RSR_

Now draw the following:

1. RSR′   2. QRS   3. QS

4. QR   5. RS   6. R

Cardiac Conduction System

The **conduction system** is a pathway of specialized cells whose job is to create and conduct the electrical impulses that tell the heart when to pump. The area of the conduction system that initiates the impulses is called the **pacemaker**. See Figure 2–6.

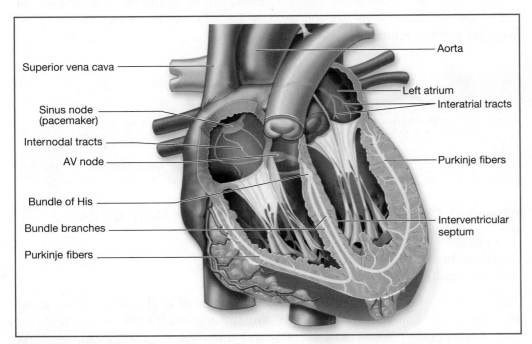

FIGURE 2–6

Cardiac conduction system.

Conduction Pathway

Let's look at the conduction pathway through the heart (see website for an animation of the conduction system):

Sinus node →→ interatrial tracts →→ atrium →→ internodal tracts →→ AV node →→ bundle of His →→ bundle branches →→ Purkinje fibers →→ ventricle

- The impulse originates in the sinus node, located in the upper right atrium just beneath the opening of the superior vena cava. The sinus node is the heart's normal pacemaker.
- From here it travels through the interatrial tracts. These special conductive highways carry the impulses through the atria to the atrial tissue. The atria then depolarize, and a P wave is written on the EKG.
- The impulse travels through the internodal tracts to the AV node, a specialized group of cells located just to the right of the septum in the lower right atrium. The AV node slows impulse transmission a little, allowing the newly depolarized atria to propel their blood into the ventricles.
- Then the impulse travels through the bundle of His, located just beneath the AV node, to the left and right bundle branches, the main highways to the ventricles.
- Then the impulse is propelled through the Purkinje fibers.
- Finally, the impulse arrives at the ventricle itself, causing it to depolarize. A QRS complex is written on the EKG paper.

Cardiac Cells

Cardiac cells have several characteristics:

- **Automaticity**   The ability to create an impulse without outside stimulation.
- **Conductivity**   The ability to pass this impulse along to neighboring cells.
- **Excitability**   The ability to respond to this stimulus by depolarizing.
- **Contractility**   The ability to contract and do work.

The first three characteristics are electrical. The last is mechanical.

Though the sinus node is the normal pacemaker of the heart, other cardiac cells can become the pacemaker if the sinus node fails. Let's look at that a little more closely. (See website for an animation showing the heart inherent rates.)

---

chapter CHECKUP

We're about halfway through this chapter. To evaluate your understanding of the material thus far, answer the following questions. If you have trouble with them, review the material again before continuing.

1. Explain *depolarization* and *repolarization*.
2. Name the EKG waves and complexes and state what each represents.
3. Track the electrical current through the conduction system.

Quick Tip

Unlike the sinus node and the ventricle, the AV node itself has no pacemaker cells. The tissue between the atria and the AV node, however—an area called the AV junction—does have pacemaking capabilities. Thus the term AV node is an anatomical term and AV junction refers to a pacemaking area.

Inherent (Escape) Rates of the Pacemaker Cells

- Sinus node: 60 to 100 beats per minute
- AV junction: 40 to 60 beats per minute
- Ventricle: 20 to 40 beats per minute

The sinus node, you'll note, has the fastest inherent rate of all the potential pacemaker cells. This means that barring any outside stimuli that speed it up or slow it down, the sinus node will fire at its rate of 60 to 100 beats per minute. The lower pacemakers (AV junction and ventricle) have slower inherent rates, each one having a slower rate than the one above it.

The fastest pacemaker at any given moment is the one in control. Thus, the lower pacemakers are inhibited, or restrained, from firing as long as some other pacemaker is faster. The lower pacemakers serve as a backup in case of conduction failure from above. The only thing that inhibits those pacemakers from escaping (taking over as the pacemaker at their slower inherent rate) is if they have been depolarized by a faster impulse. If that faster impulse never arrives, the next pacemaker in line will assume that *it* is now the fastest and should escape its restraints to become the new pacemaker.

Confused? Imagine that all the pacemaker cells have two *main* functions—to create an impulse (automaticity) and to conduct that impulse (conductivity). Normally the sinus node creates the impulse and sends it down the line. Once it arrives at the AV node, the AV junction's automaticity circuit is shut off—it doesn't need to create an impulse; it just needs to conduct it. So the AV junction sends the impulse down to the ventricle, where the ventricle's automaticity circuit is also shut off, again because there's no need to create an impulse that's already there. So the ventricle conducts the impulse through its tissue and—voila!—ventricular depolarization occurs.

Now what if the sinus node doesn't create that impulse? Maybe it was damaged by an MI (heart attack). The AV junction would never receive the anticipated impulse from above, so there'd be nothing to shut off its automaticity circuit. It should then create the impulse and send it down to the ventricle. The ventricle's automaticity circuit would then be shut off once it receives that impulse, so it would just conduct it through its tissue.

What if neither the sinus node nor the AV junction creates the impulse? (Is this guy having a bad day or what?) The ventricle would have been waiting to receive that impulse from above, so when it doesn't come, there's nothing to shut off *its* automaticity circuit. The ventricle would then create the impulse and conduct it through the ventricular tissue.

Conduction Variations

Normal conduction of cardiac impulses is dependent on the health of each part of the conduction system. Failure of any part of the system necessitates a variation in conduction. Let's look at several conductive possibilities. In the following figures, the large heart represents the pacemaker in control. See Figure 2–7.

In Figure 2–7, the sinus node fires out its impulse. When the impulse depolarizes the atrium, a P wave is written. The impulse then travels to the AV node, and on to the ventricle. A QRS is written when the ventricle is depolarized.

If the sinus node fails, however, one of the lower pacemakers will escape its restraints and take over at its slower inherent rate, thus becoming the heart's new pacemaker. If the AV junction escapes, it will fire at a rate of 40 to 60. If the ventricle takes over, the rate will be 20 to 40. Needless to say, if the ventricle has to kick in as

> **Quick Tip**
>
> Once a lower pacemaker (the AV junction or the ventricle) has received an impulse from above, its automaticity circuit is shut off, and all it has to do is conduct that impulse down the conduction pathway.

FIGURE 2–7

Normal conduction.

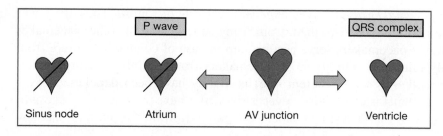

FIGURE 2–8

Sinus fails; AV junction escapes.

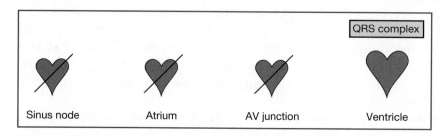

FIGURE 2–9

All higher pacemakers fail; ventricle escapes.

the pacemaker, it is a grave situation, since it means that all the pacemakers above it have failed. Remember—no pacemaker can escape unless it's the fastest at that particular time.

In Figure 2–8, the sinus node has failed. The AV junction is now the fastest escape pacemaker. It creates an impulse and sends it forward toward the ventricle and backward toward the atria, providing the P and the QRS.

In Figure 2–9, both the sinus node and AV junction have failed. The only remaining pacemaker is the ventricle, so it takes over as the pacemaker, providing the QRS. There is no P wave when the ventricle escapes.

What if the sinus node fires its impulse out but the impulse is blocked at some point along the conduction pathway? The first pacemaker below the block should escape and become the new pacemaker.

In Figure 2–10, the sinus node fires out its impulse, which depolarizes the atrium and writes a P wave. The impulse is then blocked between the atrium and the AV node. Since the faster sinus impulse never reaches the AV node, the AV junction assumes the sinus node has failed. So it escapes, creates its own new impulse, and becomes the new pacemaker, sending the impulse down to the ventricle and backward to the atria. (Backward conduction can work even when forward conduction is blocked.) If the impulse were blocked between the AV node and the ventricle, the ventricle would become the new pacemaker.

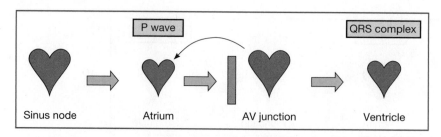

FIGURE 2–10

Block in conduction; AV junction escapes.

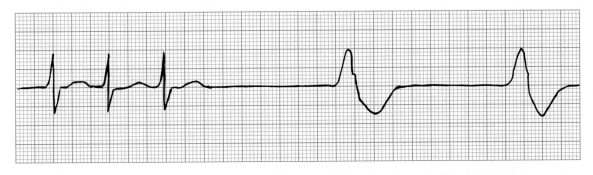

FIGURE 2–11

Escape.

Each of the pacemakers can fire at rates faster or slower than their inherent rates if there are outside stimuli. We've talked briefly about escape. Let's look at an example of escape compared with usurpation.

Escape occurs when the predominant pacemaker slows dramatically (or fails completely) and a lower pacemaker takes over at its inherent rate, providing a new rhythm that is slower than the previous rhythm. *An escape beat is any beat that comes in after a pause that's longer than the normal heartbeat-to-heartbeat cycle* (**R-R interval**). Escape beats are lifesavers. An escape rhythm is a series of escape beats.

In Figure 2–11, the normal pacemaker stops suddenly and there is a long pause, at the end of which is a beat from a lower pacemaker and then a new rhythm with a heart rate slower than before. This is escape.

Usurpation, also called irritability, means "to take control away from" and occurs when one of the lower pacemakers becomes irritable and fires in at an accelerated rate, stealing control away from the predominant pacemaker. Usurpation results in a faster rhythm than before, and it starts with a beat that comes in earlier than expected.

In Figure 2–12, the controlling pacemaker is cruising along and suddenly an impulse from a lower pacemaker fires in early, takes control, and is off and running with a new, faster rhythm. This is usurpation.

Proper function of the conduction system results in a **heart rhythm**, a pattern of successive heart beats, that originates in the sinus node. Abnormalities of the conduction system can produce **arrhythmias**, abnormal heart rhythms. Although these conduction system problems are most often related to heart disease, there are also diseases that affect the conduction system outright. Whatever the cause, conduction system abnormalities can prove harmful or fatal if not treated appropriately.

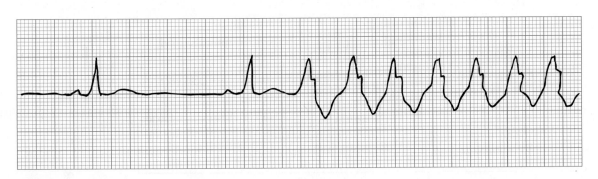

FIGURE 2–12

Usurpation.

TABLE 2–3   EKG Paper Delineations

EKG Feature	Equals
Each small block	0.04 secs (from one small line to the next)
Five small blocks	One big block
One big block	0.20 secs
25 small blocks	1 sec
Five big blocks	1 sec
1,500 small blocks	1 minute
300 big blocks	1 minute
One small block in amplitude	A millimeter

EKG Paper

EKG paper is graph paper divided into small blocks that are 1 millimeter (mm) in height and width. Dark lines are present every fifth block to subdivide the paper vertically and horizontally. Measurements of the EKG waves and complexes are done by counting these blocks. Counting horizontally measures time, or intervals. Intervals are measured in seconds. Counting vertically measures amplitude, or the height of the complexes. Amplitude is measured in millimeters.

A **12-lead EKG** is a printout of the heart's electrical activity viewed from 12 different angles as seen in 12 different leads. A lead is simply an electrocardiographic picture of the heart's electrical activity. A 12-lead EKG is typically done on special 8 × 11–inch paper, using a three-channel recorder that prints a simultaneous view of three leads at a time in sequence until all 12 leads are recorded.

A rhythm strip is a printout of one or two leads at a time and is done to assess the patient's heart rhythm. Rhythm strips are recorded on small rolls of special paper about 3 to 5 inches wide and several hundred feet in length. A 6- to 12-second strip is usually obtained, and the paper is cut to the desired length afterward. Rhythm strip paper often has lines at the top of the paper at 1- to 3-second intervals. Let's look at the EKG paper delineations. See Table 2–3.

No matter whether the EKG paper is 12-lead size or rhythm strip size, the delineations will be the same.

Figure 2–13 is an example of EKG paper. **Identifying data,** such as name, date, time, and room number, and **interpretive data,** such as heart rate, are printed at the top

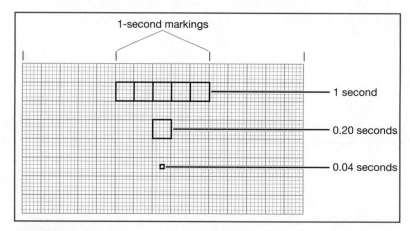

FIGURE 2–13

EKG paper.

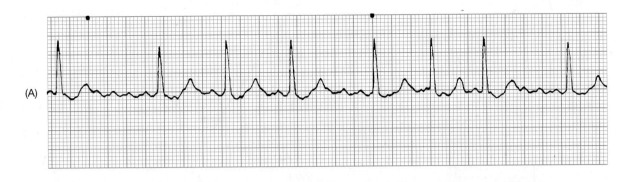

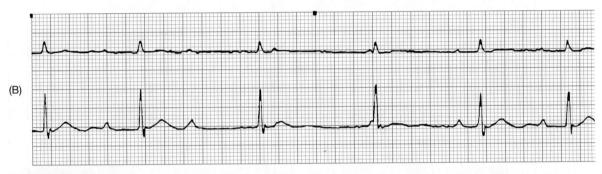

FIGURE 2–14

(A) Single- and (B) double-lead rhythm strips.

of the paper. Figure 2–14 shows single- and double-lead rhythm strips. Note that on the double-lead strip, one lead's waves and complexes show up much more clearly than on the other lead. This is typical.

See Figure 2–15 for a 12-lead EKG. Note the lead markings. Leads are arranged in four columns of three leads. Leads I, II, and III are in the first column, then aVR, aVL, and aVF in the second column, V_1 to V_3 in the third column, and V_4 to V_6 in the last column. At the bottom of the paper is a page-wide rhythm strip, usually of either Lead II or V_1.

Intervals

Now let's look at intervals, the measurement of time between the P-QRS-T waves and complexes. The heart's current normally starts in the right atrium and then spreads through both atria and down to the ventricles. Interval measurements enable a determination of the heart's efficiency at transmitting its impulses down the pathway. See Figure 2–16.

- **PR interval**   Measures the time it takes for the impulse to get from the atria to the ventricles. Normal PR interval is 0.12 to 0.20 seconds. It's measured from the beginning of the P wave to the beginning of the QRS and includes the P wave and the PR segment. The P wave itself should measure no more than 0.10 seconds in width and 2.5 mm in height.
- **QRS interval**   Measures the time it takes to depolarize the ventricles. Normal QRS interval is less than 0.12 seconds, usually between 0.06 and 0.10 seconds. It's measured from the beginning of the QRS to the end of the QRS.
- **QT interval**   Measures depolarization and repolarization time of the ventricles. The QT interval is measured from the beginning of the QRS to the end of the T wave and includes the QRS complex and the T wave. At normal heart rates of

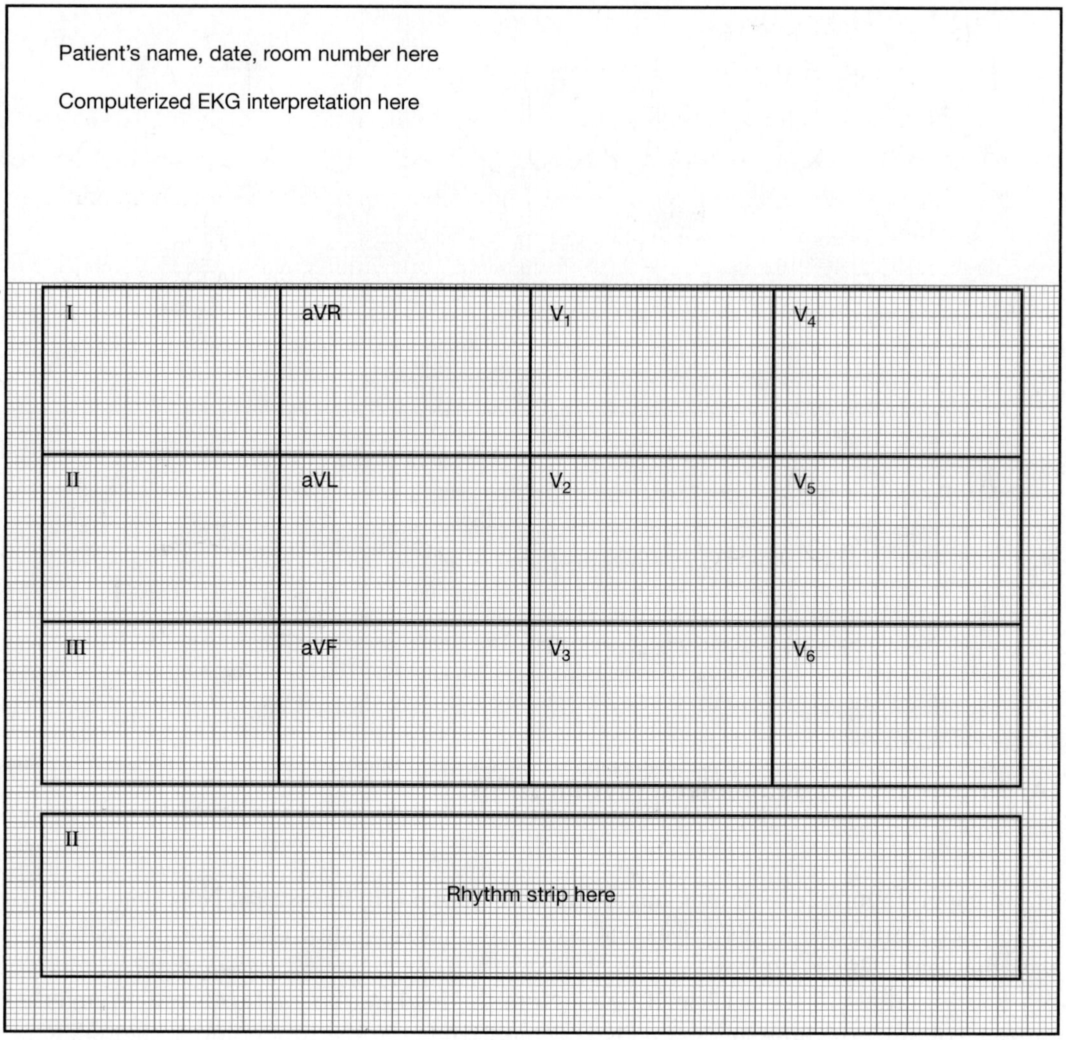

Patient's name, date, room number here

Computerized EKG interpretation here

| I | aVR | V$_1$ | V$_4$ |

| II | aVL | V$_2$ | V$_5$ |

| III | aVF | V$_3$ | V$_6$ |

| II | | | |

Rhythm strip here

FIGURE 2–15

12-lead EKG.

60 to 100, the QT interval should be less than or equal to one-half the distance between successive QRS complexes (the R-R interval). To quickly determine if the QT is prolonged, draw a line midway between QRS complexes. If the T wave ends at or before this line, the QT is normal. If it ends after the line, it is prolonged and can lead to lethal arrhythmias.

See Table 2–4 for an intervals summary.

TABLE 2–4 Intervals Summary

Interval	Represents	Normal Value
PR interval	Time traveling from atrium to ventricle	0.12–0.20 seconds
QRS interval	Ventricular depolarization time	Less than 0.12 seconds (usually between 0.06–0.10 seconds)
QT interval	Ventricular depolarization and repolarization time	Varies with heart rate—should be less than half the R-R interval if heart rate 60–100

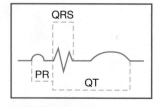

FIGURE 2–16

Intervals.

Intervals Practice

Determine the intervals on the enlarged rhythm strips that follow.

    PR interval.   Count the number of small blocks between the beginning of the P and the beginning of the QRS. Multiply by 0.04 seconds.

    QRS interval.   Count the number of small blocks between the beginning and end of the QRS complex. Multiply by 0.04 seconds.

    QT interval.   Count the number of small blocks between the beginning of the QRS and the end of the T wave. Multiply by 0.04 seconds.

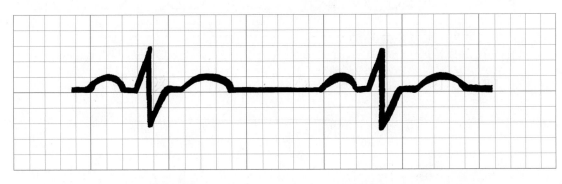

1. PR __0.12__   QRS __0.08__   QT __0.24__

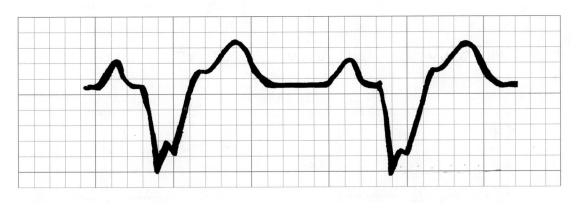

2. PR __0.12__   QRS _____   QT __0.28 0.32__

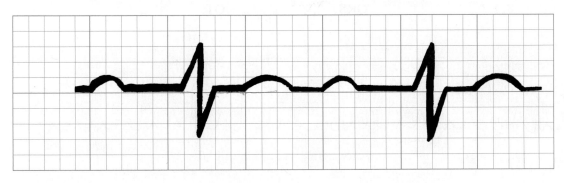

3. PR __0.24__   QRS __0.08__   QT __0.28__

Now let's practice intervals on normal-size EKG paper. Allow plus or minus 0.02 seconds for your answers. For example, if the answer is listed as 0.28, acceptable answers would be anywhere from 0.26 to 0.30. You'll note that intervals can vary slightly from beat to beat. This implies normal functioning of the sympathetic and parasympathetic nervous systems.

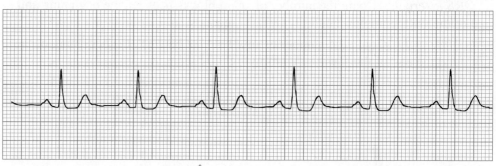

1. PR _____ 0.20 _____   QRS _____ 0.08 _____   QT _____ 0.38   0.34 _____

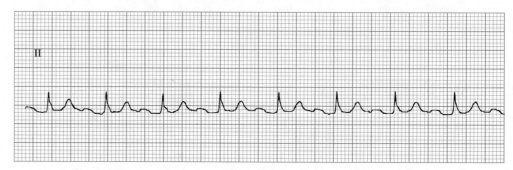

2. PR _____ 0.22 _____   QRS _____ 0.10 _____   QT _____ 0.4 _____

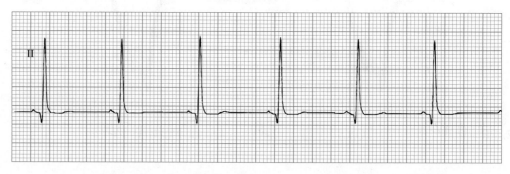

3. PR _____   QRS _____ .12 _____   QT _____ 0.36 _____

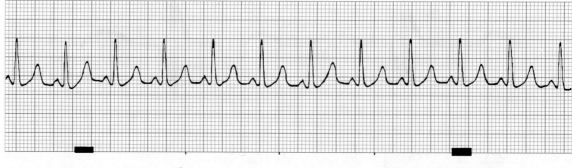

4. PR _____ 0.4 .12 _____   QRS _____ 0.06 _____   QT _____ 0.32 _____

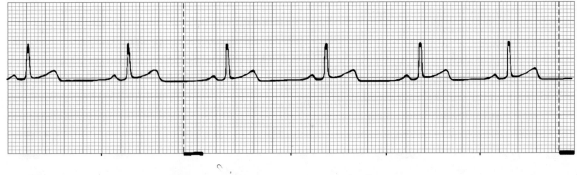

5. PR _0.16_   QRS _.12_   QT _0.32_

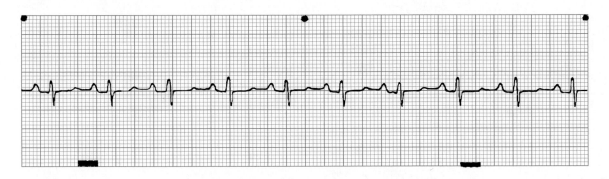

6. PR _____   QRS _____   QT _____

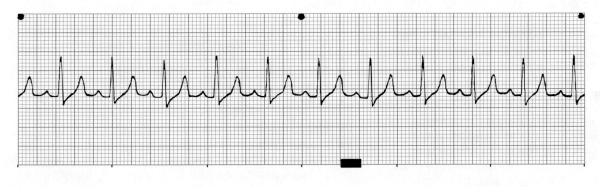

7. PR _____   QRS _____   QT _____

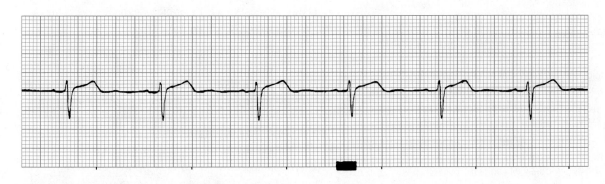

8. PR _____   QRS _____   QT _____

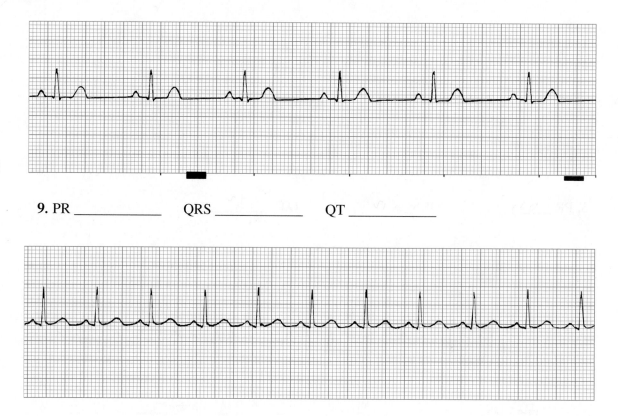

9. PR _____   **QRS** _____   **QT** _____

10. PR _____   **QRS** _____   **QT** _____

chapter two notes TO SUM IT ALL UP . . .

■ **Negatively charged resting cardiac cell is said to be polarized.**

■ **Depolarization**—Discharge of electricity—occurs when cardiac cell becomes positively charged.

■ **Repolarization**—Return of the cardiac cell to its resting negative charge.

■ **Electrical stimulus precedes mechanical response.** Cannot have myocardial contraction without first having had depolarization. **Depolarization and repolarization**—electrical events. **Contraction and relaxation**—mechanical.

■ **Action potential**—What happens to cardiac cell when stimulated by electrical charge. Several phases:

• *Phase 4*—Cardiac cell at rest. Corresponds with isoelectric line of EKG.

• *Phase 0*—depolarization. Cell becomes positively charged. Corresponds with QRS complex on EKG.

• *Phases 1 and 2*—Early repolarization. Calcium is released. Muscle contraction begins. Corresponds with ST segment of EKG.

• *Phase 3*—Rapid repolarization. Cell is returning to electrically negative state. Corresponds with T wave of EKG.

■ **Refractory periods**—Cardiac cell resists responding to/depolarizing from an impulse.

• *Absolute refractory period*—Cardiac cell cannot respond to another impulse, no matter how strong.

• *Relative refractory period*—Cell can respond only to very strong impulse.

• *Supernormal period*—Cardiac cell is "hyper," will respond to very weak stimulus.

■ **Each P-QRS-T sequence represents one heartbeat.**

■ **P wave**—Atrial depolarization.

■ **T_a wave**—atrial repolarization—usually not seen, as it occurs simultaneous with QRS.

■ **QRS complex**—Ventricular depolarization.

■ **T wave**—Ventricular repolarization.

■ **U wave**—Late ventricular repolarization—not usually seen.

■ **PR segment**—Flat line between the P wave and the QRS complex.

■ **ST segment**—Flat line between the QRS complex and the T wave.

■ **QRS complex**—A series of spiky waves. Waves have names:

• *Q wave*—Negative wave that precedes an R wave in the QRS complex; if present, always the first wave of the QRS.

• *R wave*—Any positive wave in the QRS complex.

• *S wave*—Negative wave that follows an R wave.

• *R′*—A second R wave.

■ **Cardiac conduction system**—pathway of specialized cells—job is to create and conduct impulses to tell the heart when to beat. Conduction pathway is as follows:

• Sinus node ➜ interatrial tracts ➜ atrium ➜ internodal tracts ➜ AV node ➜ bundle of His ➜ bundle branches ➜ Perkinje fibers ➜ ventricle.

- **Characteristics of cardiac cells:**
  - *Automaticity*—Electrical—ability to create an impulse.
  - *Conductivity*—Electrical—ability to pass that impulse along to neighboring cells.
  - *Excitability*—Electrical—ability to respond to that impulse by depolarizing.
  - *Contractility*—Mechanical—ability to contract and do work.
- **Inherent rates of pacemaker cells:**
  - *Sinus node*—60–100.
  - *AV junction*—40–60.
  - *Ventricle*—20–40.
- **Sinus node**—Normal pacemaker of the heart.
- **Fastest pacemaker at any given moment is the one in control.**
- **Escape**—Predominant pacemaker slows down; lower pacemaker takes over at its slower inherent rate—results in a slower heart rate than before.
- **Escape beat**—Beat that comes in after a pause longer than normal R-R interval.
- **Escape rhythm**—Series of escape beats.
- **Usurpation (irritability)**—Lower pacemaker becomes "hyper"; fires in at an accelerated rate, stealing control away from slower predominant pacemaker—results in a faster heart rate than before.
- **Heart rhythm**—Pattern of successive heart beats.
- **Arrhythmia**—Abnormal heart rhythm

- **12-lead EKG**—Printout of heart's electrical activity from 12 different angles.
- **Lead**—Electrocardiographic picture of the heart's electricity.
- **Rhythm strip**—Printout of 1 to 2 leads on small roll of graph paper.
- **EKG paper**—Graph paper divided into small vertical and horizontal blocks:
  - One small block is 0.04 seconds wide.
  - One big block is 0.20 seconds wide.
  - Five small blocks equals one big block.
  - Five big blocks equals one second.
  - 25 small blocks equals one second.
  - 300 big blocks equals one minute.
  - 1,500 small blocks equals one minute.
- **Intervals**—Measurements of time between EKG waves and complexes:
  - *PR interval*—Measures time it takes impulse to get from atrium to ventricle—measured from beginning of P wave to beginning of QRS (even if QRS does not begin with an R wave!). Normal PR interval 0.12–0.20 seconds.
  - *QRS interval*—Measures time it takes to depolarize the ventricle—measured from beginning of QRS to its end. Normal QRS interval is less than 0.12 seconds.
  - *QT interval*—Measures depolarization/repolarization time in ventricle—measured from beginning of QRS to end of T wave. QT interval varies with heart rate but should be less than or equal to half the R-R interval.

Practice Quiz

1. Cardiac cells at rest are electrically _____

2. Depolarization and repolarization are what kinds of events?_____

3. State what occurs in each of the following phases of the action potential:

   Phase 4. _____

   Phase 0. _____

   Phase 1. _____

   Phase 2. _____

   Phase 3. _____

4. State what each of the following waves/complexes represents:

   P wave. _____

   QRS complex. _____

   T wave. _____

5. What kind of impulse can result in depolarization during the absolute refractory period? _____

6. List the four characteristics of heart cells. _____
   _____
   _____

7. State the inherent rates of the pacemaker cells.

   Sinus node _____

   AV junction _____

   Ventricle _____

   _____

8. List, in order of conduction, the structures of the conduction pathway through the heart.

   _____

   _____

9. Define *escape*. _____

   _____

10. Define *usurpation*. _____

    _____

Putting It All Together—Critical Thinking Exercises

These exercises may consist of diagrams to label, scenarios to analyze, brain-stumping questions to ponder, or other challenging exercises to boost your knowledge of the chapter material.

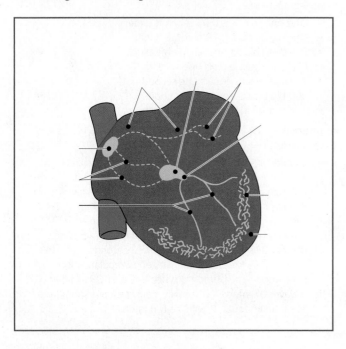

1. If the sinus node is firing at a rate of 65 and the AV node kicks in at a rate of 70, what will happen? Which pacemaker will be in control? Explain your answer.

2. Your patient's PR interval last night was 0.16 seconds. This morning it is 0.22. Which part of the conduction system is responsible for this delay in impulse transmission?

3. Explain how it is possible for the heart's pumping ability to fail but its electrical conduction ability to remain intact.

4. Label the parts of the conduction system on the diagram.

Lead Morphology and Placement

3

CHAPTER 3 OBJECTIVES

Upon completion of this chapter, the student will be able to:

- Define *electrode*.
- Name the bipolar leads and state the limbs that comprise them.
- Name the unipolar augmented leads.
- Explain what augmentation does to the EKG.
- Explain Einthoven's law.
- Draw and label Einthoven's triangle.

- Name the leads comprising the hexiaxial diagram.
- Describe the location of the precordial leads.
- Name the two leads most commonly used for continuous monitoring in the hospital.
- Explain the electrocardiographic truths.
- Describe the normal QRS complex deflections in each of the 12 leads on an EKG.

What It's All About

Mr. Hedges was admitted to the ICU after his angiogram revealed a blockage in his right coronary artery. He's scheduled to go back to the cardiac catheterization lab for a procedure to open his blocked coronary artery in the morning. "Keep an eye out for inferior wall EKG changes," his physician tells his nurse Becky. "I want to get him back to the cath lab before he has a heart attack." Becky watches Mr. Hedges all night and gives him nitroglycerine as ordered for his occasional chest pain. She notes that the routine monitor leads used in that facility, Leads I and V_1, do not look at the inferior wall. So she turns the lead selector to monitor Lead II. At 3 A.M., Mr. Hedges complains of worsening chest pain. The monitor strip shows ST segment changes in Lead II, so Becky does a 12-lead EKG, which confirms that Mr. Hedges is starting to have an inferior wall heart attack. Becky calls the physician and Mr. Hedges is taken to the cath lab immediately. His coronary artery is successfully opened up and his heart attack is aborted. Afterwards the physician thanked Becky. "I'm glad you were on last night," he told her. "I knew you knew what leads to look at. If this hadn't been picked up when it was, he would've had a big heart attack."

Introduction

Electrocardiography is the recording of the heart's electrical impulses by way of sensors, called **electrodes**, placed at various locations on the body. Willem Einthoven, inventor of the EKG machine and the "father of electrocardiography," postulated that the heart is in the center of the electrical field that it generates. He put electrodes on the arms and legs, far away from the heart. The right-leg electrode was used as a ground electrode to minimize the hazard of electric shock to the patient and to stabilize the EKG. The electrodes on the other limbs were used to create leads. A lead is simply an electrocardiographic picture of the heart. A 12-lead EKG provides 12 different views of the heart's electrical activity.

Why is it necessary to have 12 leads? The more leads, the better the chance of interpreting the heart's electrical activity. Have you ever waved to someone you saw from a distance and then realized when you got a better look that it wasn't who you thought it was? The more views you have, the better your chance of recognizing this person, right? Same thing with the heart. The more views of the heart's electrical activity, the better the chance of recognizing its patterns and abnormalities. So we have leads that view the heart from the side, the front, the bottom, and anterior to posterior (front to back).

The printed EKG is called an **electrocardiogram**.

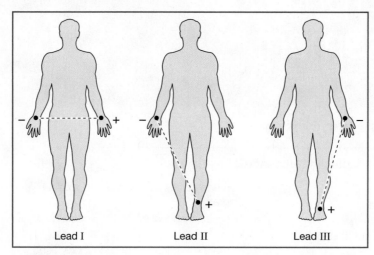

FIGURE 3–1

The bipolar leads.

TABLE 3–1   Bipolar Leads

Lead	Measures Current Traveling From	Location of Positive Pole
I	Right arm to left arm	Left arm
II	Right arm to left leg	Left leg
III	Left arm to left leg	Left leg

Bipolar Leads

Bipolar leads are so named because they require a positive pole and a negative pole. Think of the positive electrode as the one that actually "sees" the current. See Table 3–1.

Look at Figure 3–1 now. You'll notice that in the bipolar leads, the right arm is always negative and the left leg is always positive. Also note that the left arm can be positive or negative depending on which lead it is a part of. If you join Leads I, II, and III at the middle, you get the triaxial diagram seen in Figure 3–2.

If you join Leads I, II, and III at their ends, you get a triangle called Einthoven's triangle, seen in Figure 3–3.

Einthoven stated that Lead I + Lead III = Lead II. This is called Einthoven's law. It means that the height of the QRS in Lead I added to the height of the QRS in Lead III will equal the height of the QRS in Lead II. In other words, Lead II should have the tallest QRS of the bipolar leads. Einthoven's law can help determine if an EKG is truly abnormal or if the leads were inadvertently placed on the incorrect limb. See Figure 3–4.

Augmented Leads

Now let's look at the augmented leads. See Table 3–2 and Figure 3–5.

These are called **augmented leads** because they generate such small waveforms on the EKG paper that the EKG machine must augment (increase) the size of the waveforms so that they'll show up on the EKG paper. These leads are also unipolar, meaning they require only one electrode to make them. In order for the EKG machine to augment the leads, it uses a midway point between the other two limbs as a negative reference point.

Both the bipolar and augmented leads are also called frontal leads because they look at the heart from only the front of the body, and **limb leads,** as they're located on the limbs.

If you join leads aVR, aVL, and aVF in the middle, you get the triaxial diagram shown in Figure 3–6.

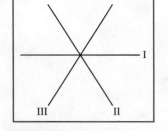

FIGURE 3–2

The triaxial diagram.

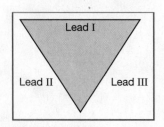

FIGURE 3–3

Einthoven's triangle.

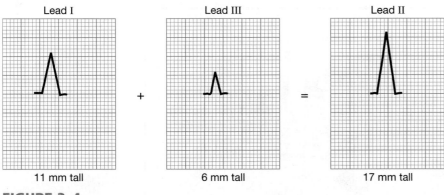

FIGURE 3–4

Einthoven's law.

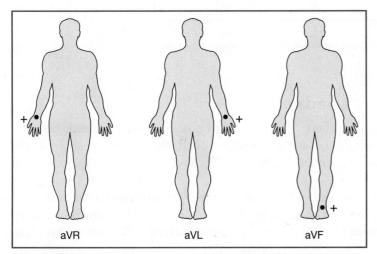

FIGURE 3–5

The augmented leads.

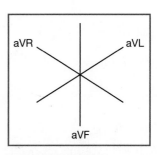

FIGURE 3–6

Triaxial diagram with augmented leads.

TABLE 3–2 Augmented Leads

Lead	Measures Current Traveling Toward	Location of Positive Pole
aVR	Right arm	Right arm
aVL	Left arm	Left arm
aVF	Left leg	Left leg

If all the frontal leads—I, II, III, aVR, aVL, and aVF—are joined at the center, the result looks like Figure 3–7. This **hexiaxial diagram** is used to help determine the direction of current flow in the heart.

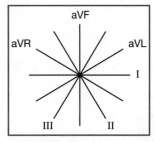

FIGURE 3–7

Hexiaxial diagram.

chapter CHECKUP

We're about halfway through this chapter. To evaluate your understanding of the material thus far, answer the following questions. If you have trouble with them, review the material again before continuing.

1. Name the bipolar leads and augmented leads and state where the positive pole of each lead is.
2. Define *electrocardiography, leads,* and *electrodes.*

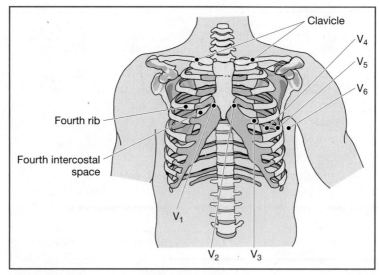

FIGURE 3–8

The precordial leads.

Precordial (Chest) Leads

These leads are located on the chest. They are also unipolar leads, and each one is a positive electrode. The precordial leads see a wraparound view of the heart from the horizontal plane. These leads are named V_1, V_2, V_3, V_4, V_5, and V_6. See Figure 3–8 and Table 3–3.

Intercostal spaces are the spaces between the ribs. The **midclavicular line** is an imaginary line down from the middle of the clavicle (collarbone). The **anterior axillary line** is an imaginary line down from the front of the axilla (armpit). The **midaxillary line** is an imaginary line down from the middle of the axilla.

TABLE 3–3   Location of the Precordial Leads

Lead	Location	Location Abbreviation
V_1	Fourth intercostal space (ICS), right sternal border (RSB): The space below the 4th rib where it joins with the sternum on the patient's right side.	4th ICS, RSB
V_2	Fourth intercostal space, left sternal border (LSB): The space below the 4th rib where it joins with the sternum on the patient's left side.	4th ICS, LSB
V_3	Between V_2 and V_4.	
V_4	Fifth intercostal space, midclavicular line (MCL): The space below the 5th rib where it joins with an imaginary line down from the middle of the clavicle on the patient's left side.	5th ICS, MCL
V_5	Fifth intercostal space, anterior axillary line (AAL): The space below the 5th rib where it joins with an imaginary line down from the front of the patient's left armpit.	5th ICS, AAL
V_6	Fifth intercostal space, midaxillary line (MAL): The space below the 5th rib where it joins with an imaginary line down from the middle of the patient's left armpit.	5th ICS, MAL

Continuous Monitoring

Hospitalized patients requiring continuous EKG monitoring are attached to either a 3-lead or a 5-lead cable connected to a remote receiver/transmitter (called telemetry) or to a monitor at the bedside (see Figure 3–9). Both of these setups send the EKG display to a central terminal where the rhythms are observed and identified (see website for an animation showing 12-lead EKG placement and a video showing electrode placement for EKG and cardiac monitoring and the electrocardiogram).

Since these patients may be on the monitor for days or longer, it is necessary to alter the placement of lead electrodes to allow for freedom of movement and to minimize artifact (unwanted jitter or interference on the EKG tracing).

Figure 3–10 shows the two most commonly used leads for continuous monitoring. Note lead placement is on the subclavicle (collarbone) area and the chest or lower abdomen instead of on the arms, legs, and chest. Also note the ground electrode may be located somewhere other than the right leg.

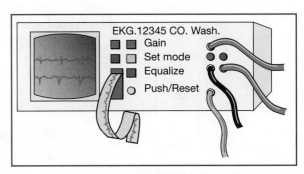

FIGURE 3–9

Bedside monitor.

Electrocardiographic Truths

- An impulse traveling toward (or parallel to) a positive electrode writes a positive complex on the EKG paper (see website for an animation showing the rule of electrical flow).
- An impulse traveling away from a positive electrode writes a negative complex.
- An impulse traveling perpendicularly to the positive electrode writes an **isoelectric** complex (one that is as much positive as it is negative).
- If there is no impulse at all, there will be no complex—just a flat line.

See Figure 3–11.

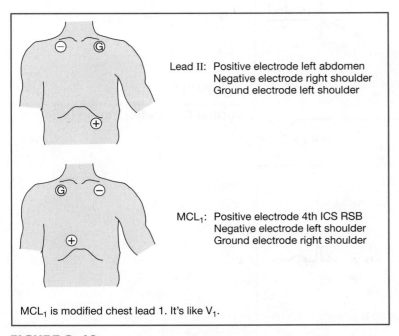

Lead II: Positive electrode left abdomen
Negative electrode right shoulder
Ground electrode left shoulder

MCL$_1$: Positive electrode 4th ICS RSB
Negative electrode left shoulder
Ground electrode right shoulder

MCL$_1$ is modified chest lead 1. It's like V$_1$.

FIGURE 3–10

Lead placement for continuous monitoring.

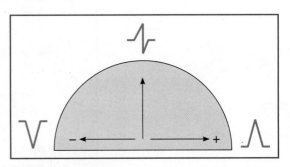

FIGURE 3–11

Electrocardiographic truths.

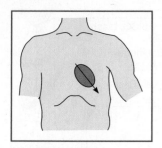

FIGURE 3–12

Normal vector.

Normal QRS Deflections

How should the QRS complexes in the normal EKG look? Let's look at the frontal leads:

Lead I should be positive.

Lead II should be positive.

Lead III should be small but mostly positive.

aVR should be negative.

aVL should be positive.

aVF should be positive.

Normal vector forces of the heart flow top to bottom, right to left. A **vector** is an arrow that points out the general direction of current flow. The current of the heart normally starts in the sinus node, which is in the right atrium, and terminates in the left ventricle. Figure 3–12 shows what the vector representing normal heart current looks like.

We've already said what the QRS complex in each lead should look like. Let's look at that a little more closely. In Figure 3–13, we have Lead I, which joins right and left arms. The positive electrode is on the left arm. Normal current of the heart flows right to left, traveling toward the left side, where Lead I's positive electrode is. This results in a positive complex in Lead I.

In Figure 3–14, we have Lead II, which connects the right arm and left leg. Recall the left leg is positive. Normal heart current flows top to bottom, right to left, parallel to Lead II. Therefore, Lead II's QRS complex should be strongly positive.

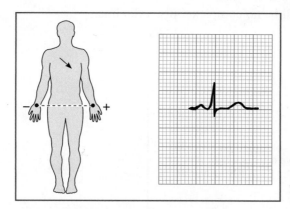

FIGURE 3–13

Normal QRS deflection in Lead I.

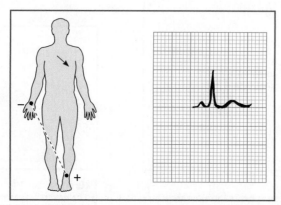

FIGURE 3–14

Normal QRS deflection in Lead II.

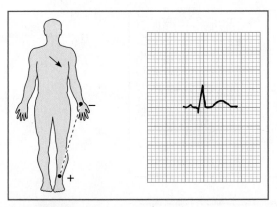

FIGURE 3–15

Normal QRS deflection in Lead III.

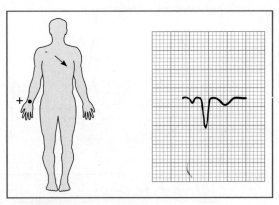

FIGURE 3–16

Normal QRS deflection in aVR.

Next is Lead III, which joins left arm and left leg. The positive electrode is on the left leg. Normal current flows toward this electrode, producing a positive complex. The QRS complex in Lead III is often small. See Figure 3–15.

In aVR, the positive electrode is on the right arm. Normal current flows right to left, away from this electrode, and aVR's QRS complex should therefore be negative. See Figure 3–16.

In aVL, the positive electrode is on the left arm. Normal current flows toward the left, producing a positive QRS complex. See Figure 3–17.

In aVF, the positive electrode is on the left leg. Normal current flows toward the left leg, so aVF should have a positive QRS complex. See Figure 3–18.

Now let's look at the precordial leads:

V_1 should be negative.

V_2 should be negative.

V_3 should be about half up, half down.

V_4 should be about half up, half down.

V_5 should be positive.

V_6 should be positive.

Quick Tip

In the frontal leads, all QRS complexes should be upright except aVR.

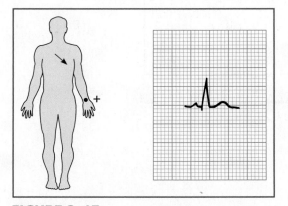

FIGURE 3–17

Normal QRS deflection in aVL.

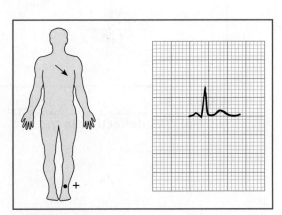

FIGURE 3–18

Normal QRS deflection in aVF.

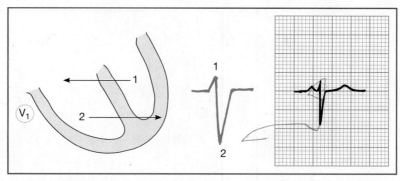

FIGURE 3–19

Normal QRS deflection in V$_1$.

The precordial leads start out negative and then go through a transition zone where they become isoelectric (half-and-half); then they become positive. For the precordial leads, we look at current flow in the *horizontal plane*. The septum depolarizes from left to right and the ventricles from right to left.

See Figure 3–19. In V$_1$, septal and right ventricular depolarization send the current toward the positive electrode, resulting in an initial positive deflection. Then the current travels away from the positive electrode as it heads toward the left ventricle. Thus, V$_1$ should have a small R wave and a deep S wave. The complex is mostly negative, since most of the heart's current is traveling toward the left ventricle, away from the V$_1$ electrode.

In V$_6$, just the opposite occurs. Initially, the impulse is heading away from the positive electrode during septal and right ventricular depolarization; then it travels toward it during left ventricular activation. See Figure 3–20.

The other leads in between show a gradual transition from negative to positive complexes.

Quick Tip

In the precordial leads, V$_1$'s and V$_2$'s QRS should be negative, V$_3$ and/or V$_4$ isoelectric, and V$_5$ and V$_6$ positive.

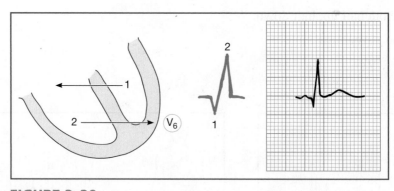

FIGURE 3–20

Normal QRS deflection in V$_6$.

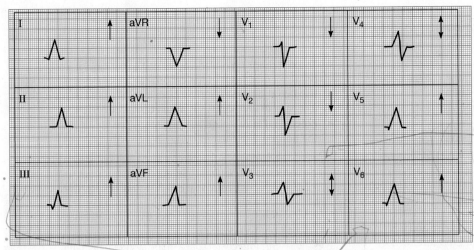

Normal 12-lead EKG. The arrows indicate the correct deflection of the QRS complexes.

Lead Morphology Practice

Determine if the following QRS morphologies are normal. If not, tell what the abnormality is.

Just by analyzing the morphology of each lead, we can get an idea of whether there is any pathology on the EKG. Three of the following four EKGs are abnormal in some way. As we continue further along in this text, we will learn the implications of this abnormality, and we'll learn more ways to analyze EKGs.

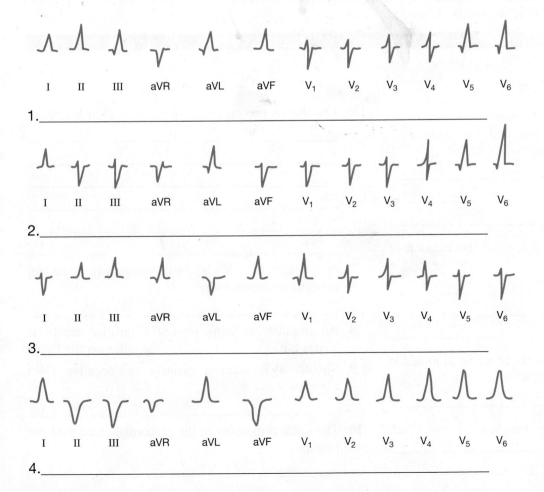

1._____

2._____

3._____

4._____

chapter three notes TO SUM IT ALL UP . . .

- **Electrocardiography**—Recording of heart's electrical impulses by way of electrodes placed at various locations on the body.
- **Electrocardiogram**—Printed EKG
- **Bipolar leads**—Placed on the limbs—require positive and negative pole:
  - *Lead I*—Measures current traveling between right and left arms. Right arm is negative pole; left arm is positive pole. QRS should be positive.
  - *Lead II*—Measures current between right arm and left leg. Right arm is negative; left leg is positive pole. Lead II's QRS should be positive.
  - *Lead III*—Measures current between left arm and left leg. Left arm is negative pole; left leg is positive. QRS should be positive.
- **Einthoven's law**—Lead I + Lead III = Lead II. This means Lead II should have the tallest QRS of the bipolar leads.
- **Augmented leads**—Require EKG machine to augment (increase) voltage—otherwise waves and complexes are too small to see. Augmented leads are a kind of unipolar lead.
  - *aVR*—On right arm. Its QRS should be negative.
  - *aVL*—On left arm. Its QRS should be positive.
  - *aVF*—On left leg. Its QRS should be positive.
- **Bipolar leads and augmented leads: also known as frontal leads, as they are located on front of the body— and limb leads, since they are located on the limbs.**

- **Triaxial diagram**—Made by joining either bipolar leads or augmented leads at the center.
- **Hexiaxial diagram**—Made by joining all frontal leads (I, II, III, aVR, aVL, and aVF) at the center.
- **Precordial leads**—Located on chest—see the heart from the horizontal plane.
  - V_1—Located at 4th intercostal space, right sternal border. QRS should be negative.
  - V_2—4th intercostal space, left sternal border. QRS should be negative.
  - V_3—Between V2 and V4. QRS should be isoelectric (half up, half down).
  - V_4—5th intercostal space, midclavicular line. QRS isoelectric.
  - V_5—5th intercostal space, anterior axillary line. QRS positive.
  - V_6—5th intercostal space, midaxillary line. QRS positive.
- **An impulse traveling toward a positive electrode → positive QRS on EKG.**
- **An impulse traveling away from a positive electrode → negative QRS.**
- **An impulse traveling perpendicularly to a positive electrode → isoelectric QRS.**
- **If there is no impulse at all → flat line.**

Practice Quiz

1. Who is Willem Einthoven? _____

2. List the three bipolar leads and the limbs they connect.

_____

_____

_____

3. List the three augmented leads and the location of their positive poles.

_____

_____

_____

4. The hexiaxial diagram consists of six leads joined at the center. List those six leads.

_____

5. The precordial leads see the heart from which plane?_____

_____

6. List the six precordial leads and state their locations.

_____

_____

_____

_____

_____

_____

7. Name the two leads most commonly used for continuous monitoring.

_____

8. An impulse traveling toward a positive electrode writes a(n) _____ complex on the EKG.

9. Should aVR have a positive or negative QRS complex?

_____

10. The QRS complexes in the precordials lead start out primarily

_____

Putting It All Together—Critical Thinking Exercises

These exercises may consist of diagrams to label, scenarios to analyze, brain-stumping questions to ponder, or other challenging exercises to boost your understanding of the chapter material.

1. What can it imply if Lead I + Lead III does not equal Lead II?

   _____

2. If the QRS complex in Lead III is isoelectric, in which direction is the heart's current traveling?

   _____

3. If your patient has a heart rhythm in which the current starts in the left ventricle and travels upward toward the sinus node, what would you expect the frontal leads to look like (i.e., indicate lead by lead whether the QRS complex in those leads would be positive or negative)?

   _____

   _____

   _____

   _____

   _____

PEARSON
myhealthprofessionskit

Use this address to access the Companion Website created for this textbook. Simply select "Basic Health Science" from the choice of disciplines. Find this book and log in using your username and password to access video clips, animations, assessment questions, and more.

4

Technical Aspects of the EKG

CHAPTER 4 OBJECTIVES

Upon completion of this chapter, the student will be able to:

- Identify the control features of an EKG machine and describe the functions of each.
- Describe what a digital converter does.
- Differentiate between *macroshock* and *microshock*.

- Describe and identify on a rhythm strip the different kinds of artifact.
- Correctly tell how to troubleshoot artifact.
- Tell how to differentiate between artifact and a real rhythm.
- Correctly identify artifact versus rhythm.

What It's All About

Monitor technicians Karen and Roxie had no patient contact and thus no way to know if Mr. McCoy's "lethal" rhythm (one that could be deadly) was a true rhythm or just artifact. So following hospital protocol, they paged a code (cardiac arrest alert). When the code team responded to his room, they expected Mr. McCoy to be unconscious and pulseless. Instead he was awake and reading the paper. "Hi, Mr. McCoy, how are you feeling? The heart monitor says you're having a problem so we're here to check it out," code team nurse Kathryn told him. "I'm fine," he replied. Kathryn attached Mr. McCoy to a monitor/defibrillator and found a normal rhythm and heart rate. His blood pressure was fine and he was having no shortness of breath or pain. The team left his room. "Let's look at that rhythm strip," Kathryn said. When she examined the strip, she could see that it looked like a flat line, which can indicate a lethal rhythm. "What's the gain setting?" Kathryn inquired of the monitor techs. "It's set on one" was the response. "Let's increase the gain and see what it looks like," Kathryn advised the techs. Once the gain was turned up, the rhythm reappeared. The setting had been so low that the waves and complexes disappeared, making it seem as if Mr. McCoy was in **cardiac arrest** (cardiac standstill).

Introduction

The heart, electrically speaking, is a transmitter, and the EKG machine is a receiver. Let's look at how the EKG machine works.

The electrical impulses generated by the heart course not only through the conduction system but also throughout the body. Electrodes, small adhesive patches with conductive gel on the skin side, are applied to the skin and pick up these impulses, sending them through **lead wires** (small wires attached to the electrodes) to a cable into the EKG machine. There an **amplifier** (an instrument that amplifies/magnifies a signal) turns up the signal and a **digital converter** converts the analog signal to a digital one so it can then be printed out on specialized paper. Some modern EKG machines are Bluetooth-capable, allowing EMS responders to send a victim's EKG to the nearest hospital so treatment can begin even before the patient arrives at the hospital. See Figure 4–1.

Control Features

EKG machines have various control features, including the following:

- **Chart speed**   This regulates the speed at which the paper prints out. Normal speed is 25 mm/s. Changing the speed to 50 mm/s doubles the width of the waves

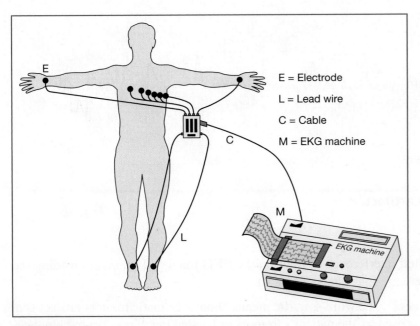

E = Electrode

L = Lead wire

C = Cable

M = EKG machine

FIGURE 4–1

Man attached to EKG machine.

and complexes. Doubling the chart speed is useful when the patient has a very fast rhythm, as widening out the rhythm separates the waves and can aid in rhythm interpretation.

- **Gain**   This regulates the height of the complexes. Normal setting is 1. Changing to 2 doubles the height of the complexes. Changing to 1/2 shrinks it. Increasing the gain is important if the rhythm printout is small and hard to read. *It is critical to check/increase the gain setting if the patient appears to be in a flat-line rhythm.* It could be true cardiac arrest or it could be that the gain is set so low that the waves and complexes aren't even visible.

Whenever any setting is changed from the norm, document this change at the top of the EKG printout to prevent misinterpretation of any EKG changes caused by the setting change.

Electrical Safety

There are two kinds of electrical shock that the patient can sustain from faulty equipment:

- **Macroshock**   A high-voltage shock resulting from inadequate grounding of electrical equipment. If there is a frayed or broken wire or cord, electrical outlet damage, or other electrical malfunction, the 110 volts of electricity running through the power line can go directly to the patient, causing burns, neurologic damage, or fatal heart rhythm disturbances. The patient's dry, intact skin will offer some resistance to the electricity, but not enough to prevent injury.
- **Microshock**   A smaller, but still dangerous, shock directly into the heart by means of a device such as a pacemaker. Normally a small **leakage current** (electrical current that escapes a device's insulation) is produced around the pacemaker and carried harmlessly away by the ground wire attaching the patient's bed to the electrical socket in the room. If the ground wire is frayed, however, a small amount of current could travel into the heart and shock it from the inside. Since the inside of the body is a wet environment, there is less protection against shock.

Precaution: Check for frayed wires or components before doing an EKG.

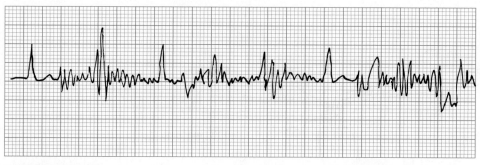

FIGURE 4–2

Somatic tremors artifact.

Artifact

Artifact is unwanted interference or jitter on the EKG tracing. This makes reading the EKG difficult. There are four kinds of artifact:

- *Somatic tremors.*   The word somatic means "body." Somatic tremors artifact is a jittery pattern caused by the patient's tremors or by shaking wires. Try to help the patient relax. Cover him or her if cold. Make sure the wires are not tangled or loose. Sometimes this artifact cannot be corrected, such as in a patient with tremors from Parkinson's disease. In that case, make a few attempts at a readable tracing and keep the best one. At the top of the EKG, write "best effort times three attempts" for example, so the physician will know this was not simply a poor tracing done by an inattentive technician. Note the shakiness of the tracing in Figure 4–2. Sometimes you can pick out the QRS complexes and sometimes not. Redo the EKG until the tracing is more easily readable.

- *Baseline sway.*   Here the baseline moves up and down on the EKG paper. It can be caused by the breathing pattern or by lotion or sweat on the skin interfering with the signal reaching the machine. Wipe off any lotion or sweat with a towel and replace the electrode patches. In Figure 4–3, the baseline looks as if someone snagged a finger under it and pulled it upward. It's not a big problem, because the waves and complexes are all still clear.

- *60-cycle interference.*   This results in a thick-looking pattern on the paper. It's caused by too many electrical devices close by. Unplug as many machines as you safely can until you finish doing the EKG. Don't forget portable phones, laptops, and pagers—they can cause interference also. In Figure 4–4, see how thick the baseline looks? It's as if someone used a thick highlighter to write it. Normally the baseline is much finer.

- *Broken recording.*   This can be caused by a frayed or fractured wire or by a loose electrode patch or cable. Check first for loose electrodes or cables. If those are OK,

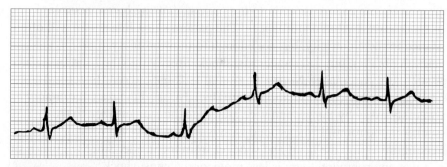

FIGURE 4–3

Baseline sway.

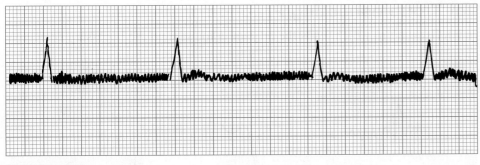

FIGURE 4–4

60-cycle interference.

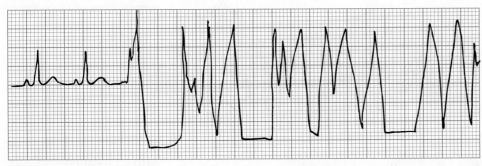

FIGURE 4–5

Broken recording.

the artifact may be from a fractured wire. If so, use a different EKG machine. Never do an EKG with a faulty machine. In Figure 4–5, note that at first the QRS complexes are easily visible; then the pattern is all over the place, going up and down trying to find the signal.

Troubleshooting

Troubleshooting involves determining and alleviating the cause of artifact and recording errors. For example, what if you saw only baseline sway in Leads I, II, and aVR? Lead I connects the right and left arms, Lead II is right arm and left leg, and aVR is right arm. The common limb is the right arm. Change that electrode, and the problem should be corrected. Always note which leads the problem is in and find the common limb. Direct your corrective efforts there. Check out Figure 4–6 to help recall which leads are where.

How do you know if the electrodes are properly placed? Remember the normal configuration of the leads. All the frontal leads except aVR should be positive, and the precordial leads start out negative and then eventually become positive. Say you do an EKG and the complexes are all messed up—I is negative, aVR is positive, and the precordial leads start out positive and become negative. The lead placement is probably wrong. Redo the EKG with the leads correctly placed. A big clue to incorrect lead placement or lead reversal is a negative P-QRS-T in Lead I. That is completely wrong unless the patient's heart is on the right side (a rare occurrence). So if you find that your Lead I is completely negative, check your lead placement. The right and left arm leads may have been inadvertently reversed.

If your patient is on a monitor in the hospital and is having artifact, another action could be to change the lead by which the patient is being monitored. For example, if he or she is in Lead II and having artifact, change the lead selector switch to a different lead without artifact, perhaps Lead I. (This is most appropriate when the patient is asleep, for example, and you don't want to awaken him or her for an electrode patch check.)

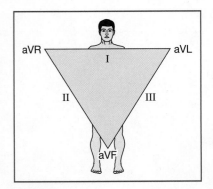

FIGURE 4–6

Leads.

Artifact Troubleshooting Practice

On these EKGs, state in which leads the artifact is found, and the necessary corrective action.

1.

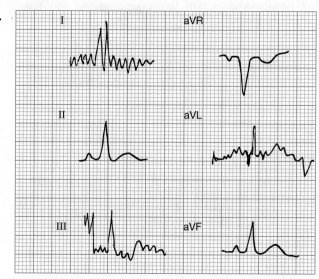

Artifact location _____

_____

Corrective action _____

_____

_____

_____

2.

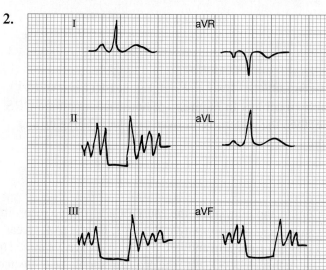

Artifact location _____

_____

Corrective action _____

_____

_____

3.

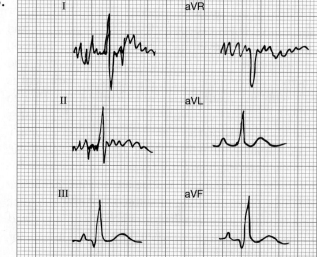

Artifact location _____

_____

Corrective action _____

_____

_____

_____

We're about halfway through this chapter. To evaluate your understanding of the material thus far, answer the following questions. If you have trouble with them, review the material again before continuing.

1. Explain the control features of an EKG machine.
2. Define *macroshock* and *microshock* and the cause of each.
3. Explain how to troubleshoot for the four types of artifact.

Artifact Masquerading as Rhythms

Artifact can mimic rhythms so convincingly that emergency teams are sometimes summoned to deal with patients with "life-threatening" rhythms that are later discovered to be nothing but artifact. The scenarios that follow will emphasize the importance of assessing the patient who has a change in rhythm. *Do not always believe what you see on the rhythm strip. Check your patient.*

Artifact Masquerading as Asystole

Figure 4–7 is a strip from an elderly man who had a myocardial infarction (heart attack) two days prior. The nurse at the monitoring station saw this rhythm on the screen and ran into the patient's room. The patient was awake and feeling fine, but his rhythm indicated that his heart had completely stopped beating. Since this obviously was not the case, the nurse checked the man's monitor patches and wires and discovered several were loose or disconnected. She reconnected them and his rhythm pattern returned to normal. Thus the rhythm in Figure 4–7 was artifact, not a real rhythm.

Now look at Figure 4–8. This is a strip of a heart that has indeed stopped beating. Notice the similarity between this strip and Figure 4–7.

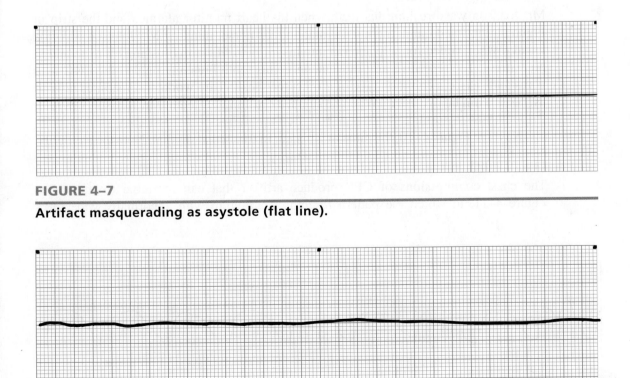

FIGURE 4–7

Artifact masquerading as asystole (flat line).

FIGURE 4–8

True asystole.

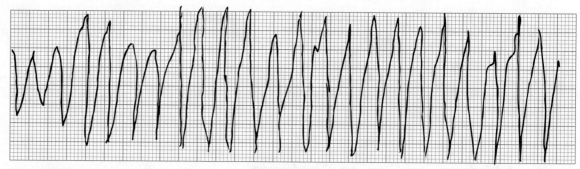

FIGURE 4–9

"Toothbrush tachycardia" masquerading as a lethal rhythm.

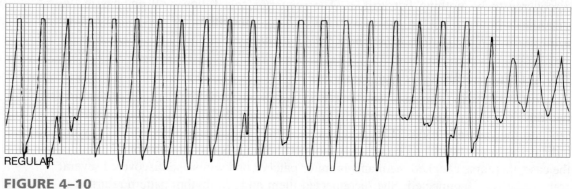

REGULAR

FIGURE 4–10

Ventricular tachycardia.

"Toothbrush Tachycardia"

Mr. Johnson was brushing his teeth when his heart monitor alarmed and the strip in Figure 4–9 printed out at the nurses' station. His nurse, thinking Mr. Johnson was in a lethal rhythm, yelled for help and ran into his room to find him brushing his teeth and in no distress. The repetitive arm movements of his tooth brushing jiggled the EKG lead wires and caused a common type of artifact that health care workers sometimes refer to as "toothbrush tachycardia." When he stopped brushing his teeth, Mr. Johnson's rhythm strip returned to normal.

Now see Figure 4–10, this time of a patient in true lethal rhythm. Note the similarity.

CPR Artifact

The chest compressions of CPR produce artifact that can resemble rhythms. See Figure 4–11, in which the pattern resembles a rhythm with abnormally wide QRS

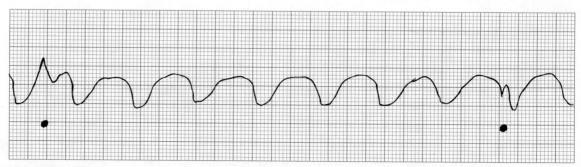

FIGURE 4–11

CPR artifact.

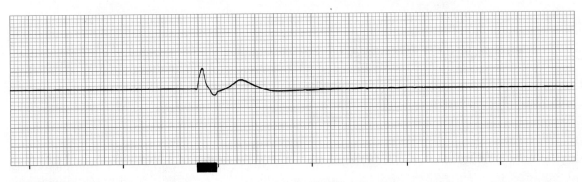

FIGURE 4–12

Rhythm without CPR artifact.

complexes. But look closer. See the dots? Look above them. See how the pattern gets a bit spiked here? Those are the patient's own QRS complexes popping out. Now look at Figure 4–12. Here CPR was stopped momentarily to allow evaluation of the rhythm without CPR artifact.

In Figure 4–12, there is one QRS complex and then flat line. This is the patient's true rhythm. The two QRS complexes in the first strip were obviously the rhythm of a dying heart. The rest of the pattern in the first strip was simply pseudo-QRS complexes produced by CPR.

Defibrillation/Cardioversion Artifact

Check out Figure 4–13. See the rhythm disappear and the baseline shoot down and up before the rhythm pattern comes back? That's the artifact produced when a patient is defibrillated or cardioverted (electrically shocked). You'll recall that the EKG records electrical current in the heart.

Defibrillation and cardioversion introduce a sudden surge of electricity into the heart, causing the EKG pattern to go wild briefly. As that electricity is dispersed, the true rhythm reappears.

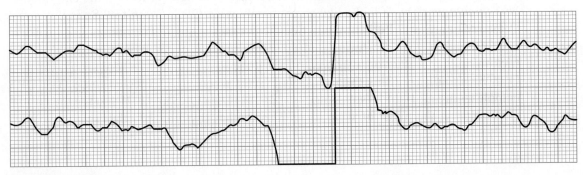

FIGURE 4–13

Defibrillation/cardioversion artifact.

Artifact in Three Leads Monitored Simultaneously

Figure 4–14 is a beautiful example of artifact masquerading as a rhythm. This patient was being monitored simultaneously in three leads—V_1, Lead II, and Lead I. *Since the three are recorded simultaneously, all three are the same rhythm, just seen in different leads.* Note that Leads II and I look alike, with multiple spiked waves scattered between the QRS complexes. But V_1 looks different, with the normal P waves preceding each QRS complex. How can that be? The strips all have to be the same rhythm. Think about this for a moment. Consider the location of the electrodes comprising each lead.

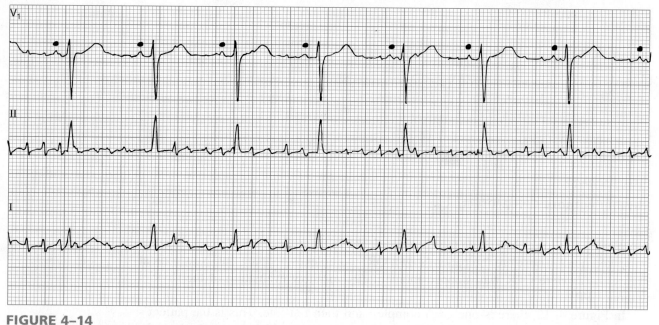

FIGURE 4–14

Artifact in three leads monitored simultaneously.

The true rhythm is seen in V_1. Leads II and I have artifact that obscures the P waves and provides what looks like spiked waves. Leads II and I are limb leads and are subject to artifact from muscle movement. Since V_1 is located on the chest, it picks up less artifact. This patient, it turns out, had tremors from Parkinson's disease. That's what was causing the spiked artifact.

Is It Real or Is It Artifact?

What do you see in Figure 4–15?

If you say it's a regular rhythm with a funny-looking beat toward the end (the 8th beat), you'd be right. It looks like an extremely wide QRS, doesn't it? So is this a real QRS or is it artifact? Let's find out. See the dot on the strip? The normal QRS spike is right beneath it. The downward and upward blips that encompass it are artifact. One trick to finding artifact on a strip is to follow the R-R intervals. Where should the next QRS be? You'll note this QRS spike is exactly where it is expected to be. The QRS complexes are all 14 to 15 small blocks apart, as is this QRS spike. If you see the normal QRS spike in the midst of what looks like another rhythm, the other rhythm is most likely artifact.

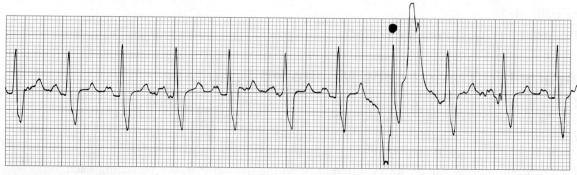

FIGURE 4–15

Is it real or is it artifact?

Real or Artifact: How to Tell the Difference

- If the rhythm is different from the patient's previous rhythm, *check your patient.* Ask how he or she feels and check vital signs (respiratory rate, heart rate, and blood pressure). This is especially important if the rhythm appears to be life-threatening. Patients with life-threatening arrhythmias will exhibit symptoms of **low cardiac output** (inadequate blood flow to meet the body's needs) and/or cardiovascular collapse. Artifact will not produce such symptoms.
- Observe the rhythm in another lead, preferably V_1 or MCL_1, which has less muscle artifact.
- Check to be sure the "rhythm" meets all its normal criteria. If it doesn't, be suspicious and check another lead.
- Check the patient's monitor wires and patches to see if they are loose or detached.
- See if the patient is having any muscle activity that could cause artifact.
- The bottom line is this: *Always check your patient, not just the monitor!*

> **Quick Tip**
>
> Do not try to interpret a strip or EKG obscured by artifact! Redo the strip or EKG until you get a readable tracing. Remember the patient's treatment depends on accurate interpretation.

 chapter four notes TO SUM IT ALL UP . . .

- **Electrically speaking, the heart is a transmitter and an EKG machine is a receiver.**
- **Chart speed**—Controls speed of paper printout. Normal chart speed—25 millimeters per second.
- **Gain**—Controls height of EKG waves and complexes. Normal setting is 1.
- **Macroshock**—High-voltage electrical shock—caused by inadequate grounding of electrical equipment.
- **Microshock**—Low-voltage shock—involves a conduit directly into the heart, such as a pacemaker.
- **Death can occur from either macroshock or microshock.** Always check your equipment. Do not use an EKG machine with frayed wires or components.
- **Artifact**—Unwanted interference or jitter on EKG tracing. Artifact can make it impossible to interpret an EKG. Four kinds of artifact:
  - *Somatic tremors*—Jittery pattern—caused by patient tremors or shaking wires.
  - *Baseline sway*—Baseline swings up and down—related to breathing pattern or lotion on skin.
- *60-cycle interference*—Thickened pattern of waves and complexes—caused by too many electrical devices close by.
- *Broken recording*—Tracing varies between flat lines and wild scribbling—caused by a frayed or broken wire.
- **To troubleshoot artifact, find the limb common to the leads showing artifact.** For example: artifact in Leads II, III, and aVF—common limb is the left leg—check wires and patches on that limb.
- **Real or artifact?**
  - *Check your patient*—If rhythm looks lethal but patient is grinning at you with a blood pressure better than yours, that "lethal rhythm" is probably artifact.
  - *Check rhythm in another lead*—Preferably V_1 or MCL_1, as those leads pick up less artifact than limb leads.
  - *See if the "rhythm" meets its normal criteria*—If it doesn't, check another lead.
  - *Check the wires and patches* to see if any are loose.
  - *Assess the patient for muscle activity* such as tremors that could cause artifact.

Practice Quiz

1. What is the function of the EKG machine? _____

_____

2. Normal chart speed for running a 12-lead EKG is

_____ millimeters per second.

3. What does the gain do? _____

4. What should the technician do if he or she changes the chart speed or gain when doing an EKG?_____

_____

5. Define *macroshock.* _____

6. Define *microshock.* _____

7. Define *artifact.* _____
   _____

8. Name the four kinds of artifact. _____
   _____
   _____
   _____

9. If there is artifact in Leads I, aVR, and II, toward which limb would you direct your troubleshooting efforts? _____
   _____

10. List three ways to determine if a rhythm is real or artifact. _____
    _____
    _____

Putting It All Together—Critical Thinking Exercises

1. Your patient, who is on telemetry monitoring, is noted to have two electrodes that have fallen off—the right arm and left leg. In which leads would you expect to see artifact?

   _____
   _____
   _____
   _____

2. Explain how you would know that your patient is having artifact and not a life-threatening arrhythmia (abnormal heart rhythm)?

   _____
   _____
   _____
   _____

PEARSON
myhealthprofessionskit™

Use this address to access the Companion Website created for this textbook. Simply select "Basic Health Science" from the choice of disciplines. Find this book and log in using your username and password to access video clips, animations, assessment questions, and more.

Calculating Heart Rate

5

CHAPTER 5 OBJECTIVES

Upon completion of this chapter, the student will be able to:

- Define *heart rate.*
- Calculate the heart rate on a variety of strips, using different methods.
- Differentiate among the three types of rhythm regularity.
- Tell which kind of heart rate to calculate for the different kinds of rhythm regularities.

What It's All About

Hattie Jefferson had a long history of an irregular heart rhythm that caused her heart rate to vary wildly—sometimes it would be in the 30s, sometimes in the 160s. She'd been on the same medication for this for years, but now that she was on dialysis, her doctor wanted her on a different medication. Hattie had been on this new medication for about a week when she began to feel faint. She called 911 and was taken to the emergency department. Her physician met her there and found Hattie's heart rate to vary from 60 to 120 with a mean rate of 90. Her blood pressure was fine. "Your heart is responding well to the new medication," her physician told a relieved Hattie. "In fact, this is the best control over your heart rate we've ever achieved. Based on your heart rate, I'm convinced it's not the medication causing the faintness. So now we just have to figure out what else could be the problem."

Introduction

Calculating heart rate involves counting the number of QRS complexes in one minute and is recorded in **beats per minute.** Heart rate is the same as **ventricular rate.** We can also determine the **atrial rate** by counting P waves, but the bottom line is this: *When we calculate heart rate, we count QRS complexes.*

Methods for Calculating Heart Rate

- *The 6-second strip method.* This is the least accurate of all the methods. Although it is considered by many experts to be the method of choice for irregular rhythms, it does not give much information and can be misleading. To use this method, count the number of QRS complexes on a 6-second rhythm strip and multiply by 10. This tells the **mean rate**, or average rate. If there are 3 QRS complexes on a 6-second strip, for example, the rate would be 30 beats per minute. (If there are 3 QRS complexes in 6 secs, there would be 30 in 60 secs, or 1 minute.) See Figure 5–1.

In Figure 5–1, both strips have 5 QRS complexes in 6 secs, so both have a mean rate of 50. Although both rhythms are irregular, with QRS complexes unevenly spaced throughout the strip, strip B shows wild swings in heart rate compared to strip A. Since treatment for rhythm disturbances depends in large part on the heart rate, it makes more sense to provide a *range* of heart rates from the slowest to the fastest, in addition to the mean rate. If a person is being treated with medication to slow down a fast heart rate, for example, it's important to know how slow and how fast the heart rate is in order to determine the effectiveness of treatment. A mean rate alone simply does not provide this

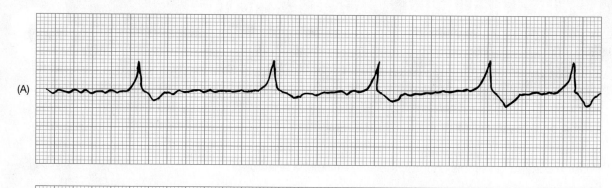

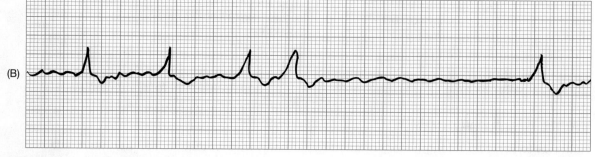

FIGURE 5–1

Two rhythms, both with mean rate of 50.

information—the heart rate range does. The heart rate range is calculated using one of the other methods. Bottom line: *The mean heart rate, as determined using the 6-second strip method, should be used only along with the heart rate range—not by itself.*

- *The memory method.* Widely used in hospitals, this is the fastest method. See Table 5–1. There are 300 big blocks every minute, so count the number of big blocks between consecutive QRS complexes and divide that number into 300. You end up with the sequence below.

  Memorize the sequence 300–150–100–75–60–50–43–37–33–30. Using this method, what would the heart rate be if there were five big blocks between QRS complexes? Go to the fifth number in the sequence. The heart rate would be 60. What if there were two big blocks between QRS complexes? Go to the second number. The heart rate is 150. Memorizing this sequence of numbers will save lots of time.

- *The little block method.* In this method, count the number of little blocks between QRS complexes and divide into 1,500, since there are 1,500 little blocks in one minute. By now you're thinking, "You've got to be kidding! Count those tiny blocks?!" (You may well be in bifocals by the end of this chapter.) Actually, it's not that bad. Remember each big block is made up of five little blocks. Simply count each big block as five and the leftover little blocks as one. See Figure 5–2.

TABLE 5–1 Memory Method of Calculating Heart Rate

Number of Big Blocks Between QRS	Heart Rate	Number of Big Blocks Between QRS	Heart Rate
1	300	6	50
2	150	7	43
3	100	8	37
4	75	9	33
5	60	10	30

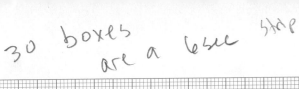

[handwritten margin notes: 30 boxes are a 6 sec strip; 1 small = .04 sec box; big box= .2]

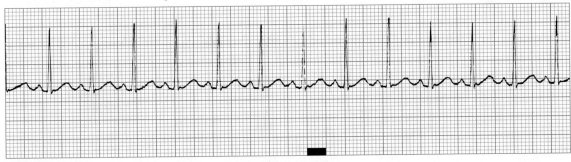

FIGURE 5–2

Little block method of calculating heart rate.

In Figure 5–2, there are 11 little blocks between QRS complexes, so the calculation is 1,500 ÷ 11 = 137. You can also use this method to calculate the heart rate range in irregular rhythms. Just find the two consecutive QRS complexes that are the farthest apart from each other and calculate that heart rate there—that's the slowest rate. Then find the two consecutive QRS complexes that are the closest together and calculate the heart rate there—that's the fastest rate.

chapter CHECKUP

We're about halfway through this chapter. To evaluate your understanding of the material thus far, answer the following questions. If you have trouble with them, review the material again before continuing.

1. Define *heart rate, ventricular rate,* and *atrial rate.*
2. Discuss the three methods of heart rate calculation.

Regularity-Based Heart Rate Calculation

Heart rate calculation is regularity based. The kind of heart rate you calculate will depend on the rhythm's regularity. **Rhythm regularity** is concerned with the spacing of the QRS complexes. Although we can also determine **atrial regularity** by examining the spacing of P waves, regularity of the QRS complexes is more important. To determine the regularity of a rhythm, compare the R-R intervals (the distance between consecutive QRS complexes). To compare R-Rs, count the number of little blocks between QRS complexes. Go from spike to spike.

Regularity Types

There are three types of regularity.

1. *Regular.* Regular rhythms are those in which the R-R intervals vary by only one or two little blocks. In regular rhythms, the QRS complexes usually look alike. Imagine these regular R-Rs as the rhythmic ticking of a clock. In Figure 5–3, the R-R intervals are all 23 to 24 little blocks apart. The rhythm is regular.
2. *Regular but interrupted.* This is a regular rhythm that is interrupted by either premature beats or pauses. At first glance, these rhythms may look irregular, but closer inspection reveals that only one or two beats, or a burst of several beats, make them look irregular, and that the rest of the R-R intervals are constant. The beats that interrupt this otherwise regular rhythm may look the same as the surrounding regular beats or may look quite different. Some texts would say that a rhythm that is interrupted by premature beats or pauses is indeed not regular and must therefore be called irregular. This text, however, makes the distinction between a rhythm that is regular except for an occasional "hiccup" and rhythms that are "all over the place" in their irregularity.

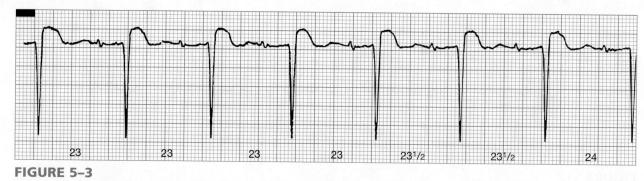

FIGURE 5–3

Regular rhythm.

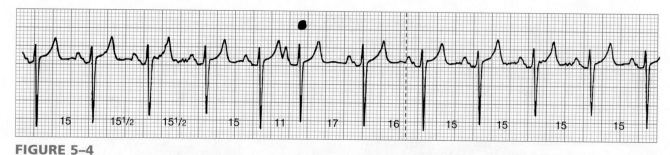

FIGURE 5–4

Regular rhythm interrupted by a premature beat.

In Figure 5–4, the rhythm is regular until the sixth QRS pops in prematurely. *Premature beats* are those that arrive early, before the next normal beat is due. Typically, after a premature beat, there is a short pause, and then the regular rhythm resumes. That's what happened on this strip. The R-R intervals are 15 to 16 little blocks apart except when beat number 6 pops in. Think of premature beats as hiccups. Imagine you're breathing normally and suddenly you hiccup. This hiccup pops in between your normal breaths and temporarily disturbs the regularity of your breathing pattern. Afterward, your breathing returns to normal. You wouldn't characterize your breathing pattern as irregular just because of one hiccup.

In Figure 5–5, the rhythm is regular until a sudden pause temporarily disturbs the regularity of the rhythm. Before and after the pause, the R-R intervals are constant—25 to 26 little blocks apart. During the pause, the R-R is 43 little blocks. Imagine these pauses are like a sudden power outage. Say you've got an electric clock ticking regularly. Suddenly, the power goes out for a few seconds and then comes back on. The outage temporarily disturbs the clock's otherwise normal, regular ticking pattern.

3. *Irregular.*   Irregular rhythms are those in which the R-R intervals vary, not just because of premature beats or pauses, but because the rhythm is intrinsically chaotic. R-R intervals will vary throughout the strip. Imagine these varying R-Rs

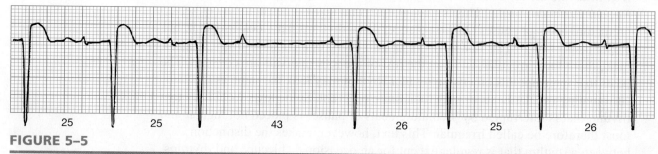

FIGURE 5–5

Regular rhythm interrupted by a pause.

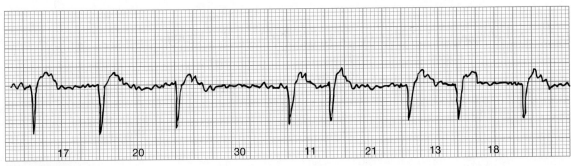

FIGURE 5–6

Irregular rhythm.

as the interval of time between rain showers. Maybe it rains once a week for two weeks in a row; then it rains again in three weeks, then after a month passes, then after a week and a half, then two months. The pattern is one of unpredictability—it happens when it happens.

In Figure 5–6, the R-R intervals are all over the place. Some QRS complexes are close together; others are farther apart. There is no sudden change, no regular pattern interrupted by a premature beat or pause. From beat to beat, the R-Rs vary. This is an intrinsically irregular rhythm. Do you see the difference between this rhythm and the strips of the regular but interrupted rhythms? *Whenever you see a rhythm that looks irregular, look closely to make sure it's not a regular but interrupted rhythm.* Let's practice a few.

Practice Strips: Regularity of Rhythms

For each of these strips, determine if it is regular, regular but interrupted, or irregular.

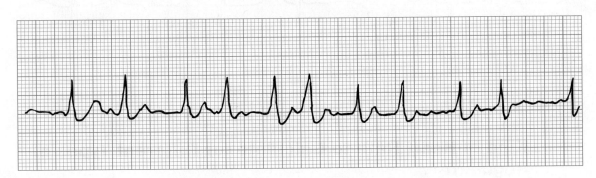

1. Answer_____

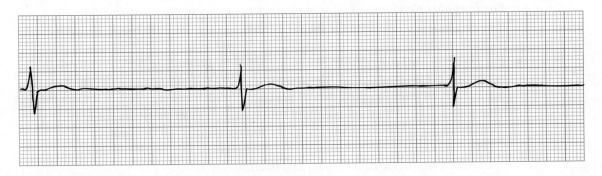

2. Answer_____

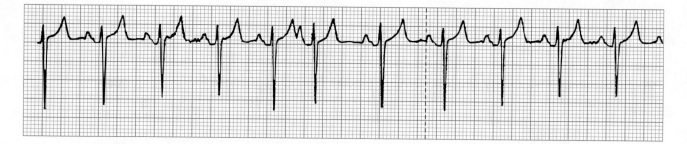

3. Answer_____

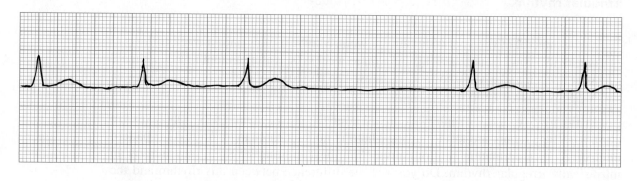

4. Answer_____

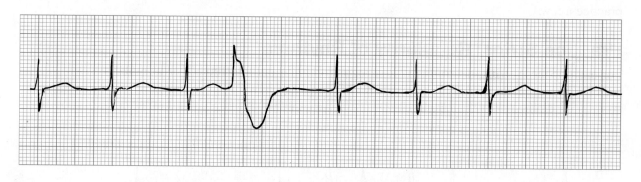

5. Answer_____

Kind of Heart Rate to Calculate for Different Types of Regularity

- *For regular rhythms.* Calculate the heart rate by choosing any two successive QRS complexes and using the little block or memory method.
- *For irregular rhythms.* Calculate the mean rate by using the 6-second strip method, and then calculate the heart rate range using the little block or memory method.
- *For rhythms that are regular but interrupted by premature beats.* Ignore the premature beats and calculate the heart rate, using the little block or memory method, on an uninterrupted part of the strip. Premature beats do not impact the heart rate much, as they are typically followed by a short pause that at least partially, if not completely, makes up for the prematurity of the beat. In Figure 5–7, the fifth QRS is a premature beat. Ignore this premature beat for purposes of heart rate calculation. The heart rate is 100.

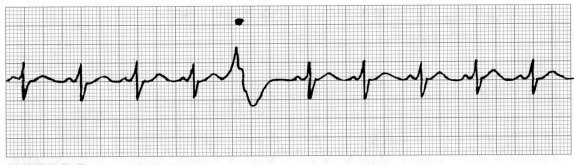

FIGURE 5–7

Regular rhythm interrupted by a premature beat.

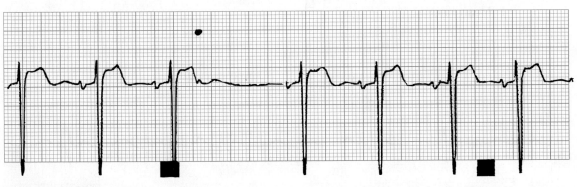

FIGURE 5–8

Regular rhythm interrupted by a pause.

■ *For rhythms that are regular but interrupted by pauses.*   Calculate the heart rate range slowest to fastest, along with the mean rate. Since pauses can be lengthy, they can greatly impact the heart rate; it's important to take them into account when calculating heart rate. See Figure 5–8.

In Figure 5–8, the regular rhythm is interrupted by a pause. Here the mean rate is 70, since there are 7 QRS complexes on this 6-second strip. There are 34 little blocks between the third and fourth QRS complexes, giving a rate of 44. There are 20 little blocks between the remainder of QRS complexes, for a heart rate of 75. The heart rate range is 44 to 75.

To sum up, see Table 5–2.

Calculating heart rate is a basic skill you will use throughout this book, and indeed throughout your work with EKGs. With practice, you will become expert at it. Let's get to the practice.

TABLE 5–2   Kind of Heart Rate to Calculate for Different Types of Regularity

Rhythm Regularity	Kind of Heart Rate to Calculate
Regular	One heart rate
Irregular	Range slowest to fastest, plus mean rate
Regular but interrupted by premature beats	One heart rate (ignoring premature beats)
Regular but interrupted by pauses	Range slowest to fastest, plus mean rate

Practice Strips: Calculating Heart Rate

Calculate the heart rate on these strips.

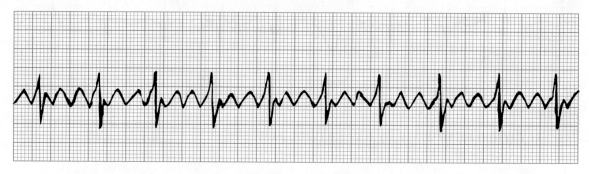

1. Heart rate _____100___ or 94

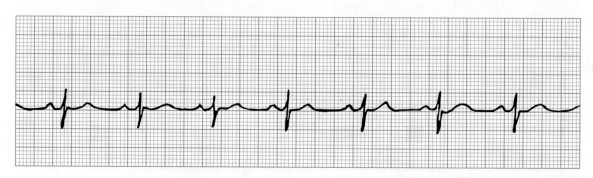

2. Heart rate _____75 b/m

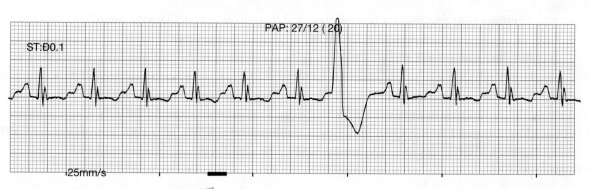

3. Heart rate _____107 b/m

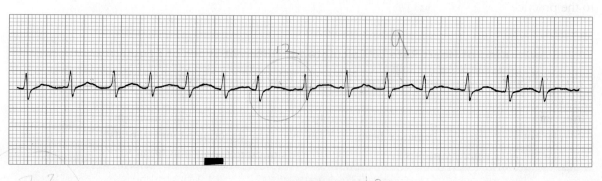

(107?)

4. Heart rate _____140_____125 – 115

120 → 155

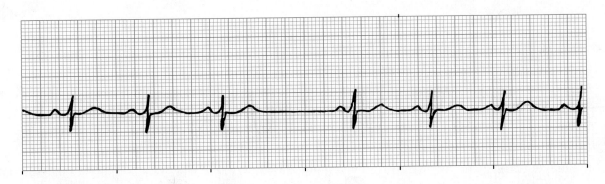

5. Heart rate _____

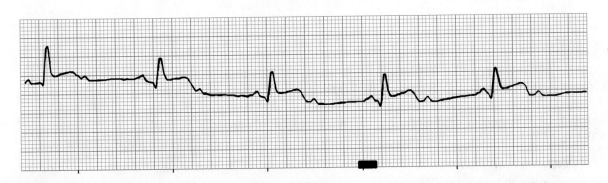

6. Heart rate _____

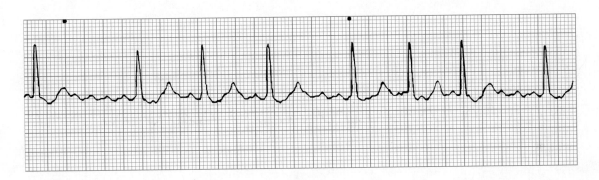

7. Heart rate _____

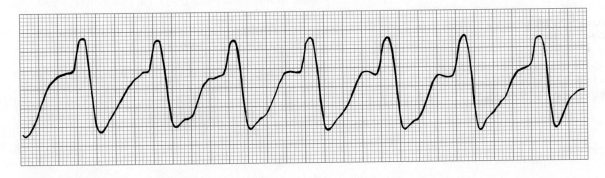

8. Heart rate _____

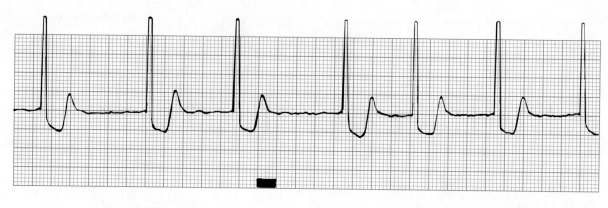

9. Heart rate _____

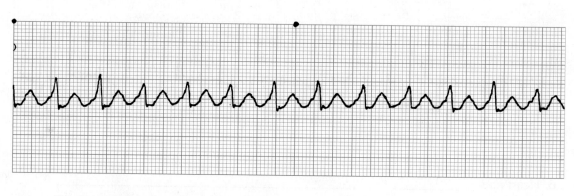

10. Heart rate _____

chapter five notes TO SUM IT ALL UP . . .

- **Heart rate**—Number of QRS complexes in one minute.
- **Heart rate is same as ventricular rate.**
- **Atrial rate**—Number of P waves in one minute.
- **Three methods of calculating heart rate:**
  - *6-second strip method*—Least accurate. Count QRS complexes on a 6-second strip and multiply by 10—provides **mean heart rate.**
  - *Memory method*—Memorize the chart.
  - *Little block method*—Count number of little blocks between consecutive QRS complexes and divide into 1,500.
- **Heart rate calculations are regularity based.**
- **Regularity**—Refers to the constancy of QRS complexes and/or P waves.
- **R-R interval**—Distance between consecutive QRS complexes. Count number of little blocks between QRS complexes and that's the R-R interval.

- **Three kinds of regularity:**
  - *Regular*—R-R intervals vary by only one or two little blocks.
  - *Regular but interrupted*—R-R intervals are regular until interrupted by a premature beat or a pause.
  - *Irregular*—R-R intervals are all over the place—completely unpredictable.
- **Regularity-based heart rate calculation:**
  - *Regular rhythm*—Choose method of choice and calculate one heart rate.
  - *Irregular rhythm*—Calculate heart rate range slowest to fastest, along with mean rate.
  - *Regular rhythm interrupted by premature beat*—Ignore premature beat and the short pause that usually follows it. Go to uninterrupted part of the strip—calculate heart rate there using method of choice.
  - *Regular rhythm interrupted by pause*—Calculate heart rate range slowest to fastest, along with mean rate.

Practice Quiz

1. Name the three methods for calculating heart rate.

   _____

   _____

   _____

2. The least accurate method of calculating heart rate is the _____

3. When using the little block method, count the number of little blocks between QRS complexes and divide into _____

4. Write the sequence of the memory method. _____

   _____

5. With regular rhythms interrupted by premature beats, how is the heart rate calculated? _____

   _____

6. Name the three types of regularity. _____

   _____

   _____

   _____

7. A rhythm with R-R intervals that vary throughout the strip is a(n) _____ rhythm.

8. A rhythm that is regular except for premature beats or pauses is a(n) _____ rhythm.

9. A rhythm in which the R-R intervals vary by only one or two little blocks is a(n) _____ rhythm.

10. Define *R-R interval*. _____

    _____

Putting It All Together—Critical Thinking Exercises

These exercises may consist of diagrams to label, scenarios to analyze, brain-stumping questions to ponder, or other challenging exercises to boost your understanding of the chapter material.

1. A rhythm whose R-R intervals are 23, 24, 23, 23, 12, 24, 23, 24, 23, 23 would be considered which kind of regularity? _____ What's the heart rate? _____

2. A rhythm with R-R intervals of 12, 17, 22, 45, 10, and 18 would be considered which type of regularity? _____ What's the heart rate? _____

3. A rhythm with R-R intervals of 22, 23, 22, 22, 23, 22, 22, 22 would be considered which kind of regularity? _____ What's the heart rate? _____

How to Interpret a Rhythm Strip

CHAPTER 6 OBJECTIVES

Upon completion of this chapter, the student will be able to:

- Use the five steps to interpret a variety of rhythms.

What It's All About

"I'll never learn this stuff," Erica, a new ICU nurse, moaned to her preceptor (trainer) Kimla while staring at a rhythm strip. "It's like trying to read hieroglyphics on Egyptian tombs. It just looks like squiggly lines to me. Do you actually understand this stuff?" "I do," Kimla replied. "It took a lot of practice but eventually I caught on. Find a good textbook and try this method step by step and you'll get it." So Erica studied her textbook and practiced the rhythms there. She asked her fellow nurses to explain things to her that she didn't understand. She collected rhythm strips to practice on. About a month later, Kimla and Erica were discussing a patient and examining a rhythm strip. "So what do you think this is, Erica?" Kimla asked. "Well," Erica answered, "it looks like third degree AV block to me. Look at all those P waves not followed by a QRS. And the rhythm is regular." Kimla looked up over her glasses at a grinning Erica. "Go, girl, look at you! You're ALMOST as good as me now."

Introduction

When we analyze a rhythm strip, we are looking for pathology in the form of arrhythmias. Arrhythmias can originate in any of the heart's pacemakers. Some of these rhythms are benign, causing no problem, and others are lethal, killing almost instantly. It's important to know not just what rhythm the patient is in now, but what rhythm preceded it and what's normal for this particular patient. Even so-called normal rhythms or heart rates can be cause for concern. For example, if a patient has a heart rate of 110 (abnormally fast) for two consecutive days, and it suddenly drops to 66, which is normal, it may be a sign of trouble—the heart rate may be at 66 on its way to 0. *Always look at the trend.* Only so much information can be obtained from a single rhythm strip. Comparing the present rhythm strip to previous ones paints a better picture of the patient's condition.

The Five Steps to Rhythm Interpretation

It's important to have a plan of attack in analyzing EKG rhythms. In the previous chapters, you learned how to identify the waves and complexes on rhythm strips, and how to calculate the heart rate and measure intervals. Let's put all that together now. Asking the following questions for each rhythm strip will help identify the rhythm (see website for a video showing arrhythmia):

1. Are there QRS complexes? There are a few rhythms that have no QRS complexes at all, so look for the QRS complexes first. It can save you some time and trouble.
   - If yes, are they the same shape, or does the shape vary?
   - If no, skip to question 4.

2. Is the rhythm regular, regular but interrupted, or irregular?
   - Compare the R-R intervals.

3. What is the heart rate?
   - If the heart rate is greater than 100, the patient is said to have a **tachycardia**.
   - If the heart rate is less than 60, the patient has a **bradycardia**.

4. Are there P waves?
   - If so, what is their relationship to the QRS? In other words, are the Ps always in the same place relative to the QRS, or are the Ps in different places with each beat?
   - Are any Ps not followed by a QRS?
   - Are the Ps all the same shape, or does the shape vary?
   - Is the **P-P interval** (the distance between consecutive P waves) regular?

5. What are the PR and QRS intervals?
   - Are the intervals within normal limits, or are they too short or too long?
   - Are the intervals constant on the strip, or do they vary from beat to beat?

Quick Tip

Treat the patient, not just the rhythm. Any significant change in rhythm or heart rate should prompt an immediate assessment of the patient's condition. Two patients can have the same rhythm and heart rate, but differ drastically in their tolerance of it. If the patient has a rhythm you cannot immediately identify, but it's a change from previous ones, *check on the patient and come back to the strip later.* The patient's life may well depend on your prompt action.

What Is Normal?

You'll recall that the heart's normal pacemaker is the sinus node. The normal rhythm originating from the sinus node is called **sinus rhythm.** Normal sinus rhythms have the following:

- Narrow QRS complexes of uniform shape.
- Regularly spaced QRS complexes.
- Heart rate between 60 and 100.
- Upright, rounded, matching P waves "married to" the QRS complexes (in the same place preceding each QRS) in Lead II.
- PR interval between 0.12 to 0.20 seconds, constant from beat to beat.
- QRS interval less than 0.12 secs.

   Arrhythmias, on the other hand, will exhibit some combination of the following:

- QRS complexes that are absent or abnormally shaped.
- P waves that are absent, multiple in number, or abnormally shaped.
- Abnormally prolonged or abnormally short PR intervals.
- Abnormally prolonged QRS intervals.
- Heart rate that is abnormally slow or fast.
- Irregular rhythm or a rhythm that has interruptions by premature beats or pauses.

The Five Steps Practice

Let's practice the five steps on the five rhythm strips that follow:

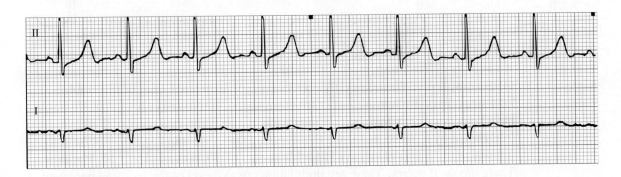

1. Note that this is a double-lead strip. The top strip is labeled Lead II, and the bottom is Lead I. Use either lead (whichever one is clearer to you) to gather your data about the strips. **QRS complexes:** There are QRS complexes on the strip. They are all shaped the same (in each lead). **Regularity:** The rhythm is regular, as evidenced by the R-R

intervals all measuring about 18 small blocks. **Heart rate:** Since the rhythm is regular, we choose any two successive QRS complexes and calculate the heart rate there: 1,500 divided by 18 equals a heart rate of 83. **P waves:** There are upright matching P waves preceding each QRS. P waves are "married" to the QRS complexes—they are in the same place relative to the QRS. All P waves are followed by a QRS. P-P interval is regular, meaning the P waves are regularly spaced. **PR interval:** PR interval is about 0.12 secs (normal) and is constant from beat to beat. **QRS interval:** QRS interval is about 0.08 secs (normal, constant beat to beat).

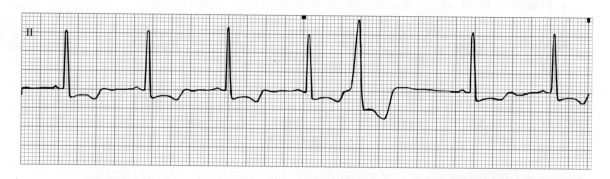

2. **QRS complexes:** There are QRS complexes, all but one of which is narrow and shaped the same. The fifth QRS is taller and wider than the others. **Regularity:** Regular but interrupted by a premature beat. The R-R intervals are 21, 21½, 21, 13 (the premature beat), 30 (the normal pause following a premature beat), and 21. **Heart rate:** 1,500 divided by 21 equals 71. **P waves:** Upright and matching preceding all but the fifth QRS. That QRS has no P wave. The P waves are married to the QRS—they are in the same place relative to their QRS complexes. P-P interval is constant except for the wide QRS beat that has no P wave. **PR interval:** 0.12 secs (normal), constant from beat to beat. **QRS interval:** 0.06 (normal) on the narrow beats, 0.12 (abnormally wide) on the wide beat.

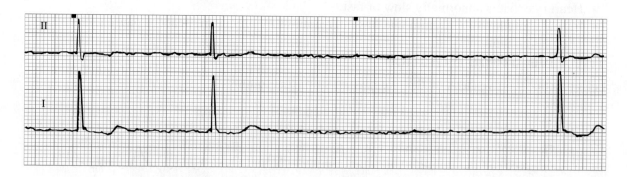

3. **QRS complexes:** There are only 3 QRS complexes in each lead of this double-lead strip. They are narrow and of uniform shape. **Regularity:** Irregular. (It would have been helpful to have had a longer strip to see if this is a regular rhythm interrupted by a pause, but since this is all we have, we must call it irregular). R-R intervals are 34 and 91. **Heart rate:** Mean rate of 30, range is 16 to 44. **P waves:** There are no P waves. There are undulations (waviness) of the baseline between QRS complexes. We cannot assess P-P interval since there are no P waves. Absence of P waves is abnormal. **PR interval:** Since there are no P waves, there can be no PR interval. **QRS interval:** 0.08 (normal), constant from beat to beat.

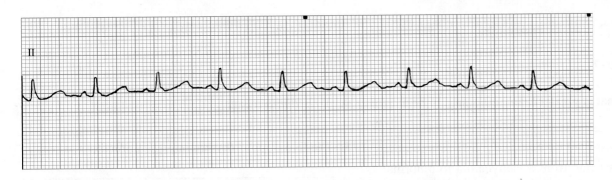

4. **QRS complexes:** All QRS complexes are narrow and of uniform shape.
Regularity: Regular, as evidenced by the R-R intervals of about 16 small blocks.
Heart rate: 1,500 divided by 16 equals 94. **P waves:** Upright and matching
preceding each QRS. P waves are married to the QRS. P-P interval is regular. **PR
interval:** 0.12 secs (normal), constant. **QRS interval:** 0.08 secs (normal), constant.

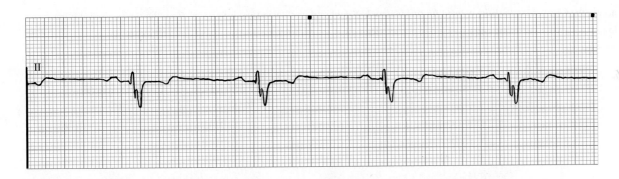

5. **QRS complexes:** All QRS complexes are wide and of uniform shape. **Regularity:**
Regular, as evidenced by the R-R intervals of about 33 little blocks. **Heart rate:**
1,500 divided by 33 equals 45. **P waves:** P waves are upright, matching, and
married to the QRS complexes. P-P interval is regular. **PR interval:** 0.20 secs
(abnormally long). **QRS interval:** 0.16 secs (abnormally long).

You now should have a feel for what to look for on rhythm strips. In Chapters 7 to 11,
you'll learn about the different rhythms themselves. Let's get to it.

chapter six notes TO SUM IT ALL UP . . .

- **Five steps to rhythm interpretation:**
  - Are there QRS complexes? Are they the same shape?
  - What's the regularity?
  - What's the heart rate?
  - Are there P waves? Are they the same shape? Are they in the same place relative to the QRS? Are any P waves not followed by a QRS?
  - What are the PR and QRS intervals?
- **The only normal rhythm is sinus rhythm. Characteristics:**
  - QRS narrow, uniform shape.
  - Regular.
  - Heart rate 60–100.
  - Upright uniform shape P waves married to the QRS.
  - PR 0.12–0.20 secs, constant. QRS <0.12 secs.
- **Arrhythmia characteristics:**
  - QRS absent or abnormally shaped.
  - Irregular or regular-but-interrupted.
  - Heart rate varies from zero to tachycardias.
  - P waves may be absent, multiple in number, or abnormally shaped.
  - Intervals abnormal.

Practice Quiz

1. A heart rate that is greater than 100 is said to be a
_____

2. A heart rate less than 60 is a _____

3. A drop in heart rate from a tachycardia to a normal heart rate (is/is not) cause for concern.

4. *Arrhythmia* means_____
_____

5. The five steps to rhythm interpretation are_____
_____
_____

Rhythms Originating in the Sinus Node

7

CHAPTER 7 OBJECTIVES

Upon completion of this chapter, the student will be able to:

- State the criteria for each of the sinus rhythms.
- Using the five steps, correctly interpret a variety of sinus rhythms on single- and double-lead strips.
- State the adverse effects for each of the sinus rhythms.
- State the possible treatment for the sinus rhythms.

What It's All About

Paula, Donna, and Jackie were in their nursing fundamentals class learning how to check pulses. They were practicing on one another and were surprised to find that their heart rates were so different. Paula's was 106, Donna's was 88, and Jackie's was 54. Knowing that the normal heart rate is between 60 and 100, the girls were concerned that Paula and Jackie had some exotic medical condition that was affecting their heart. (A little knowledge can be a dangerous thing, can't it?) The girls approached their instructor Stella, all of them now worried that something was wrong. Stella chuckled when she checked the girls' pulses. *All of them* now had a heart rate over 100. "You all worry too much," she told them. "You're all worked up now so your heart rate is up. Remember adrenalin? It pours out of your adrenal gland whenever you're excited, worried, scared, and so on. And you all had different heart rates to start off with because you're all different. Jackie is an athlete, so her pulse was slower because of her excellent conditioning. Donna, your heart rate was normal, and Paula is excited that her husband is coming back from overseas tonight—you thought I didn't hear that, huh?—so her heart rate was higher than normal. Relax, girls. I'm sure you're all in sinus rhythms. You'll live . . . at least until you see my final exam."

Introduction

Sinus rhythms originate in the sinus node, travel through the atria to depolarize them, and then head down the normal conduction pathway to depolarize the ventricles. You'll recall the sinus node is the normal pacemaker of the heart. See Figure 7–1.

In Figure 7–1, the sinus node fires its impulse, which travels throughout the atria, causing atrial depolarization and writing the P wave on the EKG. The impulse then heads down through the AV node to the ventricle. The QRS is written when ventricular depolarization occurs.

The Word on Sinus Rhythms

The sinus node is the acknowledged king of the conduction system's pacemaker cells. There are only two ways for the sinus node king to relinquish its throne:

1. By illness or death of the sinus node, requiring a lower pacemaker to step in for it (escape).
2. By being overthrown by a lower pacemaker (usurpation/irritability).

Although they can be irregular at times, sinus rhythms are, for the most part, regular. They're like the ticking of a clock—predictable and expected. You'll recall the inherent rate of the sinus node is 60 to 100. But also remember that this rate can go higher or lower if the

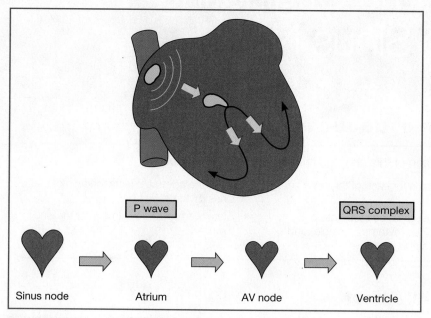

FIGURE 7–1

Conduction in sinus rhythms.

sinus node is acted on by the sympathetic or parasympathetic nervous system. The individual's tolerance of these rhythms will depend in large part on the heart rate. Heart rates that are too fast or too slow can cause symptoms of decreased cardiac output (inadequate blood flow to the body). Such symptoms can include pallor, dizziness, chest pain, shortness of breath, confusion, decreased urine output, hypotension (low blood pressure), and diaphoresis (cold sweat; also referred to as cold and clammy).

Treatment is not needed unless symptoms develop. At that time, the goal is to return the heart rate to normal levels.

Sinus rhythms are the standard against which all other rhythms are compared. Since most of the rhythms you will see in real life will be sinus rhythms, you'll need a thorough understanding of them. Let's look at the criteria for sinus rhythms. *All these criteria must be met for the rhythm to be sinus in origin:*

- Upright matching P waves in Lead II followed by a QRS *and*
- PR intervals constant *and*
- Heart rate less than or equal to 160 at rest

All matching upright P waves in Lead II are considered sinus P waves until proven otherwise. The width and deflection of the QRS complex is irrelevant in determining whether a rhythm originates in the sinus node. The QRS is normally narrow (<0.12 seconds) in sinus rhythms, but it can be wide (≥0.12 secs) if conduction through the bundle branches is altered. *The deflection of the QRS will depend on the lead in which the patient is being monitored. For example, you'll recall from Chapter 3 that the QRS in Lead II should be upright but in V_1 should be inverted.* Now let's look at the sinus rhythms.

Sinus Rhythm

Sinus rhythm is *the* normal rhythm. The impulse is born in the sinus node and heads down the conduction pathway to the ventricle. Every P wave is married to a QRS complex, and the heart rate is the normal 60 to 100. The QRS complex can be positive, negative, or isoelectric depending on the lead being monitored.

Rate	60-100
Regularity	Regular
P waves	Upright in most leads, although may be normally inverted in V_1. One P to each QRS. All P waves have the same shape. *All matching upright P waves are sinus P waves until proven otherwise* (this is the most crucial criterion to identifying rhythms originating in the sinus node); P-P interval is regular.
Intervals	PR 0.12 to 0.20 secs, constant from beat to beat QRS <0.12 secs
Cause	Normal
Adverse effects	None (unless the heart rate is a drastic change from previously— always look at the trend).
Treatment	None

Figure 7–2 shows QRS complexes, all the same shape. The rhythm is regular. Heart rate is 88. P waves are present, one before each QRS complex, and they are all matching and upright. *Remember—all matching upright P waves in Lead II are sinus P waves until proven otherwise.* P-P interval is regular. PR interval is 0.20, QRS interval is 0.10, both normal. Interpretation: sinus rhythm.

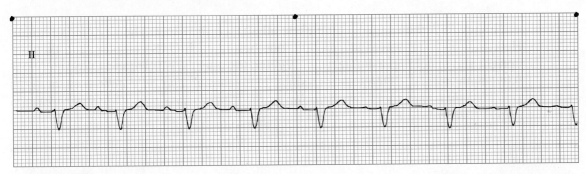

FIGURE 7–2

Sinus rhythm.

Sinus Bradycardia

Sinus bradycardia is a slower-than-normal rhythm from the sinus node. The impulse originates in the sinus node and travels the conduction system normally. The QRS complex can be positive, negative, or isoelectric depending on the lead being monitored.

Rate	Less than 60
Regularity	Regular
P waves	Upright in most leads, although may be inverted in V_1. One P to each QRS. P waves shaped the same. P-P interval regular.
Intervals	PR 0.12 to 0.20 secs, constant from beat to beat QRS <0.12 secs
Cause	Vagal stimulation such as vomiting or straining to have a bowel movement, **myocardial infarction** (MI), **hypoxia** (low blood oxygen level), **digitalis toxicity** (an overabundance of the medication digitalis in the bloodstream), and other medication side effects.

Sinus bradycardia is common in athletes because their well-conditioned heart pumps more blood out with each beat and therefore doesn't need to beat as often.

Adverse effects

Too slow a heart rate can cause signs of decreased cardiac output. Many individuals, however, tolerate a slow heart rate and do not require treatment.

Treatment

None unless the patient is symptomatic. A medication called *atropine* can be used if needed to speed up the heart rate. Atropine increases the rate at which the sinus node propagates (creates) its impulses and speeds up impulse conduction through the AV node. Thus, it causes an increase in heart rate. If atropine is unsuccessful, an electronic pacemaker or medications such as epinephrine and dopamine can be utilized, although they are not usually necessary for sinus bradycardia unless the individual is in shock. Consider starting oxygen. If the heart does not receive adequate oxygen, conduction system cells become **ischemic** (oxygen starved) and may respond by firing at rates above or below their norm. Providing supplemental oxygen can help these stricken cells return to more normal functioning and a more normal heart rate.

Figure 7–3 shows QRS complexes, all shaped the same. The rhythm is regular. Heart rate is 54. P waves are present, one before each QRS complex, and they are upright and matching. P-P interval is regular. PR interval is 0.16, and QRS interval is 0.09, both normal. Interpretation: sinus bradycardia. *The only difference between sinus rhythm and sinus bradycardia is the heart rate—the other interpretation criteria are the same.*

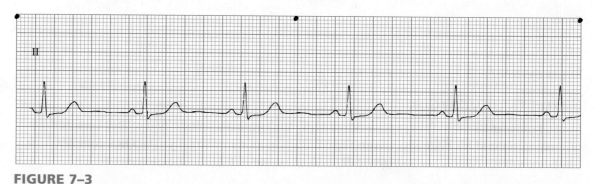

FIGURE 7–3

Sinus bradycardia.

chapter CHECKUP

We're about halfway through this chapter. To evaluate your understanding of the material thus far, answer the following questions. If you have trouble with them, review the material again before continuing.

Mrs. Spock calls you to her hospital room—she's having crushing chest pain, nausea, and shortness of breath. You check her vital signs—pulse, blood pressure, and respiratory rate—and find that her heart rate, which had been 78, is now 34. Her blood pressure is also lower, as is her respiratory rate. She is cold and clammy. You note her rhythm has a narrow (<0.12 secs) QRS and matching upright P waves in Lead II.

1. What is her rhythm?
2. What's the likely cause?
3. What treatment would be indicated?

Sinus Tachycardia

Sinus tachycardia is a rhythm in which the sinus node fires at a heart rate faster than normal. The impulse originates in the sinus node and travels down the conduction pathway normally. The QRS complex can be positive, negative, or isoelectric depending on the lead being monitored.

Rate	101 to 160. According to most experts, the sinus node does not fire at a rate above 160 in *supine resting adults.* Although this is somewhat controversial, we will adopt 160 as the upper limit of the sinus node. *All strips in this text are from supine resting adults unless otherwise specified.*
Regularity	Regular
P waves	Upright in most leads, although may be inverted in V_1. One P to each QRS. P waves shaped the same. P-P interval regular.
Intervals	0.12 to 0.20 secs, constant from beat to beat QRS <0.12 secs
Cause	Medications such as atropine or bronchodilators (medications used to open up narrowed respiratory passages in patients with asthma or chronic obstructive pulmonary disease [COPD]); emotional upset, **pulmonary embolus** (blood clot in the lung), MI, **congestive heart failure** (CHF), fever, inhibition of the vagus nerve, hypoxia, and **thyrotoxicosis** (thyroid storm—an emergent medical condition in which the thyroid gland overproduces thyroid hormones so that the heart rate, blood pressure, and temperature all rise to dangerously high levels)
Adverse effects	Increased heart rate causes increased cardiac workload. The faster a muscle works, the more blood and oxygen it requires. This can stress an already weakened heart. Cardiac output can drop. This is especially true in the patient with an acute MI, as the increased blood and oxygen demand taxes the already damaged heart muscle.
Treatment	Treat the cause. For example, if the patient in sinus tachycardia has a fever, give medications to decrease the fever. If the tachycardia is caused by anxiety, consider sedation. For cardiac patients with persistent sinus tachycardia, a class of medications called *beta-blockers* may be used to slow the heart rate. Consider starting oxygen to decrease the heart's workload.

Quick Tip

Every one degree increase in body temperature causes the heart rate to rise by about 10 beats per minute.

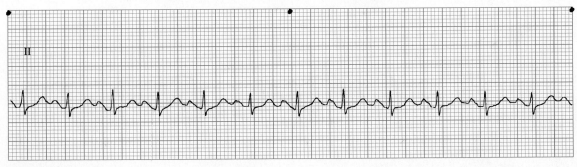

FIGURE 7–4

Sinus tachycardia.

Figure 7–4 shows QRS complexes, all shaped the same. The rhythm is regular. Heart rate is about 125. P waves are present, one before each QRS, and they are all upright and matching. P-P interval is regular. PR interval is 0.14, and QRS interval is 0.06, both within normal limits. Interpretation: sinus tachycardia. *Just as in sinus rhythm and sinus bradycardia, all the criteria for interpretation are the same for sinus tachycardia—the only difference is the heart rate.*

Sinus Arrhythmia

Sinus arrhythmia is the only *irregular* rhythm from the sinus node, and it has a pattern that is cyclic and usually corresponds with the breathing pattern. The QRS complex can be positive, negative, or isoelectric depending on the lead being monitored.

Rate	Varies with respiratory pattern—faster with inspiration, slower with expiration. The negative pressure in the chest during inspiration sucks up blood from the lower extremities, causing an increase in blood returning to the right atrium. The heart rate speeds up to circulate this extra blood. Sinus arrhythmia is especially common during sleep, especially among those with **sleep apnea** (a temporary, often repetitive cessation of breathing during sleep).
Regularity	Irregular in a repetitive pattern; longest R-R cycle exceeds the shortest by ≥0.16 secs (four or more little blocks).
P waves	Upright in most leads, although may be inverted in V_1. P waves shaped the same. One P to each QRS. P-P interval is irregular.
Intervals	PR 0.12 to 0.20 secs, constant from beat to beat QRS <0.12 secs
Cause	Usually caused by the breathing pattern, but can be caused by heart disease
Adverse effects	Usually no ill effects
Treatment	Usually none required

Figure 7–5 shows QRS complexes, all the same shape. The rhythm is irregular. Heart rate is 62 to 88, with a mean rate of 80. The longest R-R interval (24 little blocks) exceeds the shortest (17 blocks) by 7 little blocks. P waves are present, one before each QRS, and all are upright and shaped the same. P-P interval varies. PR interval is 0.24 secs (abnormally long), and QRS interval is 0.10 (normal). Interpretation: sinus arrhythmia with a prolonged PR interval.

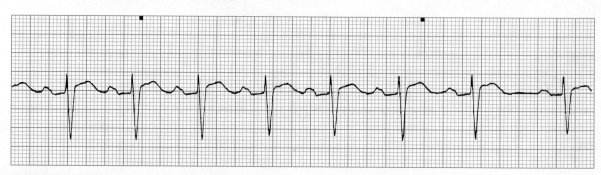

FIGURE 7–5

Sinus arrhythmia.

Sinus Arrest

Sinus arrest is a pause that occurs when the regularly firing sinus node suddenly stops firing for a brief period. One or more P-QRS-T sequences will be missing. An escape beat from a lower pacemaker may then take over for one or more beats. The sinus node may resume functioning after missing one or more beats, or the lower pacemaker may continue as the pacemaker, creating a new escape rhythm. The pause is not a multiple of the previous R-R intervals. The escape beat or rhythm resumes whenever it can. The QRS complex can be positive, negative, or isoelectric depending on the lead being monitored.

Rate	Can occur at any heart rate
Regularity	Regular but interrupted (by a pause). In any rhythm with a pause, always measure the length of the pause in seconds.
P waves	Normal sinus P waves before the pause, normal or different-shaped Ps (if even present) on the beat ending the pause. P-P interval is usually regular before the pause and may vary after the pause, depending on whether the sinus node regains pacemaking control.
Intervals	PR 0.12 to 0.20 secs before the pause, may be shorter or absent after the pause. QRS on the sinus beats will be <0.12 secs. On the escape beat(s), the QRS may be narrow (<0.12 secs) or wide (>0.12 secs) depending on which pacemaker of the heart resumes following the pause.
Cause	Sinus node ischemia, hypoxia, digitalis toxicity, excessive vagal tone, other medication side effects.
Adverse effects	Frequent or very long sinus arrests can cause decreased cardiac output.
Treatment	Occasional sinus arrests may not cause a problem—the patient has no ill effects. Frequent sinus arrests may require that the medication causing it be stopped and can require atropine and/or a pacemaker to speed up the heart rate. Consider starting oxygen.

In Figure 7–6, the first three beats are sinus beats firing along regularly. Suddenly there is a long pause, at the end of which is a beat from a lower pacemaker. How do we know the beat that ends the pause (the escape beat) is not a sinus beat? Sinus beats all have matching upright P waves. This beat has no P wave at all, plus its QRS complex is huge, completely unlike the other QRS complexes. Note the pause is not a multiple of the

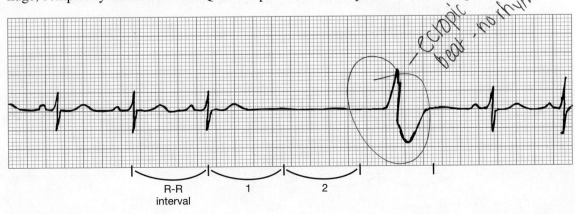

— ectopic beat - no rhythm

R-R interval   1   2

FIGURE 7–6

Sinus arrest.

R-R intervals. Going through our steps: There are QRS complexes, all but one having the same shape. Regularity is regular but interrupted. Heart rate is 30 to 75, with a mean rate of 60. P waves are upright, matching, one before all QRS complexes except the escape beat. PR interval is 0.16, and QRS interval is 0.08 on the sinus beats and 0.14 on the escape beat. Interpretation: sinus rhythm interrupted by a 2-second sinus arrest (you'll recall every 5 big blocks equals 1 second; there are 10 big blocks between these QRS complexes) and a wide-QRS-complex escape beat. Note that the sinus node resumes functioning after one escape beat.

Sinus Block (Also Called Sinus Exit Block)

Sinus block is a pause that occurs when the sinus node fires its impulse on time, but the impulse's exit from the sinus node to the atrial tissue is blocked. *In other words, the beat that the sinus node propagated is not conducted anywhere.* This results in one or more P-QRS-T sequences being missing, creating a pause, the length of which will depend on how many sinus beats are blocked. When conduction of the regularly firing sinus impulses resumes, the sinus beats return on time at the end of the pause. The pause will be a multiple of the previous R-R intervals—that is, exactly 2 or more R-R cycles will fit into the pause. The QRS complex can be positive, negative, or isoelectric depending on the lead being monitored.

Rate	Can occur at any heart rate
Regularity	Regular but interrupted (by a pause)
P waves	Normal sinus Ps both before and after the pause; P waves shaped the same
Intervals	PR 0.12 to 0.20 secs QRS <0.12 secs.
Cause	Medication side effects, hypoxia, or strong vagal stimulation
Adverse effects	Same as sinus arrest
Treatment	Same as sinus arrest

Figure 7–7 shows a pause that lasts 8 big blocks. This is exactly twice the R-R interval of the sinus beats that precede and follow the pause. The pause is therefore a multiple of the R-R intervals. The pause ends with a sinus beat. Going through our steps: There are QRS complexes, all shaped the same. Regularity is regular but interrupted. Heart rate is 37 to 75, with a mean rate of 60. P waves are upright, matching, one before each QRS complex. PR interval is 0.16, and QRS interval is 0.08. Interpretation: sinus rhythm with a 1.6-second sinus block.

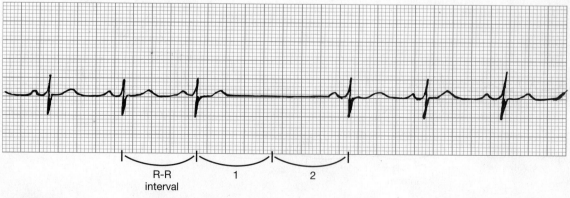

FIGURE 7–7

Sinus block.

Practice Strips: Sinus Rhythms

Following are 25 rhythm strips, the first 10 on single-lead strips, most of the remainder on double-lead strips.

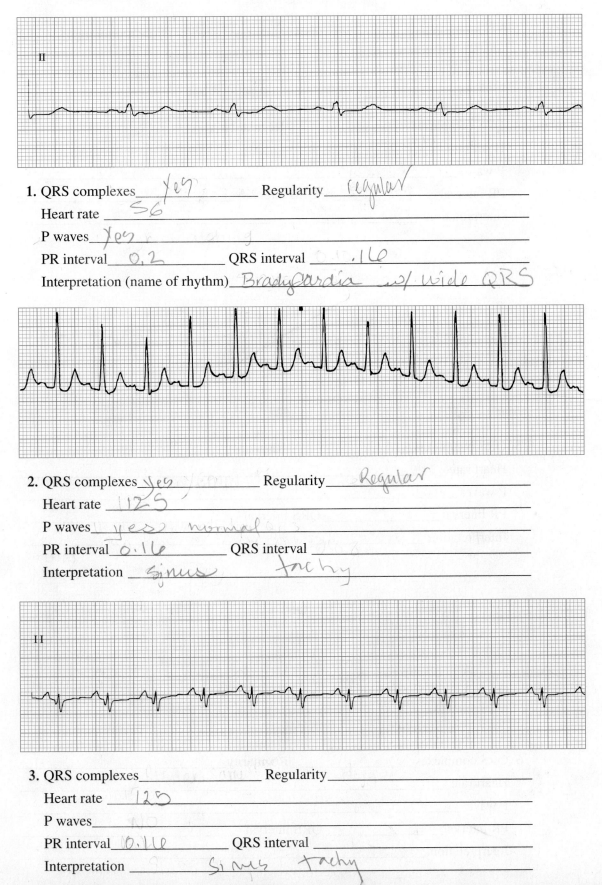

1. QRS complexes____Yes_____ Regularity____regular____
   Heart rate ____56____
   P waves____Yes_____
   PR interval____0.2_____ QRS interval ____.16____
   Interpretation (name of rhythm)____Bradycardia___w/ wide QRS____

2. QRS complexes__yes_____ Regularity____Regular____
   Heart rate ____125____
   P waves____yes____normal_____
   PR interval____0.16_____ QRS interval _____
   Interpretation ____Sinus_____tachy____

3. QRS complexes_____ Regularity_____
   Heart rate ____125____
   P waves____NO____
   PR interval____0.16_____ QRS interval _____
   Interpretation ____Sinus____tachy____

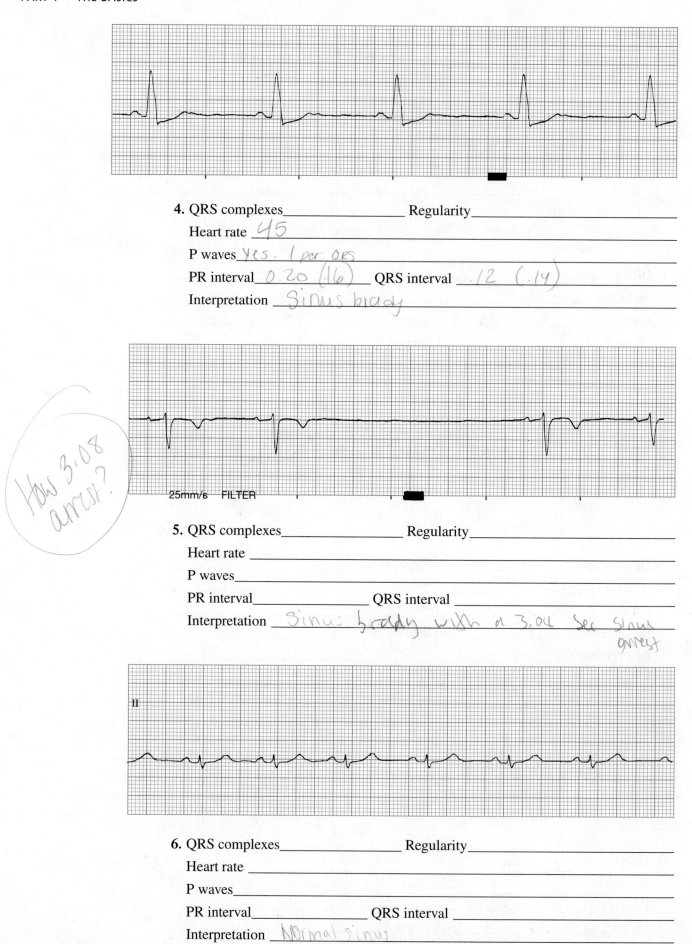

4. QRS complexes_____ Regularity_____

Heart rate _45_

P waves_Yes. 1 per QRS_

PR interval_0.20 (.16)_ QRS interval _.12 (.14)_

Interpretation _Sinus brady_

How 3.08 arrest?

25mm/s   FILTER

5. QRS complexes_____ Regularity_____

Heart rate _____

P waves_____

PR interval_____ QRS interval _____

Interpretation _Sinus brady with a 3.04 sec sinus arrest_

II

6. QRS complexes_____ Regularity_____

Heart rate _____

P waves_____

PR interval_____ QRS interval _____

Interpretation _Normal sinus_

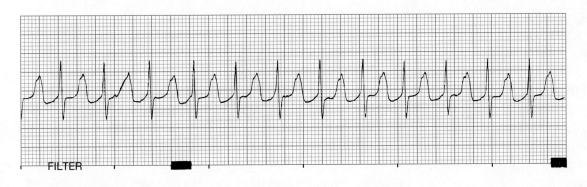

FILTER

7. QRS complexes_____ Regularity_____

Heart rate _____

P waves_____

PR interval_____ QRS interval _____

Interpretation _____ Sinus Tachycardia _____

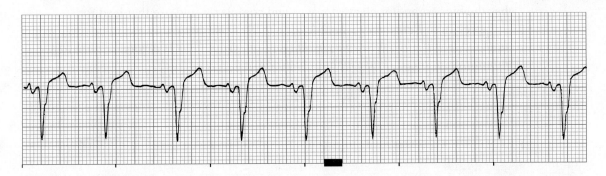

8. QRS complexes_____ Regularity_____

Heart rate _____

P waves_____

PR interval_____ QRS interval _____

Interpretation _____ Sinus rhythm _____

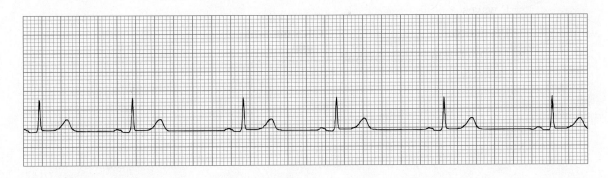

9. QRS complexes_____ Regularity_____

Heart rate _____

P waves_____

PR interval_____ QRS interval _____

Interpretation _____ Sinus arrhythmia _____

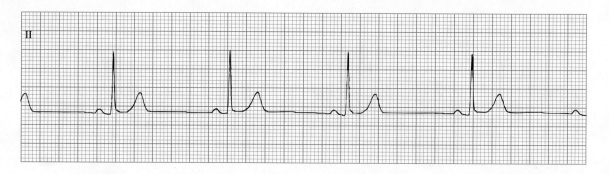

10. QRS complexes_____ Regularity_____

Heart rate _____

P waves_____

PR interval_____ QRS interval _____

Interpretation ___Sinus brady_____

Most of the remaining are double-lead strips. On each strip, choose the lead that has the biggest and/or clearest waves and complexes and use that lead for interpretation. *Remember—both leads are the same patient at the same time, so both leads will have the same rhythm and intervals. This is a good chance to see how different these sinus rhythms can look in different leads.*

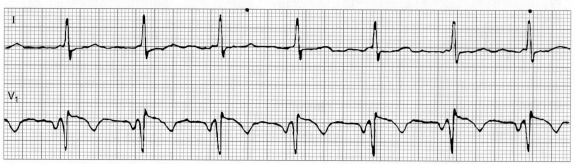

11. QRS complexes_____ Regularity_____

Heart rate _____

P waves_____

PR interval_____ QRS interval _____

Interpretation ___Sinus rhythm_____

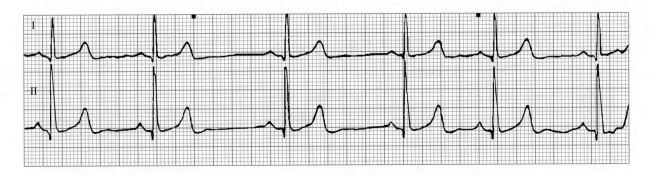

12. QRS complexes_____ Regularity_____

    Heart rate _____

    P waves_____

    PR interval_____ QRS interval _____

    Interpretation _Sinus arrhythmia_____

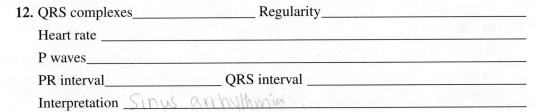

Manual   I : 10mm/mv   II : 10mm/mv

13. QRS complexes_____ Regularity_____

    Heart rate _____

    P waves_____

    PR interval_____ QRS interval _____

    Interpretation _____ Sinus rhythm_____

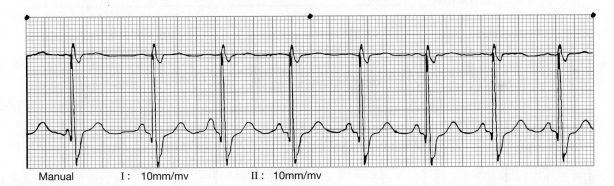

Manual   I : 10mm/mv   II : 10mm/mv

14. QRS complexes_____ Regularity_____

    Heart rate _71_____

    P waves_____

    PR interval_____ QRS interval _____

    Interpretation _Normal Sinus_____

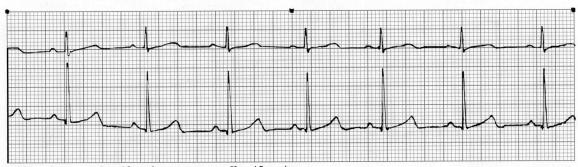

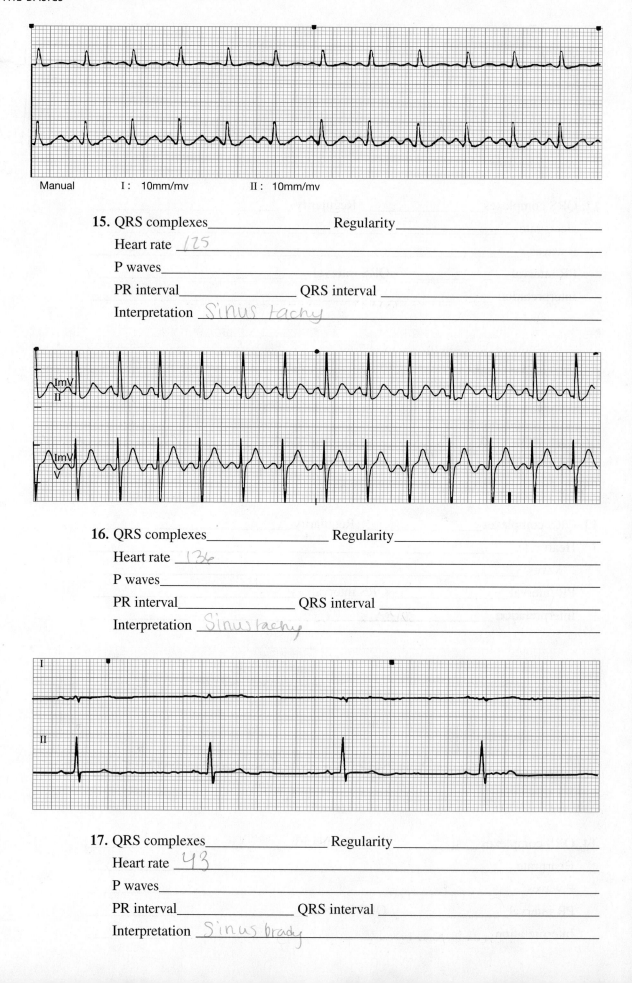

Manual   I : 10mm/mv   II : 10mm/mv

15. QRS complexes_____ Regularity_____

Heart rate _/25_____

P waves_____

PR interval_____ QRS interval _____

Interpretation _Sinus tachy_____

16. QRS complexes_____ Regularity_____

Heart rate _136_____

P waves_____

PR interval_____ QRS interval _____

Interpretation _Sinus tachy_____

17. QRS complexes_____ Regularity_____

Heart rate _43_____

P waves_____

PR interval_____ QRS interval _____

Interpretation _Sinus brady_____

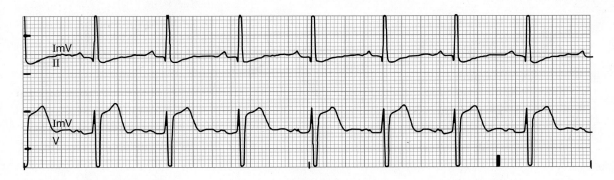

18. QRS complexes_____ Regularity_____

　　　Heart rate _83 79_____

　　　P waves_____

　　　PR interval_____ QRS interval _____

　　　Interpretation _Sinus rhythm_____

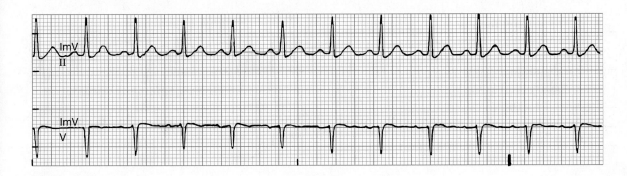

19. QRS complexes_____ Regularity_____

　　　Heart rate _115_____

　　　P waves_____

　　　PR interval_____ QRS interval _____

　　　Interpretation _Sinus tachy_____

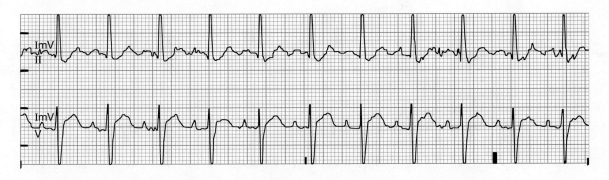

20. QRS complexes_____ Regularity_____

　　　Heart rate _115_____

　　　P waves_____

　　　PR interval_____ QRS interval _____

　　　Interpretation _Sinus tachy_____

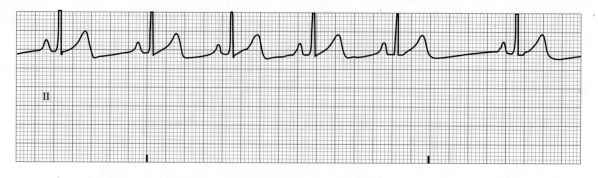

II

21. QRS complexes_____ Regularity_____

Heart rate _48-71_

P waves_____

PR interval_____ QRS interval _____

Interpretation _Sinus arrhythmia_____

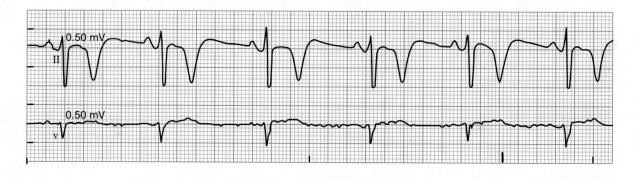

22. QRS complexes_____ Regularity _____

Heart rate _____

P waves_____

PR interval_____ QRS interval _____

Interpretation _____Sinus brady_____

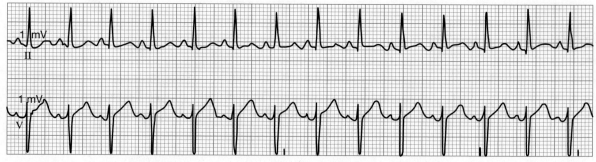

23. QRS complexes_____ Regularity_____

Heart rate _____

P waves_____

PR interval_____ QRS interval _____

Interpretation ___~~tachy~~____Sinus Tachycardia_____

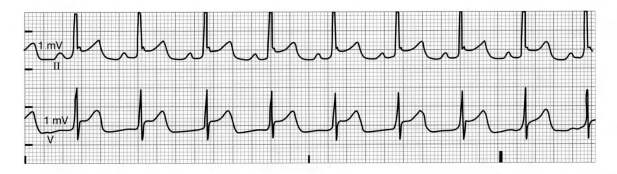

24. QRS complexes_____ Regularity _____

Heart rate _____

P waves_____

PR interval_____ QRS interval _____

Interpretation _____No Sinus rhythm_____

25. QRS complexes_____ Regularity _____

Heart rate _____

P waves_____

PR interval_____ QRS interval _____

Interpretation _____Sinus rhythm_____

chapter seven notes TO SUM IT ALL UP . . .

- **All matching upright P waves in Lead II are sinus P waves until proven otherwise.**
- **QRS interval should be <0.12 secs, but width and deflection of QRS is irrelevant in determining whether or not a rhythm is sinus in origin.** QRS width is determined by the state of conduction through the bundle branches. QRS deflection depends on lead being monitored. Lead II's QRS should be positive; V_1's should be negative.
- **Sinus rhythm criteria:**
  - *Heart rate*—60–100
  - *Regularity*—Regular
  - *P waves*—Matching upright P waves in Lead II; P-P interval regular
  - *Intervals*—PR interval 0.12–0.20 secs constant; QRS <0.12 secs
  - *Causes*—Normal rhythm
  - *Adverse effects*—none
  - *Treatment*—none needed

- **Sinus bradycardia criteria:**
  - *Heart rate*—<60
  - *Regularity*—Regular
  - *P waves*—Matching upright P waves in Lead II; P-P interval regular
  - *Intervals*—PR interval 0.12–0.20 secs constant; QRS <0.12 secs
  - *Causes*—Vagal stimulation, hypoxia, medication side effects, MI, athletic conditioning
  - *Adverse effects*—Can cause decreased cardiac output
  - *Treatment*—Atropine if symptoms; oxygen, pacemaker if necessary

- **Sinus tachycardia criteria:**
  - *Heart rate*—101–160
  - *Regularity*—Regular
  - *P waves*—Matching upright P waves in Lead II; P-P interval regular
  - *Intervals*—PR interval 0.12–0.20 secs; QRS <0.12 secs

- *Causes*—Medications, anxiety, pain, MI, pulmonary embolus, fever, CHF, hypoxia
- *Adverse effects*—Decreased cardiac output
- *Treatment*—Oxygen, treat the cause, beta blockers if persistent in presence of acute MI

■ **Sinus arrhythmia criteria:**

- *Heart rate*—Varies with respirations
- *Regularity*—Irregular
- *P waves*—Matching upright P waves in Lead II; P-P interval varies
- *Intervals*—PR interval 0.12–0.20 secs; QRS <0.12 secs
- *Causes*—Normal during sleep; follows respiratory pattern
- *Adverse effects*—Usually none
- *Treatment*—None

■ **Sinus arrest criteria:**

- *Heart rate*—Can occur at any heart rate
- *Regularity*—Regular but interrupted by a pause. Pause is not a multiple of R-Rs.

- *P waves*—Matching upright Ps before the pause; may have different or absent Ps after lower pacemaker takes over
- *Intervals*—PR interval 0.12–0.20 secs before pause, may change after; QRS <0.12 secs.
- *Causes*—Sinus node ischemia, hypoxia, medication side effects, excessive vagal tone
- *Adverse effects*—Decreased cardiac output
- *Treatment*—Atropine if symptoms; oxygen, pacemaker if needed.

■ **Sinus exit block criteria:**

- *Heart rate*—Can occur at any heart rate
- *Regularity*—Regular but interrupted by a pause. Pause is a multiple of R-Rs.
- *P waves*—Matching upright P waves in Lead II; P-P interval varies
- *Intervals*—PR interval 0.12–0.20 secs, QRS <0.12 secs
- *Causes*—Same as sinus arrest
- *Adverse effects*—Same as sinus arrest
- *Treatment*—Same as sinus arrest

Practice Quiz

1. True or false: All rhythms from the sinus node are irregular.

2. The only difference in interpretation between sinus rhythm, sinus bradycardia, and sinus tachycardia is *Heart rate*

3. Sinus arrhythmia is typically caused by *breathing pattern*

4. In what way does a sinus exit block differ from a sinus arrest? *it's a multiple of R-Rs*

5. True or false: Atropine is a medication that is useful in treating sinus tachycardia.

6. What rhythm would be expected in an individual with a fever of 103°F? *tachy*

7. A regular rhythm from the sinus node that has a heart rate of 155 is called *tachy*

8. True or false: All rhythms originating in the sinus node have matching P waves that are upright in most leads.

9. What effect does atropine have on the heart rate? *Speeds it up*

10. True or false: Anyone with a heart rate of 45 should be given atropine, whether or not he/she is symptomatic.

Putting It All Together—Critical Thinking Exercises

These exercises may consist of diagrams to label, scenarios to analyze, brain-stumping questions to ponder, or other challenging exercises to boost your understanding of the chapter material.

Let's play with sinus rhythms a bit. The following scenario will provide you with information about a fictional patient and ask you to analyze the situation, answer questions, and decide on appropriate actions.

Mr. Cavernum, age 62, is admitted to your telemetry floor with a diagnosis of pneumonia. He has a past medical history of sleep apnea and an "irregular heartbeat." On admission, his vital signs are as follows: blood pressure (BP) normal at 132/84, heart rate 94 (normal), temperature 98.9 degrees (normal),

respirations normal at 20. His rhythm strip is shown in Figure 7–8.

1. What is this rhythm? *Sinus rhythm*

At 3 A.M., Mr. Cavernum calls his nurse, saying he feels awful. The nurse notes his skin to be very hot and his face flushed. His vitals are as follows: BP 140/90 (slightly high), respirations 26 (rapid), temp 101.1 degrees (high). See his rhythm strip in Figure 7–9.

2. What is the rhythm and heart rate? *tachy - 115*

3. What do you suspect is causing this change in heart rate? *fever*

Your coworker brings three medications—atropine,

a beta-blocker called diltiazem, and acetaminophen (Tylenol)—into Mr. Cavernum's room.

4. Which of the three medications is indicated in this situation? _Acetaminophen_

After receiving his medication, Mr. Cavernum falls asleep and within two hours his rhythm is as shown in Figure 7–10.

5. What is this rhythm? _Sinus arrhythmia_

6. Does this rhythm require emergency treatment? _NO_

7. What in Mr. Cavernum's past medical history is a possible cause of this rhythm? _Sleep apnea_

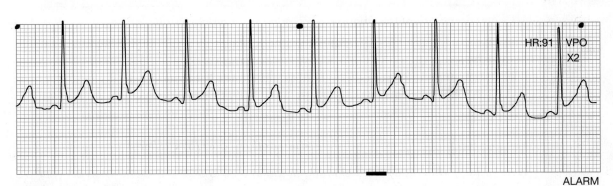

FIGURE 7–8

Admission rhythm strip.

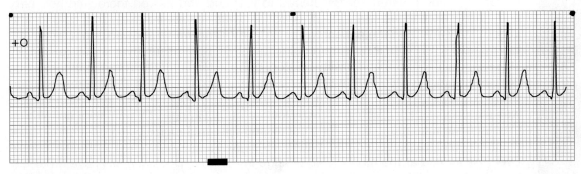

FIGURE 7–9

Second rhythm strip.

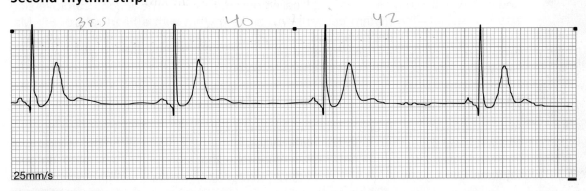

FIGURE 7–10

Final rhythm.

Rhythms Originating in the Atria

Upon completion of this chapter, the student will be able to:

- State the criteria for each of the atrial rhythms.
- Using the criteria and other rhythm analysis tools, interpret a variety of atrial rhythms.
- State the adverse effects for each rhythm.
- State the possible treatment for each rhythm.

What It's All About

Nurses Terry and Lacey were chatting at the intensive care unit desk when 87-year-old Ms. Avis was brought in by Monica and Lee from a medical floor. Monica and Lee reported that Ms. Avis was very pale, unresponsive to verbal commands, and drenched in a cold sweat, but she was breathing fine so far on oxygen. Her physician Dr. Granger had ordered her transferred to ICU and had arrived there with her. Terry and Lacey exchanged glances—this patient was in big trouble—and sprang into action. Terry attached the patient to the heart monitor, which showed supraventricular tachycardia (SVT) with a heart rate in the 190s. Blood pressure was 68/36 (extremely low, especially for this patient with a history of hypertension). Lacey ran to get the code cart. She removed Ms. Avis's shirt and wiped her chest dry with it. Terry attached defibrillation pads to Ms. Avis's chest and back. They double-checked that the IV line was working properly. Terry and Lacey looked at Dr. Granger. "Now?" they asked him. "Yes—hit her with 100 joules." Terry depressed the synchronize button, charged up the machine, and cardioverted the patient. Ms. Avis's chest lurched from the shock. Everyone looked at the monitor. No change in rhythm. "Does she still have a pulse?" somebody asked. By then all the ICU staff had come into the room to help. "Yes, she's still pulsating but it's weak and her blood pressure is really low. Let's shock her again. And call the cardiology resident out," called out Dr. Granger. The second cardioversion was successful—the rhythm converted to sinus rhythm with a heart rate of 88. Ms. Avis's blood pressure improved and she woke up. It was discovered later that Ms. Avis had a history of SVT and could not refill her medication for several days because she was waiting for her social security check to come in.

Introduction

Atrial rhythms originate in one or more irritable **foci** (locations) in the atria, then depolarize the atria and head down the conduction pathway to the ventricles. Atrial rhythms, and indeed all rhythms that originate in a pacemaker other than the sinus node, are called **ectopic rhythms.** See Figures 8–1 and 8–2. In Figure 8–1, a single atrial impulse depolarizes the atria and writes a P wave on the EKG. The impulse then heads down the pathway normally, and a QRS is written once the impulse depolarizes the ventricle. In Figure 8–2, there are multiple atrial impulses. They write a P wave (or an alternate form of atrial wave) and then head down the pathway normally and write a QRS once the ventricles have been depolarized.

The Word on Atrial Rhythms

Although the atrium is not considered an inherent pacemaker like the sinus node, AV junction, and ventricle (it is highly unusual for the atrium to fire in an escape capacity), the atrium is indeed another pacemaker of the heart. It is best known for usurping the

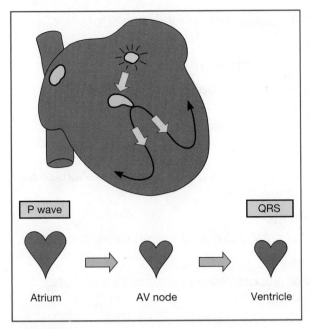

FIGURE 8–1

Conduction of a single atrial focus.

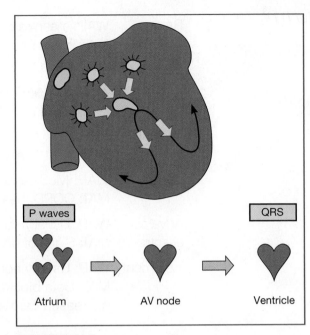

FIGURE 8–2

Conduction of multiple atrial foci.

underlying sinus rhythm and producing rhythms with rapid heart rates. Because of these rapid heart rates, patients are often symptomatic. Every now and then the atrium will fire more slowly and produce rhythms with rates less than 100.

Treatment is aimed at converting the rhythm back to sinus rhythm or, if that is not possible, returning the heart rate to more normal levels.

Atrial rhythms are extremely variable in their presentation. Some rhythms have obvious P waves. Others have no Ps at all—instead, they have a wavy or fluttery baseline between the QRS complexes. Some atrial rhythms are regular and others are completely irregular, even chaotic. Although most atrial rhythms are rapid; a few are slower.

Unlike sinus rhythms, which have a common set of criteria, atrial rhythms have multiple and variable possible criteria. If the rhythm or beat in question meets *any* of these criteria, it is atrial in origin. Let's look at these criteria now:

- Matching upright Ps, atrial rate (the heart rate of the P waves) >160 at rest *or*
- No Ps at all; wavy or sawtooth baseline between QRSs present instead *or*
- P waves of ≥ 3 different shapes *or*
- Premature abnormal P wave (with or without QRS) interrupting another rhythm, *or*
- Heart rate ≥ 130, rhythm regular, P waves not discernible (may be present, but can't be sure)

It's important to note that atrial rhythms can have a positive QRS or a negative QRS depending on the lead in which the patient is being monitored. For example, in Lead II the QRS should be positive, but in V$_1$ it should be negative. Reread Chapter 3 to review this if needed.

Now let's look at these rhythms in detail.

Wandering Atrial Pacemaker/Multifocal Atrial Tachycardia

Wandering atrial pacemaker (WAP) and *multifocal atrial tachycardia* (MAT) are rhythms that occur when the pacemaking impulses originate from at least 3 different foci in the atria. Each focus produces its own unique P wave, resulting in a rhythm with at least 3 different shapes of P waves. WAP is an example of a slow atrial arrhythmia. MAT is rapid. *WAP and MAT are exactly the same rhythm, just with differing heart rates.*

Rate	WAP: mean rate <100, usually a mean rate in the 50s to 60s
	MAT: mean rate >100
Regularity	Irregular
P waves	At least 3 different shapes. Some beats may have no visible P waves at all.
Intervals	PR varies
	QRS <0.12 seconds
Cause	WAP: Medication side effects, hypoxia, vagal stimulation, or MI
	MAT: COPD, heart disease
Adverse effects	WAP: Usually no ill effects
	MAT: Signs of decreased cardiac output if heart rate is too fast
Treatment	WAP: Usually none needed
	MAT: Beta blockers or calcium channel blockers if signs of decreased cardiac output exist

Figure 8–3A shows QRS complexes, all shaped the same. Regularity is irregular. Heart rate is 50 to 60, with a mean rate of 50. At least 3 different shapes of P waves precede the QRS complexes. P-P interval varies. PR interval varies from 0.24 to 0.32. QRS interval is 0.08. Interpretation: wandering atrial pacemaker.

Figure 8–3B shows QRS complexes of uniform shape. Regularity is irregular. Heart rate is 107 to 187, with a mean rate of 120. P waves vary in shape. P-P interval varies. PR interval varies. QRS interval is 0.06. Interpretation: multifocal atrial tachycardia.

Remember: *To differentiate between WAP and MAT, check the heart rate!*

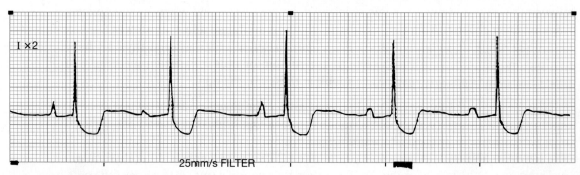

FIGURE 8–3A

Wandering atrial pacemaker.

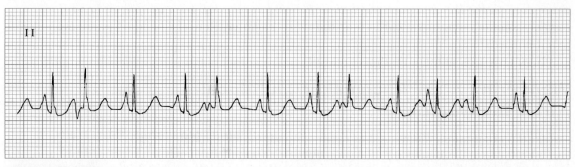

FIGURE 8–3B

Multifocal atrial tachycardia.

Premature Atrial Complexes (PACs)

Premature atrial complexes (PACs) are premature beats that are fired out by irritable atrial tissue before the next sinus beat is due. The premature P wave may or may not be followed by a QRS, depending on how premature the PAC is. If the PAC is very premature, it will not be conducted to the ventricle because it will arrive during the ventricle's refractory period.

Rate	Can occur at any rate
Regularity	Regular but interrupted (by the PACs)
P waves	Shaped differently from sinus P waves. The premature P waves of PACs may be hidden in the T wave of the preceding beat. If so, they will deform the shape of that T wave. Always be suspicious when a T wave suddenly changes shape. If the QRS complexes look the same, then the T waves that belong to them should also look the same. If one T wave is different, there's probably a P wave hiding in it. If the PAC's P wave is inverted, the PR interval should be the normal 0.12 to 0.20 secs.
Intervals	PR 0.12 to 0.20 secs QRS <0.12 secs QRS will be absent after a nonconducted PAC. *The most common cause of an unexplained pause is a nonconducted PAC.* If you see a pause and you're tempted to call it a sinus arrest or sinus block, make sure there's no P hiding in the T wave inside the pause. It might just be a nonconducted PAC.
Cause	The atria become "hyper" and fire early, before the next sinus beat is due. This can be caused by medications (stimulants, caffeine, bronchodilators), tobacco, hypoxia, or heart disease. Occasional PACs are normal.
Adverse effects	Frequent PACs can be an early sign of impending heart failure or impending atrial tachycardia or atrial fibrillation. Patients usually have no ill effects from occasional PACs.
Treatment	Usually none needed. Omit caffeine, tobacco, and other stimulants. Can give digitalis, calcium channel blockers, or beta blockers to treat PACs if needed. These medications all slow the heart rate and can decrease atrial irritability, decreasing PACs and other atrial arrhythmias. Treat heart failure if present. Consider starting oxygen.

In Figure 8–4, the fourth beat is premature, as evidenced by the shorter R-R interval there. Recall that premature beats are followed by a short pause immediately afterward. The QRS complexes are all the same shape. Regularity is regular but interrupted (by a premature beat). Heart rate is 54. P waves precede each QRS complex, and all but the fourth P wave are the same shape. Thus the matching upright P waves are sinus Ps, and the premature P wave is *not* a sinus P since it has a different shape. P-P interval is irregular because of the premature P wave. PR interval is 0.16, and QRS interval is 0.08. Interpretation: sinus bradycardia with a PAC.

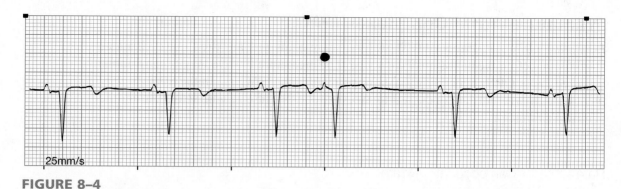

FIGURE 8–4

PAC.

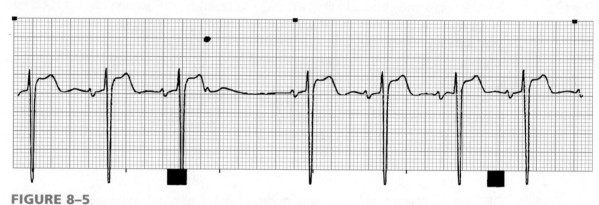

FIGURE 8–5

Nonconducted PAC.

Figure 8–5 shows QRS complexes, all the same shape. Regularity is regular but interrupted (by a pause). Heart rate is 43 to 75, with a mean rate of 70. P waves are biphasic (half up, half down) and matching, except for the P wave that's at the end of the third beat's T wave. See the little hump there under the dot? That's a P wave. That P wave is shaped differently from the sinus P waves, and it is premature. How do we know it's premature? Look at the P-P intervals, the distance between consecutive P waves. All the sinus P waves are about 4 big blocks apart. This abnormal P wave is only 2¹/₂ blocks from the P wave that precedes it. Thus it is premature. A premature P wave that is not followed by a QRS complex is a nonconducted PAC. Note the long pause that this noncoducted PAC causes. *Nonconducted PACs are the most common cause of otherwise unexplained pauses.* It is important to note that many nonconducted PACs do not have such easily noticeable P waves. Much of the time the premature P wave is hidden inside the T wave of the preceding beat, deforming that T wave's shape. PR interval here is 0.16, and QRS interval is 0.10. Interpretation: sinus rhythm with a nonconducted PAC.

chapter CHECKUP

We're about halfway through this chapter. To evaluate your understanding of the material thus far, answer the following questions. If you have trouble with them, review the material again before continuing.

Mr. Sulu's rhythm is very irregular, with a heart rate in the 130s and multiple P wave shapes. His QRS is narrow (<0.12 secs). Medication is given and the heart rate slows to the 50s but the multiple P wave shapes continue. His blood pressure with this new rhythm is good and he feels fine now.

1. What was his rhythm before the medication?
2. What's his rhythm after?
3. What treatment, if any, is indicated for this new rhythm?

Paroxysmal Atrial Tachycardia (PAT)

Paroxysmal atrial tachycardia (PAT) is a sudden burst of 3 or more PACs in a row that usurps the underlying rhythm and then becomes its *own* rhythm for a period of time. The term **paroxysmal** refers to a rhythm that starts and stops suddenly. PAT resembles sinus tach, but with a faster heart rate. *In order to diagnose PAT, the PAC that initiates it must be seen.*

Rate	160 to 250 on the atrial tachycardia itself. The rhythm it interrupts will have a different rate.
Regularity	The atrial tachycardia itself is regular; but since it interrupts another rhythm, the rhythm strip as a whole will be regular but interrupted.
P waves	The atrial tachycardia Ps will be shaped the same as each other, but differently from sinus P waves.
Intervals	PR 0.12 to 0.20 secs, constant QRS <0.12 secs
Cause	Same as PACs or sinus tach
Adverse effects	Prolonged runs of PAT can cause decreased cardiac output. Healthy people can tolerate this rhythm for a while without symptoms, but those with heart disease may develop symptoms rapidly.
Treatment	Digitalis, calcium channel blockers, beta-blockers, sedation, amiodarone (a medication that helps abolish atrial and ventricular arrhythmias), adenosine (another medication to slow the heart rate), and oxygen. Elective cardioversion (a small electrical shock to the heart to restore sinus rhythm) can be done if the patient is unstable because of the rhythm.

   Figure 8–6 shows 4 sinus beats and then a run of 5 PACs. This run of PACs is called PAT. There are QRS complexes, all the same shape. Regularity is regular but interrupted (by a run of premature beats). Heart rate is 75 for the sinus rhythm, and 187 for the atrial tachycardia. P waves precede each QRS complex but are not all the same shape. The sinus beats have one shape of P wave, and the atrial tachycardia has a different shape P that is deforming the T waves. Note the dots over the premature P waves. Wait a minute, you say! What P waves? We can't see them! Here's a rule to help you: *If the QRS complexes on the strip look alike, the T waves that follow them*

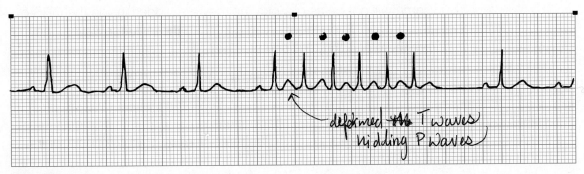

deformed the T waves
hidding P waves

FIGURE 8–6

Paroxysmal atrial tachycardia.

should also look alike. A T wave that changes shape when the QRSs don't is hiding a P wave inside it. Look at the T waves of the first 4 beats. They have rather broad sloping T waves. The PAT's T waves are pointy—totally different in shape. They're hiding a P wave. Now to continue with our interpretation: P-P interval is regular during the sinus rhythm, and regular, though different, during the atrial tachycardia. PR interval of the sinus beats is 0.16. We cannot measure the PR interval of the PAT beats, since the P wave is hidden. QRS 0.08. Interpretation: sinus rhythm with a 5-beat run of PAT.

Atrial Flutter

Atrial flutter is a rhythm that results when one irritable atrial focus fires out regular impulses at a rate so rapid that a fluttery pattern is produced instead of P waves. The atrium is firing out its impulses so fast that the AV node, bombarded with all these impulses, lets some through but blocks others. Imagine a tennis ball machine firing out tennis balls so fast that there's no way you can hit them all. You end up ducking to protect yourself. The AV node is the gatekeeper—the protector—of the ventricles. Impulses must pass through it to reach the ventricles. Impulses that are too fast would provide a dangerously fast heart rate, so the AV node selectively blocks out some of the impulses, letting only some through.

Rate	Atrial rate 250 to 350. Ventricular rate depends on the conduction ratio.
Regularity	Regular if the conduction ratio (ratio of flutter waves to QRS complexes) is constant; irregular if the conduction ratio varies; can look regular but interrupted at times
P waves	No P waves present. Flutter waves are present instead. These are sawtooth-shaped waves between the QRS complexes. Flutter waves are also described as picket-fence-shaped, V-shaped, or upside-down-V shaped. There will be 2 or more flutter waves to each QRS. All flutter waves march out—they're all the same distance apart. Flutter waves are regular. They do not interrupt themselves to allow a QRS complex to pop in. Some flutter waves will therefore be hidden inside QRS complexes or T waves. The easiest way to find all the flutter waves is to find 2 flutter waves back-to-back and note the distance between them (go from top to top of the flutter waves or bottom to bottom). Then march out where the rest of the flutter waves should be using this interval. Although most flutter waves will be easily visible using this method, some will not be as obvious, as they are hidden inside the QRS or the T wave. Even though you can't see these flutter waves, they are there and they still count.
Intervals	PR not measured, since there are no real P waves QRS <0.12 secs
Cause	Almost always implies heart disease; other causes include pulmonary embolus, valvular heart disease, thyrotoxicosis, or lung disease

Adverse effects	Can be well tolerated at normal heart rates; at higher or lower rates, signs of decreased cardiac output can occur. Cardiac output is influenced not by the atrial rate, but by the heart rate.
Treatment	Digitalis, calcium channel blockers, beta-blockers, adenosine, **carotid sinus massage** (rubbing the carotid artery in the neck to stimulate the vagus nerve) to slow the ventricular rate. Electrical cardioversion can be done if medications are ineffective or the patient is unstable.

Figure 8–7 shows QRS complexes, all shaped the same. Regularity is regular. Atrial rate is 250; heart rate is 65. P waves are not present; flutter waves are present instead, as evidenced by the V-shaped waves between the QRS complexes. Flutter waves are all regular. PR interval is not measured in atrial flutter. QRS interval is approximately 0.08, although it's difficult to measure as the flutter waves distort the QRS complex. Interpretation: atrial flutter with 4:1 conduction (4 flutter waves to each QRS). See the dots under the flutter waves? There are 4 dots for each QRS. What if we measured from the top of the flutter waves instead of the bottom? Same thing. See the asterisks above the flutter waves? There are 4 of them (the fourth flutter wave is *inside* the QRS, but it still counts) to each QRS complex.

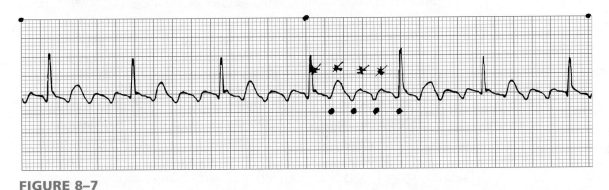

FIGURE 8–7

Atrial flutter.

Atrial Fibrillation

During *atrial fibrillation,* hundreds of atrial impulses from different locations all fire at the same time. As a result, the atria depolarize not as a unit as they usually do, but rather in small sections. This causes the atria to wiggle instead of contract. The AV node is bombarded with all these impulses and simply cannot depolarize fast enough to let them all through. Every now and then one of these impulses does get through to the ventricle and provides a QRS.

Rate	Atrial rate is 350 to 700; ventricular rate varies. Atrial fibrillation with a mean ventricular rate >100 is said to have RVR (rapid ventricular response). Remember ventricular rate is the same as heart rate.
Regularity	Irregularly irregular, completely unpredictable

P waves	No P waves are present. Fibrillatory waves are present instead. These are undulations or waviness of the baseline between QRSs. *If there are P waves, the rhythm is not atrial fibrillation.*
Intervals	Since there are no P waves, there is no PR interval. QRS <0.12 secs
Cause	MI, lung disease, valvular heart disease, hyperthyroidism
Adverse effects	Atrial fibrillation can cause a drop in cardiac output because of the loss of the atrial kick, which accounts for 15% to 30% of the cardiac output. One possible complication of atrial fibrillation is blood clots, which can collect in the sluggish atria. This can result in MI, strokes, or blood clots in the lung.
Treatment	Depends on the duration of atrial fibrillation. Since the atria are wiggling, not contracting, blood flow is stagnant and clots can develop. If there are atrial clots and the rhythm is converted back to sinus, the restored atrial contraction (atrial kick) can dislodge these clots, propelling them out of the atrium into the circulation.

If atrial fibrillation duration is less than 48 hours, the goal is to convert the rhythm back to sinus. Digitalis, calcium channel blockers, beta-blockers, amiodarone, or electrical cardioversion can be utilized. In atrial fibrillation less than 48 hours old, the likelihood that there are blood clots in the atria is low, so there is minimal chance of showering clots to the brain, heart, lungs, and other organs once the atrial kick is reestablished in sinus rhythm.

In stable patients who have been in atrial fibrillation for greater than 48 hours, the risk of blood clots is greater, so initial treatment is aimed at controlling the heart rate rather than converting the rhythm back to sinus. Anticoagulants (blood thinners) are given to prevent any more blood clots from forming, and cardioversion is delayed 2 to 3 weeks to allow any clots that are there to dissolve on their own. Meanwhile, medications can be given to regulate the heart rate to a more normal level. In emergencies, patients in atrial fibrillation greater than 48 hours will be started on heparin (an anticoagulant) intravenously, given a transesophageal echocardiogram (TEE—a sonarlike test using a probe inserted into the esophagus) to rule out blood clots in the atria, then electrically cardioverted. Consider starting oxygen.

Figure 8–8 shows QRS complexes, all the same shape. Regularity is irregular. Heart rate is 65 to 100, with a mean rate of 90. P waves are absent; fibrillatory waves are present instead. PR interval is not applicable, and QRS interval is 0.10. Interpretation: atrial fibrillation.

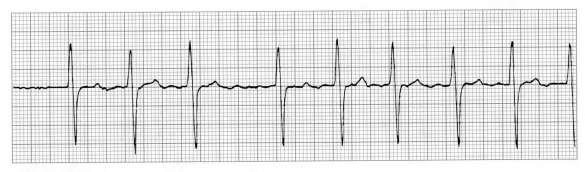

FIGURE 8–8

Atrial fibrillation.

Supraventricular Tachycardia (SVT)

Supraventricular tachycardia (SVT) is a catchall term given to tachycardias that are supraventricular; that is, they originate above the ventricles (the prefix *supra-* means "above") in either the sinus node, the atrium, or the AV junction, but whose exact origin cannot be identified because P waves are not discernible.

Rate	About 130 or higher (usually > 150)
Regularity	Regular
P waves	Not discernible
Intervals	PR cannot be measured since P waves cannot be positively identified. QRS <0.12 secs
Cause	Same as PAT
Adverse effects	Decreased cardiac output secondary to the rapid heart rate
Treatment	Adenosine, digitalis, ibutilide (a medication to control atrial arrhythmias), calcium channel blockers, beta-blockers. Consider starting oxygen. Elective cardioversion can also be done if the patient is unstable.

Figure 8–9 shows QRS complexes, all shaped the same. Rhythm is regular. Heart rate is 150. P waves are not identifiable. PR interval is not measurable. QRS interval is 0.08. Interpretation: SVT. The origin of this rhythm is not clear, but we know that it originated in a pacemaker above the ventricle, since the QRS complex is narrow, less than 0.12 secs. (Rhythms that originate in the ventricle have a wide QRS complex, greater than 0.12 secs.) Bottom line: *If the QRS is <0.12 secs, the heart rate is around 130 or higher, the rhythm is regular, and you can't pick out the P waves, call the rhythm SVT.*

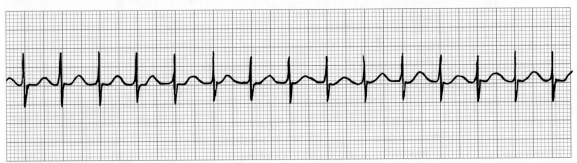

FIGURE 8–9

SVT (supraventricular tachycardia).

Practice Strips: Atrial Rhythms

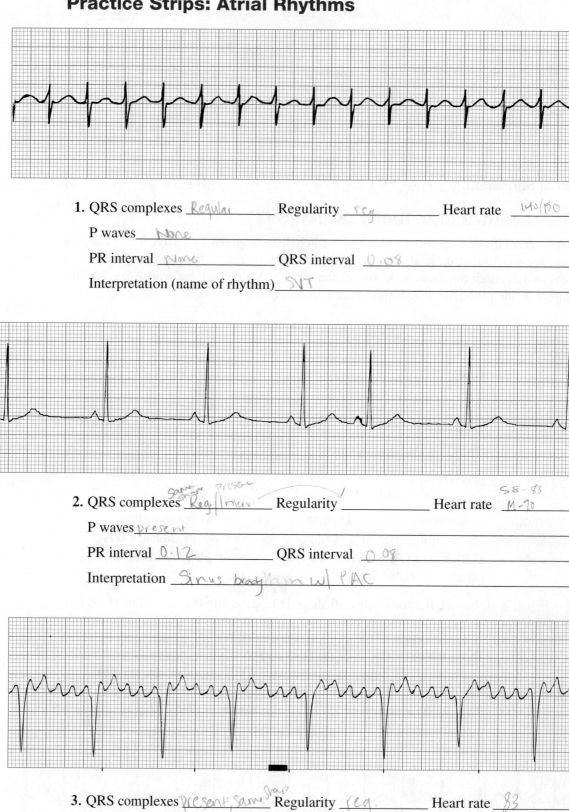

1. QRS complexes _Regular_____ Regularity _reg_____ Heart rate _140/50_

P waves_None_____

PR interval _None_____ QRS interval _0.08_____

Interpretation (name of rhythm)_SVT_____

2. QRS complexes _Reg./Irreg._ Regularity _____ Heart rate _M-70_

P waves_present_____

PR interval _0.12_____ QRS interval _0.08_____

Interpretation _Sinus bradythm w/ PAC_____

3. QRS complexes_present, same shap_ Regularity _reg._ Heart rate _83_

P waves_—_____

PR interval _—_____ QRS interval _0.08_____

Interpretation _Atrial Flutter 5:1; 6:1   conduction_____

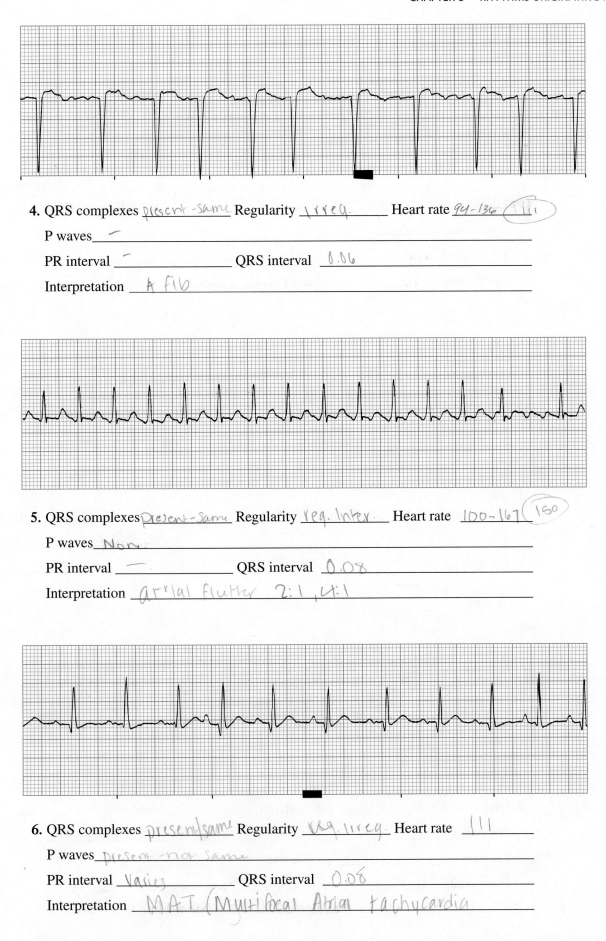

4. QRS complexes _present -same_ Regularity _irreg._   Heart rate _94-136_ (_111_)

P waves _—_

PR interval _—_   QRS interval _0.06_

Interpretation _A fib_

5. QRS complexes _Present-Same_ Regularity _reg. Inter._   Heart rate _100-167_ (_150_)

P waves _None_

PR interval _—_   QRS interval _0.08_

Interpretation _atrial flutter 2:1, 4:1_

6. QRS complexes _present/same_ Regularity _reg. irreg_ Heart rate _111_

P waves _present - not same_

PR interval _Varies_   QRS interval _0.08_

Interpretation _MAT (Multifocal Atrial Tachycardia_

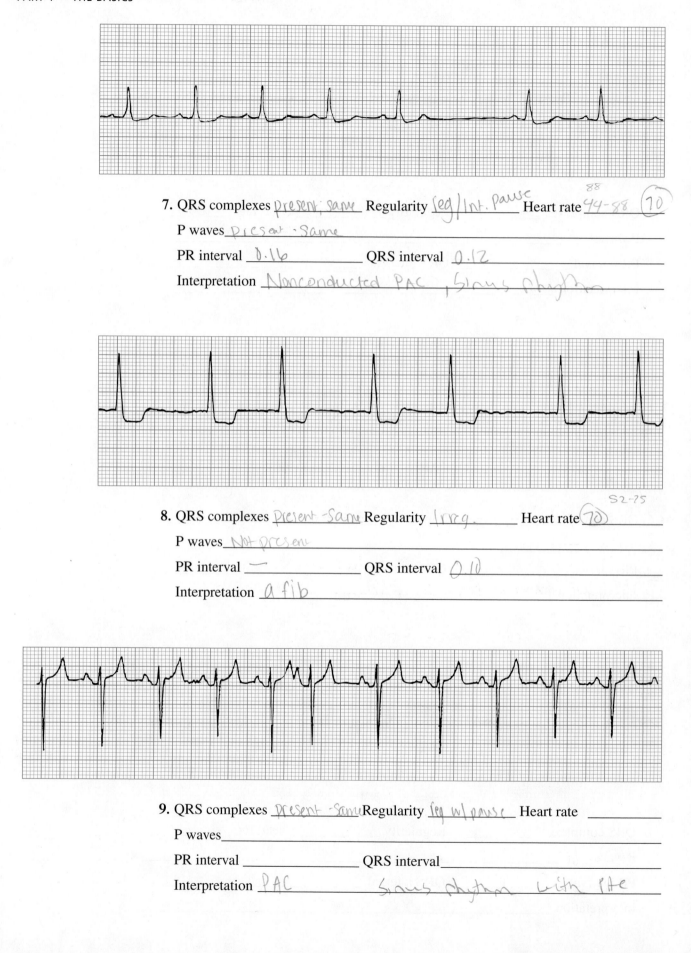

7. QRS complexes _Present, same_ Regularity _reg/Int. pause_ Heart rate _44-88_ ⁸⁸ ⑺⁰

P waves _Present · Same_

PR interval _0.16_   QRS interval _0.12_

Interpretation _Nonconducted PAC , Sinus rhythm_

8. QRS complexes _Present -Same_ Regularity _Irreg._ Heart rate ⑺⁰   S2-25

P waves _Not present_

PR interval _—_   QRS interval _0.10_

Interpretation _a fib_

9. QRS complexes _Present -Same_ Regularity _reg w/ pause_ Heart rate _____

P waves _____

PR interval _____   QRS interval _____

Interpretation _PAC_   _Sinus rhythm with PAC_

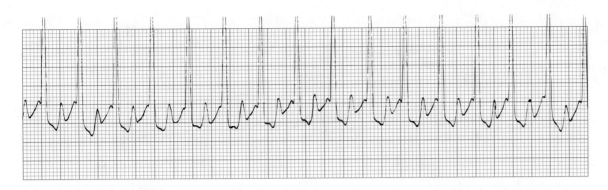

10. QRS complexes _____ Regularity _____ Heart rate _____

P waves_____

PR interval _____ QRS interval _____

Interpretation ___SVT_____

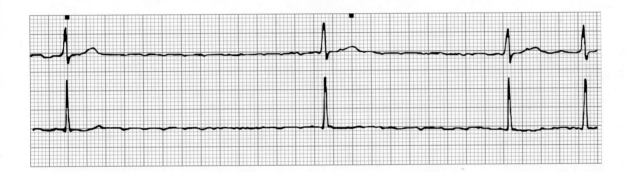

11. QRS complexes _____ Regularity _____ Heart rate _____

P waves_____

PR interval _____ QRS interval _____

Interpretation (name of rhythm)___A-Fib_____

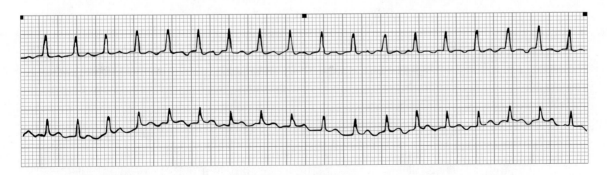

12. QRS complexes _____ Regularity _____ Heart rate _____

P waves_____

PR interval _____ QRS interval _____

Interpretation ___SVT_____

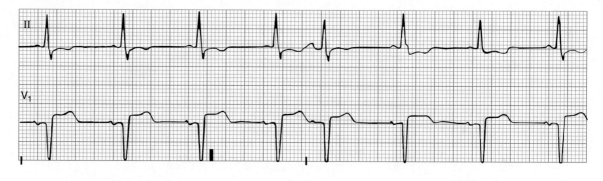

13. QRS complexes _____ Regularity _____ Heart rate _____

P waves_____

PR interval _____ QRS interval _____

Interpretation _PAC_____   _Sinus rhythm with a PAC_

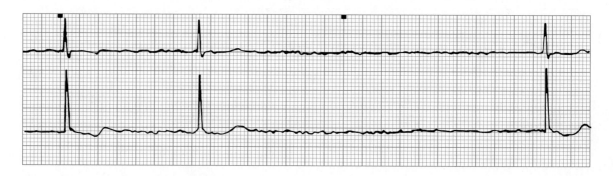

14. QRS complexes _____ Regularity _____ Heart rate _____

P waves_____

PR interval _____ QRS interval _____

Interpretation _A fib_____

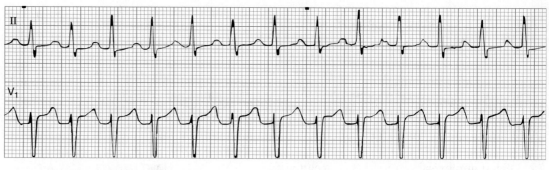

15. QRS complexes _____ Regularity _____ Heart rate _____

P waves_____

PR interval _____ QRS interval _____

Interpretation _SVT____   _may be sinus Tachy_

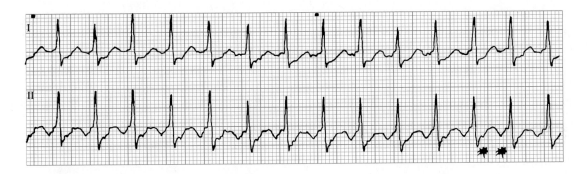

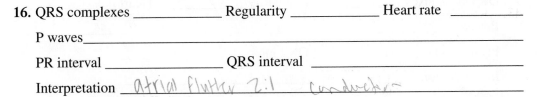

16. QRS complexes _____ Regularity _____ Heart rate _____

P waves_____

PR interval _____ QRS interval _____

Interpretation ___atrial flutter 2:1   conduction_____

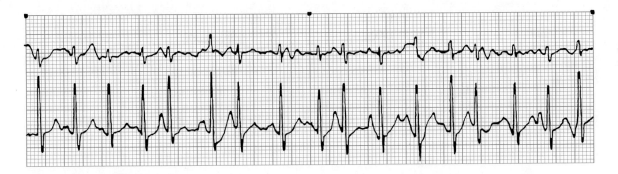

17. QRS complexes _____ Regularity _____ Heart rate _____

P waves_____

PR interval _____ QRS interval _____

Interpretation ___MAT_____

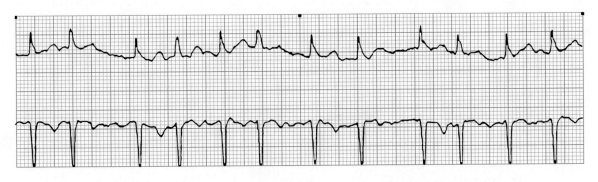

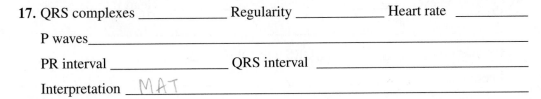

18. QRS complexes _____ Regularity _____ Heart rate _____

P waves_____

PR interval _____ QRS interval _____

Interpretation ___A fib_____

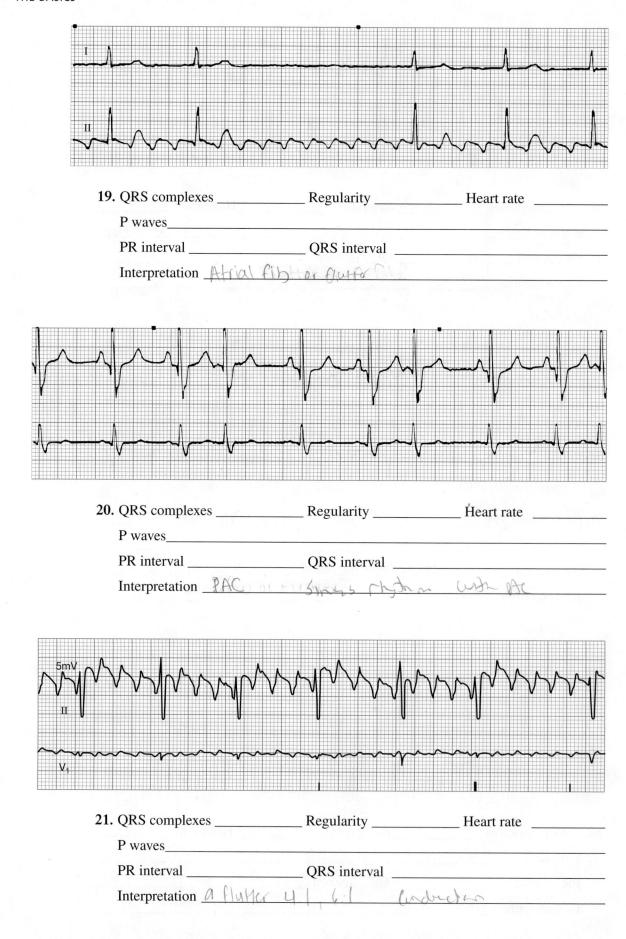

19. QRS complexes _____ Regularity _____ Heart rate _____

   P waves_____

   PR interval _____ QRS interval _____

   Interpretation _Atrial fib? or Aflutter _____

20. QRS complexes _____ Regularity _____ Heart rate _____

   P waves_____

   PR interval _____ QRS interval _____

   Interpretation _PAC   Sinus rhythm   with PAC _____

21. QRS complexes _____ Regularity _____ Heart rate _____

   P waves_____

   PR interval _____ QRS interval _____

   Interpretation _a flutter 4:1 6:1   conduction _____

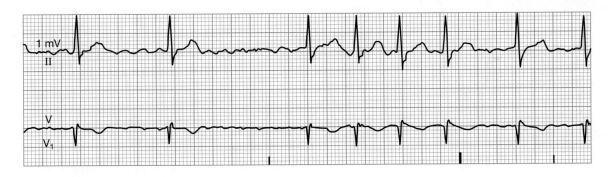

22. QRS complexes _____ Regularity _____ Heart rate _____

P waves_____

PR interval _____ QRS interval _____

Interpretation __a fib_____

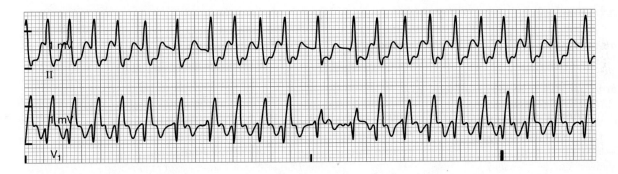

23. QRS complexes _____ Regularity _____ Heart rate _____

P waves_____

PR interval _____ QRS interval _____

Interpretation __a fib_____

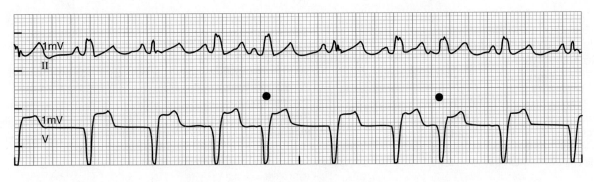

24. QRS complexes _____ Regularity _____ Heart rate _____

P waves_____

PR interval _____ QRS interval _____

Interpretation __PAC_____ Sinus rhythm with a PAC

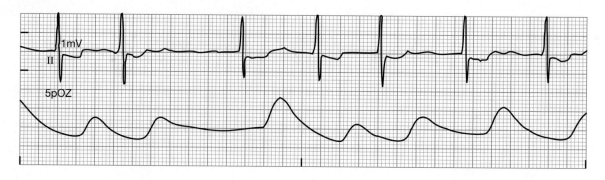

25. QRS complexes _____ Regularity _____ Heart rate _____

P waves_____

PR interval _____ QRS interval _____

Interpretation ___Afb_____wide QRS_____

chapter eight notes TO SUM IT ALL UP . . .

- **Atrial rhythms can have positive or negative QRS complexes depending on the lead being monitored.** In Lead II, the QRS should be positive; in V$_1$ they'll be negative.
- **Wandering atrial pacemaker (WAP) / Multifocal atrial tachycardia (MAT):**
  - *Heart rate*—WAP—mean rate <100
                          MAT—mean rate >100
  - *Regularity*—Irregular
  - *P waves*—At least 3 different shapes
  - *Intervals*—PR varies; QRS <0.12 secs
  - *Causes*—WAP—medication side effects, MI, vagal stimulation
                 MAT—typically COPD
  - *Adverse effects*—WAP—usually none
                 MAT—signs of decreased cardiac output if heart rate too fast
  - *Treatment*—WAP—usually none needed
                 MAT—beta blockers, calcium channel blockers
- **PACs:**
  - *Heart rate*—Can occur at any rate
  - *Regularity*—Cause the rhythm to be regular but interrupted by a premature beat
  - *P waves*—Different shape than sinus P waves. Ps may be hidden inside T waves.
  - *Intervals*—PR 0.12–0.20 secs; QRS <0.12 secs
  - *Causes*—Stimulants, medications, hypoxia, heart disease
  - *Adverse effects*—Usually none
  - *Treatment*—Oxygen, calcium channel blockers, beta blockers, omit stimulants, treat CHF if present
- **PAT:**
  - *Heart rate*—160–250. Rhythm it interrupts will have a different heart rate.
  - *Regularity*—The atrial tach itself is regular, but it will cause the whole strip to look regular but interrupted since it interrupts another rhythm.
  - *P waves*—Different from sinus Ps; uniform shape
  - *Intervals*—PR 0.12–0.20 secs; QRS <0.12 secs

- *Causes*—Same as PACs
- *Adverse effects*—Decreased cardiac output
- *Treatment*—Digitalis, calcium channel blockers, beta blockers, adenosine, oxygen, electrical cardioversion
- **Atrial flutter:**
  - *Heart rate*—Atrial rate 250–350; ventricular rate varies depending on conduction ratio
  - *Regularity*—Regular, irregular, or regular but interrupted—depends on conduction ratio
  - *P waves*—No P waves. Flutter waves are present (zigzag waves of uniform shape).
  - *Intervals*—No PR interval since no P waves; QRS <0.12 secs
  - *Causes*—Heart disease, pulmonary embolus, lung disease, heart valve disease
  - *Adverse effects*—Decreased cardiac output if heart rate too fast or too slow
  - *Treatment*—Oxygen, calcium channel blockers, beta blockers, adenosine, digitalis
- **Atrial fibrillation:**
  - *Heart rate*—Atrial rate 350–700; ventricular rate varies
  - *Regularity*—Irregularly irregular
  - *P waves*—No P waves. Fibrillatory waves present (undulating baseline).
  - *Intervals*—No PR interval since no P waves; QRS <0.12 secs
  - *Causes*—MI, lung disease, heart valve disease, hyperthyroidism
  - *Adverse effects*—Decreased cardiac output, blood clots that can cause strokes, pulmonary emboli, or MI
  - *Treatment*—If duration <48 hours—digitalis, calcium channel blockers, beta blockers, amiodarone, or electrical cardioversion; if duration >48 hours—anticoagulants for 2–3 weeks, then cardioversion. In emergencies—start on heparin, do a TEE to check for blood clots in the atria, then cardiovert.

- **SVT:**
  - *Heart rate*—130 or higher
  - *Regularity*—Regular
  - *P waves*—None seen
  - *Intervals*—No PR interval since can't see P waves; QRS <0.12 secs

- *Causes*—Same as PAT
- *Adverse effects*—Decreased cardiac output
- *Treatment*—Adenosine, digitalis, ibutilide, calcium channel blockers, beta blockers, oxygen, electrical cardioversion

Practice Quiz

1. What common complication of atrial fibrillation can be prevented by the use of anticoagulant medications?
   Blood clots

2. The rhythm that is the same as wandering atrial pacemaker except for the heart rate is
   Multifocal Atrial Tachy

3. The rhythm that produces V-shaped waves between QRS complexes is
   Atrial flutter

4. Atrial rhythms take which path to the ventricles?
   Normal conduction pathway to vent after depolar atria

5. All rhythms that originate in a pacemaker other than the sinus node are called *ectopic rhythms*

6. Treatment for atrial fibrillation is dependent on which factor? *duration*

7. True or false: All PACs conduct through to the ventricles.

8. The classic cause of multifocal atrial tachycardia is
   Chronic lung disease

9. Which test can be used in emergencies to determine if atrial blood clots are present?
   TEE

10. If the rhythm is regular, heart rate is 130 or greater, and P waves cannot be identified, the rhythm is called
    SVT

Putting It All Together—Critical Thinking Exercises

These exercises may consist of diagrams to label, scenarios to analyze, brain-stumping questions to ponder, or other challenging exercises to boost your knowledge of the chapter material.

Let's play with atrial rhythms a bit. The following scenario will provide you with information about a fictional patient and ask you to analyze the situation, answer questions, and decide on appropriate actions.

Mr. Baldo, a 20-year-old college student, awoke feeling palpitations in his chest. He arrives at your emergency department an hour later with the following vital signs: BP normal at 130/78, respirations 22, temp 98.0 degrees. Skin is warm and dry. No pain, shortness of breath, or other distress aside from feeling the palpitations off and on. He denies ever having felt anything like this before. His rhythm strip is shown in Figure 8–10.

1. What is Mr. Baldo's rhythm and heart rate?
   A fib   110

2. Is his situation an emergency? Why or why not?
   No

3. Since Mr. Baldo's rhythm started this morning, what medication do we *not* need to consider as a part of his treatment? *Heparin / coumadin*

4. What treatment would be appropriate for Mr. Baldo's rhythm? *B blockers, Ca Blocker, amiodarone Dig.*

   Mr. Baldo is given medication and, within the hour, the nurse records the rhythm strip shown in Figure 8–11.

5. What's happening on this strip?
   A fib → NS

Mr. Baldo is watched in your emergency department for 2 more hours and then discharged with the rhythm shown in Figure 8–12. He is sent home with medication and told to follow up with a cardiologist for more studies.

6. What is Mr. Baldo's rhythm on discharge?

Normal Sinus

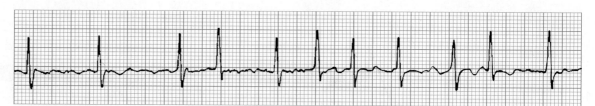

FIGURE 8–10

Mr. Baldo's initial strip.

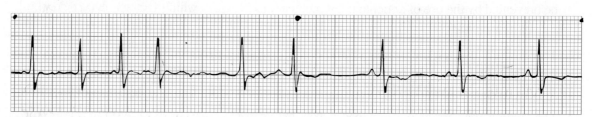

FIGURE 8–11

Rhythm after medication.

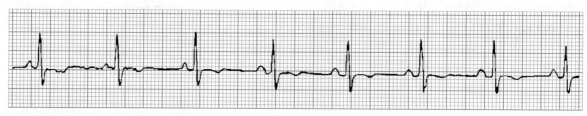

FIGURE 8–12

Discharge rhythm.

Rhythms Originating in the AV Junction

9

CHAPTER 9 OBJECTIVES

Upon completion of this chapter, the student will be able to:

- State the criteria for each junctional rhythm.
- Differentiate among *high, low,* and *midjunctional* impulses.
- Correctly identify the junctional rhythms on a variety of strips.

- State the adverse effects of each junctional rhythm.
- State the possible treatment for the junctional rhythms.
- State which junctional rhythms occur mostly because of escape and which imply usurpation.

What It's All About

Mr. Alvin felt lousy. He thought maybe he was getting the flu, so he took a sick day from work and stayed in bed. "Where is that darned cold medicine?" he mumbled, fumbling around on the bedside table. "I can't see a thing without my glasses." He took some cold medicine but didn't feel any better. So he took another dose. When his wife came home from work, she found Mr. Alvin still in bed. He complained to his wife that he had thought at first he had the flu but now he wasn't so sure because now he was getting chest pain. Mr. Alvin thought he'd better get to the hospital. His wife scooped up all of his medications, put them in a paper bag, and drove Alvin to the hospital. In the emergency department, Mr. Alvin had labs drawn and had an EKG, which showed *junctional tachycardia* with a heart rate of 160. He was not having a heart attack, the physician told him—he had a toxic amount of digitalis in his system. "How did that happen? I take only one digitalis a day," Mr. Alvin said. "Show me which medicine you took this morning," his nurse Sam said on a hunch. Alvin reached into the paper bag and showed the nurse his bottle of cold pills. Yep—you guessed it. The "cold medicine" was actually his digitalis. Because of Mr. Alvin's poor vision, he'd grabbed the wrong medication and had taken several doses of digitalis over and above his normal daily dose. The chest pain he experienced was caused by the fast heart rate and went away once Mr. Alvin's heart rate returned to normal.

Introduction

Junctional rhythms arise from the **AV junction**, the tissue located between the right atrium and ventricle and surrounding the AV node.

The impulse originates around the AV node and travels **antegrade**, or forward, toward the ventricle, and **retrograde**, or backward, toward the atria. Thus, the impulse travels in two directions. The AV junctional area can be divided into regions—high, mid, and low—and whichever of these regions initiates the impulse will determine the location of the P wave. If the impulse originates high in the AV junction, close to the atria, it will arrive at the atria first and write an **inverted** (upside down) P wave. The P wave is inverted because the impulse is going in a backward direction to reach the atria. Then the forward impulses reach the ventricle and write the QRS complex. The PR interval is short, less than 0.12 seconds. Because the impulse starts out in the AV junction, halfway to the ventricle, it simply doesn't have as far to go as sinus impulses would. Bottom line: *If the impulse originates high in the AV junction, the resultant rhythm or beat will have an inverted P wave preceding the QRS, and the PR interval should be less than 0.12 secs.*

If the impulses originate midway in the AV junction, the impulses will reach the atria and ventricles simultaneously because both are the same distance from the AV junction.

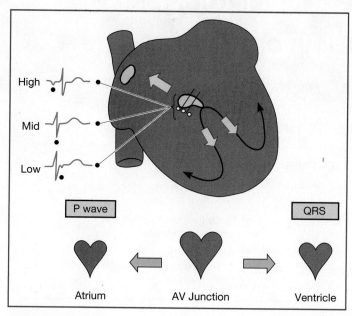

FIGURE 9–1

Conduction and P wave location in junctional rhythms.

Therefore, the P wave will be swallowed up by the QRS complex. Bottom line: *Midjunctional impulses have no visible P waves.*

If the impulses originate low in the AV junction, the impulses will reach the ventricle first, writing a QRS complex, and then reaching the atria and writing the P wave. Thus, the P wave will follow the QRS and, since the impulses must travel backward to reach the atria, the P wave will be inverted. Bottom line: *Impulses originating from low in the AV junction have inverted P waves following the QRS complex.* See Figure 9–1.

The Word on Junctional Rhythms

Junctional rhythms are seen less often than sinus or atrial rhythms. Although the inherent rate of the AV junction is 40 to 60, the heart rate could actually be much faster or slower, which can result in symptoms. More normal heart rates are less likely to cause symptoms.

Treatment is aimed at alleviating the cause of the junctional rhythm. More active treatment is not usually necessary unless symptoms develop, at which time the goal is to return the sinus node to control or to return the heart rate to more normal levels.

Junctional rhythms are easy to identify. Let's look at the criteria, which dictate a regular rhythm or premature beat with narrow QRS along with one of the following:

- Absent P waves
- Inverted P waves following the QRS
- Inverted P waves with short PR interval preceding the QRS

It's important to note that the QRS in junctional rhythms can be positive (upright) or negative (downward) depending on the lead the patient is being monitored in. For example, the QRS in Lead II should be positive, but in V_1 should be negative. Look back to Chapter 3 for a refresher on this if needed. Now let's look at the junctional rhythms in detail.

Premature Junctional Complexes (PJCs)

Premature junctional complexes (PJCs) are premature beats that originate in the AV junction before the next sinus beat is due. This is caused by irritable tissue in the AV junction firing and usurping the sinus node for that beat.

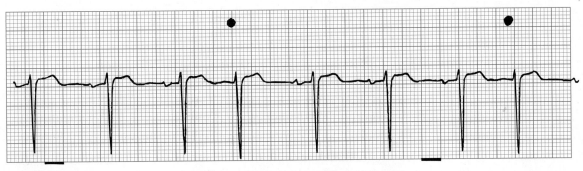

FIGURE 9–2

PJC.

Rate	Can occur at any rate
Regularity	Regular but interrupted
P waves	Inverted before or after the QRS, or hidden inside the QRS
Intervals	PR <0.12 secs if the P wave precedes the QRS
	QRS <0.12 secs
Cause	Stimulants (such as caffeine or drugs), nicotine, hypoxia, heart disease
Adverse effects	Usually no ill effects
Treatment	Usually none required aside from removal of the cause

Figure 9–2 shows QRS complexes, all shaped the same. Regularity is regular but interrupted (by 2 premature beats). Heart rate is 71. P waves are matching and biphasic except for the fourth and eighth beats, which are premature and have no P waves. PR interval is 0.16, and QRS is 0.10. Interpretation: sinus rhythm with 2 PJCs.

---

chapter CHECKUP

We're about halfway through this chapter. To evaluate your understanding of the material thus far, answer the following questions. If you have trouble with them, review the material again before continuing.

Mr. Chekhov has been in a sinus rhythm but he's now having narrow-QRS (<0.12 secs) premature beats that interrupt the rhythm. These beats resemble the sinus beats but have no P waves. He has no symptoms and feels fine.

1. What are these premature beats?
2. What treatment, if any, is required?
3. From which part of the AV junction do these premature beats originate?

Junctional Bradycardia

Junctional bradycardia is a junctional rhythm with a heart rate slower than usual. A higher pacemaker has failed, and the AV junction has to escape to save the patient's life.

Rate	<40
Regularity	Regular
P waves	Inverted before or after the QRS, or hidden inside the QRS
Intervals	PR <0.12 secs if the P precedes the QRS
	QRS <0.12 secs

Cause	Vagal stimulation, hypoxia, ischemia of the sinus node, heart disease
Adverse effects	Slow heart rate can cause decreased cardiac output.
Treatment	Prepare for immediate transcutaneous pacing (attaching a pacemaker to the patient's skin). If the pacemaker is not immediately available and the patient is symptomatic, give atropine or consider starting an epinephrine or dopamine infusion to increase the heart rate. Start oxygen. Stop any heart rate–slowing medications.

Figure 9–3 shows QRS complexes, all shaped the same. Regularity is regular. Heart rate is 25. P waves are absent, or at least not visible. PR interval is not applicable. QRS interval is 0.08. Interpretation: junctional bradycardia.

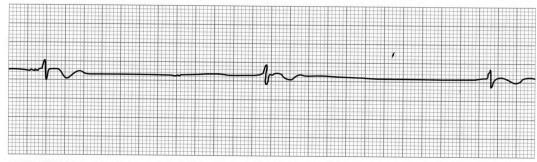

FIGURE 9–3

Junctional bradycardia.

Junctional Rhythm

Junctional rhythm is a rhythm that originates in the AV junction at its inherent rate of 40 to 60. It is usually an escape rhythm.

Rate	40 to 60
Regularity	Regular
P waves	Inverted before or after the QRS, or hidden inside the QRS
Intervals	PR <0.12 secs if the P precedes the QRS QRS <0.12 secs
Cause	Vagal stimulation, hypoxia, sinus node ischemia, heart disease
Adverse effects	Usually none if the heart rate is closer to the 50s to 60s range. Signs of decreased cardiac output are possible at slower heart rates.
Treatment	Transcutaneous pacing, atropine, dopamine or epinephrine infusion if symptomatic from the slow heart rate. Withdraw or decrease any medications that can slow the heart rate. Consider starting oxygen.

Figure 9–4 shows QRS complexes, all the same shape. Regularity is regular. Heart rate is 58. P waves are absent. (Those are not P waves after the QRS; those are S waves, a part of the QRS.) PR interval is not applicable. QRS interval is 0.12. Interpretation: junctional

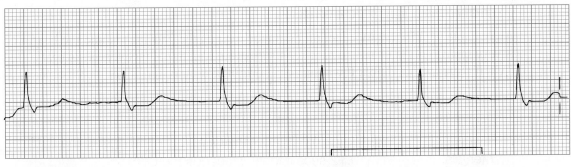

FIGURE 9–4

Junctional rhythm.

rhythm with a wide QRS. Although this example of junctional rhythm has no visible P waves, it could just as easily have had an inverted P wave with a short PR interval preceding the QRS, or an inverted P wave following the QRS. Remember, *the location of the P wave is dependent on the region of the AV junction in which the impulse originates.*

Accelerated Junctional Rhythm

Accelerated junctional rhythm can occur because of escape or usurpation. If the sinus node slows down, the AV junction can escape and take over as the pacemaker. Or an irritable spot in the AV junction can usurp control from the slower sinus node and become the heart's pacemaker at a faster-than-normal rate.

Rate	60 to 100
Regularity	Regular
P waves	Inverted before or after the QRS, or hidden inside the QRS
Intervals	PR <0.12 secs if the P precedes the QRS
	QRS <0.12 secs
Cause	Heart disease, stimulant drugs, and caffeine
Adverse effects	Usually none because the heart rate is within normal limits
Treatment	Usually none required aside from removal of the cause

Figure 9–5 shows QRS complexes, all the same shape. Regularity is regular. Heart rate is 75. P waves are absent. PR interval is not applicable. QRS interval is 0.08. Interpretation: accelerated junctional rhythm.

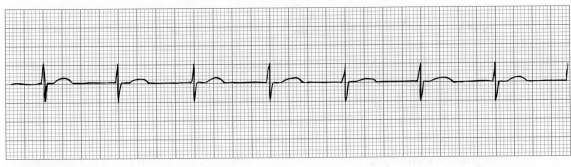

FIGURE 9–5

Accelerated junctional rhythm.

Junctional Tachycardia

An irritable spot in the AV junction has taken over as the pacemaker, and the heart rate is very rapid. This is usually a result of usurpation. Junctional tachycardia is best called SVT if there are no visible P waves, as the origin of the rhythm is not identifiable.

Rate	>100
Regularity	Regular
P waves	Inverted before or after the QRS, or hidden inside the QRS
Intervals	PR <0.12 secs if the P precedes the QRS
	QRS <0.12 secs
Cause	Most often caused by digitalis toxicity, but can be caused by heart disease, stimulants, or sympathetic nervous system stimulation
Adverse effects	Decreased cardiac output possible if the heart rate is fast enough
Treatment	Beta-blockers, calcium channel blockers, adenosine. Consider starting oxygen. Electrical cardioversion can be done if the patient is unstable.

Figure 9–6 shows QRS complexes, all the same shape. Regularity is regular. Heart rate is 125. P waves are present, inverted, following the QRS complex. PR interval is not applicable. QRS interval is 0.08. Interpretation: junctional tachycardia.

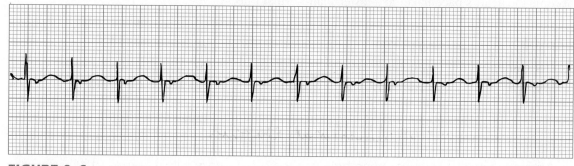

FIGURE 9–6

Junctional tachycardia.

Practice Strips: Junctional Rhythms

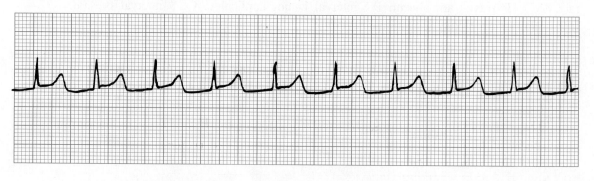

1. QRS complexes ___Reg___ Regularity ___Yes___ Heart rate ___100___
   P waves ___absent___
   PR interval ___N/A___   QRS interval ___0.08___
   Interpretation (name of rhythm) ___accelerated mid Junctional Rhythm___

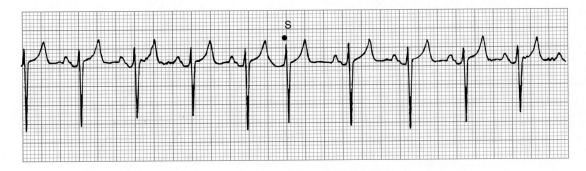

2. QRS complexes _____ Regularity _Yes__ Heart rate _100_
P waves _yes before QRS_
PR interval _____ QRS interval __08_
Interpretation _Sinus Rhythm w/ a PJC_

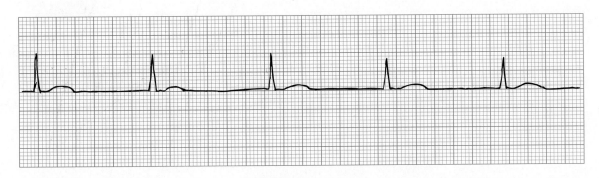

3. QRS complexes _____ Regularity _Yes_ Heart rate _50_
P waves _None_
PR interval _N/A_ QRS interval _0.08_
Interpretation _Mid AV Junctional Rhythm_

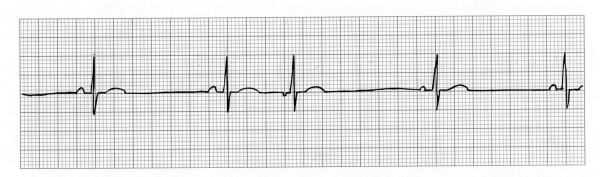

4. QRS complexes _____ Regularity _____ Heart rate _50_
P waves _Yes. Regular except 3rd beat has inverted P wave_
PR interval _____ QRS interval _____
Interpretation _Sinus Bradycardia w/ Low Level PJC_

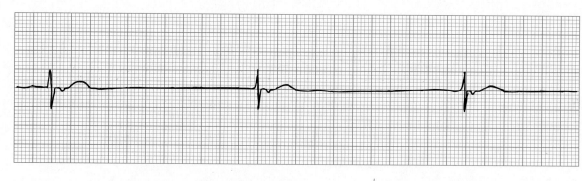

60~100
40~60
20~40

5. QRS complexes _Yes_ _____ Regularity _Yes_ _____ Heart rate _____ 30 _____
P waves _inverted 3 after SQRS_ _____
PR interval _———_ _____ QRS interval _0.08_ _____
Interpretation _Low level AV Junction Bradycardia_ _____

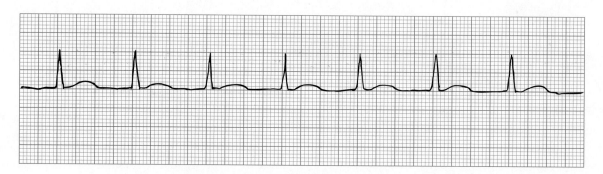

6. QRS complexes _____ Regularity _Yes_ _____ Heart rate _____ 70 _____
P waves _None_ _____
PR interval _N/A_ _____ QRS interval _0.08_ _____
Interpretation _Accelerated mid AC Junal Rhythm_ _____

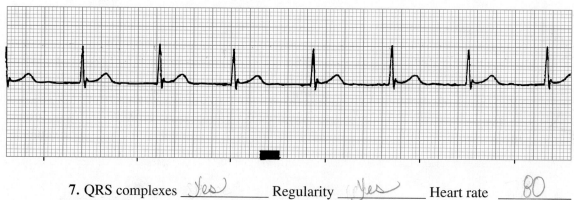

7. QRS complexes _Yes_ _____ Regularity _Yes_ _____ Heart rate _____ 80 _____
P waves _none_ _____
PR interval _N/A_ _____ QRS interval _0.08_ _____
Interpretation _accelerated mid AC Junctional Rhythm_ _____

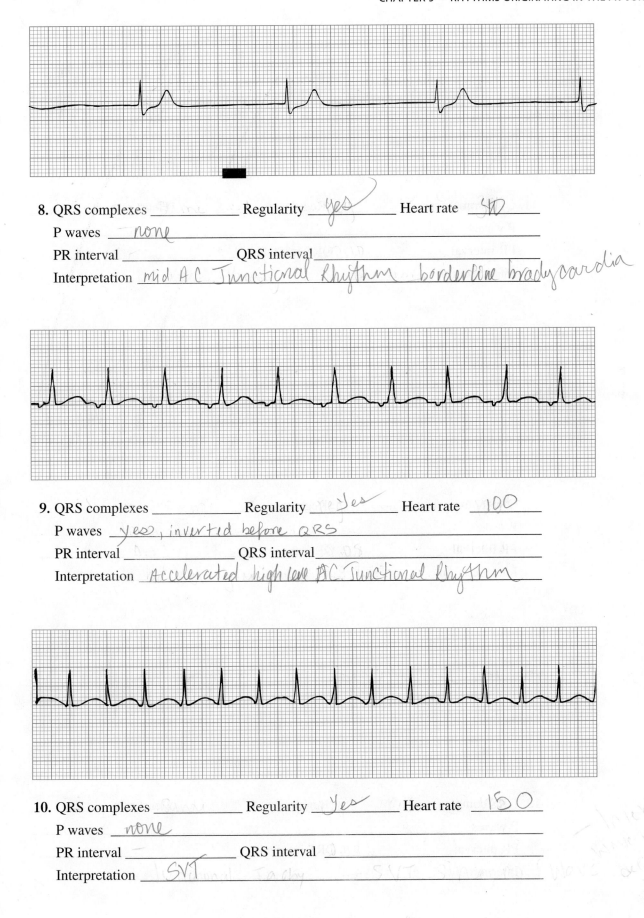

8. QRS complexes _____ Regularity __*yes*__ Heart rate __*50*__

   P waves __*none*__

   PR interval _____ QRS interval _____

   Interpretation __*mid AC Junctional Rhythm   borderline bradycardia*__

9. QRS complexes _____ Regularity __*yes*__ Heart rate __*100*__

   P waves __*yes, inverted before QRS*__

   PR interval _____ QRS interval _____

   Interpretation __*Accelerated high leve AC Junctional Rhythm*__

10. QRS complexes _____ Regularity __*Yes*__ Heart rate __*150*__

    P waves __*none*__

    PR interval _____ QRS interval _____

    Interpretation __*SVT*__

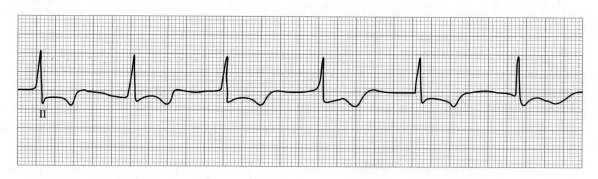

11. QRS complexes _Same_   Regularity _reg._   Heart rate _60_

P waves_ ⁻ _

PR interval _ ⁻ _   QRS interval _0.16_

Interpretation _Junctional_

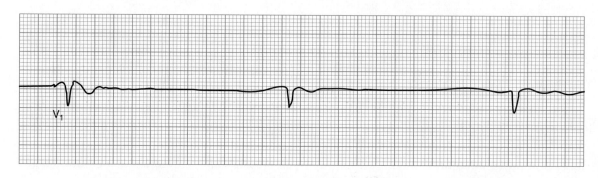

12. QRS complexes _Same_   Regularity _reg_   Heart rate _25_

P waves_ ⁻ _

PR interval _ ⁻ _   QRS interval _0.08_

Interpretation _Junctional Brady_

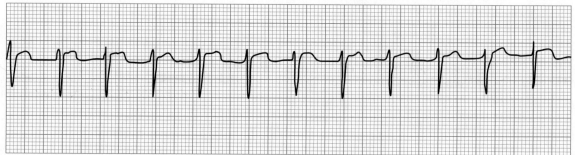

Why not SVT

13. QRS complexes _Same_   Regularity _reg_   Heart rate _125_

P waves_ ⁻ _

PR interval _ ⁻ _   QRS interval_

Interpretation _Junctional tachy_

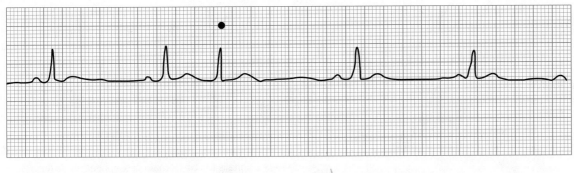

14. QRS complexes ___Same___ Regularity ___reg. Int.___ Heart rate ___50___
P waves ___yes - except 3rd___
PR interval ___0.16___ QRS interval ___0.08___
Interpretation ___PJC - Sinus brady___

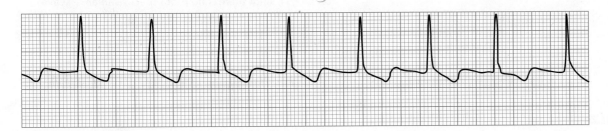

15. QRS complexes ___Same___ Regularity ___reg___ Heart rate ___88___
P waves ___—___
PR interval ___—___ QRS interval ___0.08___
Interpretation ___accelerated junctional___

---

chapter nine notes TO SUM IT ALL UP . . .

- **Junctional rhythms**—Arise from tissue located between the right atrium and right ventricle, an area known as the AV junction.
- **In junctional rhythms, the impulse travels antegrade toward the ventricles and retrograde toward the atria.**
- **P waves in junctional rhythms can be inverted preceding the QRS, inverted following the QRS, or hidden inside the QRS (invisible).**
- **The QRS in junctional rhythms will be positive or negative depending on the lead being monitored.** In Lead II, for example, the QRS should be positive; in V$_1$ it should be negative.
- **PJCs:**
  - *Heart rate*—Can occur at any heart rate
  - *Regularity*—Regular but interrupted by a premature beat
  - *P waves*—Inverted preceding or following the QRS, or hidden inside the QRS
  - *Intervals*—PR <0.12 secs if P wave precedes QRS; QRS <0.12 secs
  - *Causes*—Stimulants such as caffeine or drugs, nicotine, hypoxia, heart disease

- *Adverse effects*—Usually none
- *Treatment*—None except treat the cause
- **Junctional bradycardia:**
  - *Heart rate*—<40
  - *Regularity*—Regular
  - *P waves*—Inverted preceding or following the QRS, or hidden inside QRS
  - *Intervals*—PR <0.12 secs if P wave precedes QRS; QRS <0.12 secs
  - *Causes*—Vagal stimulation, hypoxia, sinus node ischemia, heart disease
  - *Adverse effects*—Decreased cardiac output
  - *Treatment*—Atropine, pacemaker, epinephrine or dopamine infusions, oxygen, stop any heart rate–slowing medications
- **Junctional rhythm:**
  - *Heart rate*—40–60
  - *Regularity*—Regular
  - *P waves*—Inverted preceding or following the QRS, or hidden inside QRS

- *Intervals*—PR <0.12 secs if P wave precedes QRS; QRS <0.12 secs
- *Causes*—Vagal stimulation, hypoxia, sinus node ischemia, heart disease
- *Adverse effects*—Usually none if heart rate closer to 50–60; decreased cardiac output possible at slower rates
- *Treatment*—Atropine, pacemaker, epinephrine or dopamine infusion, oxygen, stop heart rate–slowing medications

■ **Accelerated junctional rhythm:**

- *Heart rate*—60–100
- *Regularity*—Regular
- *P waves*—Inverted preceding or following the QRS, or hidden inside QRS
- *Intervals*—PR <0.12 secs if P wave precedes QRS; QRS <0.12 secs
- *Causes*—Heart disease, stimulant drugs, caffeine

- *Adverse effects*—Usually none
- *Treatment*—None except to treat the cause

■ **Junctional tachycardia:**

- *Heart rate*—>100
- *Regularity*—Regular
- *P waves*—Inverted preceding or following the QRS, or hidden inside QRS
- *Intervals*—PR <0.12 secs if P wave precedes QRS; QRS <0.12 secs
- *Causes*—Digitalis toxicity is main cause; heart disease, stimulants
- *Adverse effects*—Decreased cardiac output if heart rate too fast
- *Treatment*—Stop digitalis; start beta blockers, calcium channel blockers, or adenosine; consider cardioversion

■ **Junctional tachycardia with no visible P waves is best called SVT, since there is no proof there even *are* P waves there.** So no way to know the rhythm's origin for sure.

Practice Quiz

1. What are the three possible locations for the P waves in junctional rhythms? *before or after qrs or hidden*

2. Why is the P wave inverted in junctional rhythms? *Impulse travels backward to reach atria*

3. A junctional rhythm with a heart rate greater than 100 is *@ junctional tachy*

4. True or false: PJCs are a sign that the heart is going to develop a lethal arrhythmia.

5. A junctional rhythm with a heart rate less than 40 is *junctional brady*

6. Treatment for junctional bradycardia could consist of *transcutaneal pacing epi, dopamine*

7. PJCs cause the regularity to be *interrupted*

8. Is junctional bradycardia usually a result of escape or usurpation? *escape*

9. Junctional tachycardia is best called SVT if the P waves are located where? *Not located / hidden*

10. Is junctional tachycardia a result of escape or usurpation? *usurpation*

Putting It All Together—Critical Thinking Exercises

These exercises may consist of diagrams to label, scenarios to analyze, brain-stumping questions to ponder, or other challenging exercises to boost your understanding of the chapter material.

Let's play with junctional rhythms a bit. The following scenario will provide you with information about a fictional patient and ask you to analyze the situation, answer questions, and decide on appropriate actions.

Mrs. Dubos, age 86, is to be admitted to your intensive care unit. The ER nurse reports the following: Mrs. Dubos came to the ER complaining of shortness of breath and chest pain. Examination in the ER found her to be in sinus bradycardia with a heart rate of 47. BP at that time was 76/43 (very low), respirations 34 (fast), and temperature was normal. She was cool and clammy and appeared a bit dazed

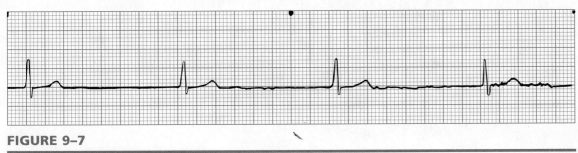

FIGURE 9–7

Mrs. Dubos's ER rhythm strip.

and confused. After appropriate medication, the heart rate came up to 86, her BP came up to 132/74 (normal), and her respirations slowed to a normal 20. Chest pain and shortness of breath subsided.

1. What medication do you believe was given in the ER to speed up Mrs. Dubos's heart rate? _atropine_

When Mrs. Dubos arrives on your floor, you look at the ER rhythm strip. See Figure 9–7.

2. What is the rhythm and rate? _____

38   Junctional Brady

_____

3. Was the ER nurse correct in her interpretation of this rhythm and rate? Explain. _NO — No p waves_

_____

_____

_____

4. Do you agree that the treatment rendered in the ER was appropriate for this patient? Why or why not?

Yes

_____

_____

_____

5. Did Mrs. Dubos have signs of decreased cardiac output in the ER? If yes, what were they?

low BP, ↑ RR, ↓ pulse

cool clamy, dazed

chest pain

Rhythms Originating in the Ventricles

CHAPTER 10 OBJECTIVES

Upon completion of this chapter, the student will be able to:

- State the criteria for each of the ventricular rhythms.
- Correctly identify ventricular rhythms on a variety of strips.
- State the adverse effects for each ventricular rhythm.
- State the possible treatment for the ventricular rhythms.
- Explain fusion beats and Wolff-Parkinson-White Syndrome (WPW).

What It's All About

Chris was at the gas station when he heard a groan and saw an elderly man collapse in cardiac arrest. An experienced ICU nurse, Chris hollered for bystanders to call 911 and began doing CPR. Soon there was a crowd surrounding Chris and the victim. "Find his family's phone number—somebody call his family," Chris yelled. "Check his cell phone for numbers!" The paramedics soon arrived and were briefed by Chris, who told them he suspected the patient was in V-fib. Seeing that Chris was doing effective CPR, the paramedics attached the patient to the heart monitor and evaluated the man's heart rhythm. He was indeed in ventricular fibrillation—Chris recognized the telltale pattern on the monitor immediately. He knew what was coming next. The paramedics ordered Chris out of the way and immediately defibrillated the heart. The rhythm converted to sinus rhythm for a few beats, then slowed dramatically and the QRS widened. There was no pulse. Paramedics quickly resumed CPR, inserted an IV line, and gave medications. Soon the pulse returned and the man was loaded into the ambulance and taken to a nearby hospital, where it was discovered that he'd had a heart attack that had caused his arrhythmia. At work the next day, his coworkers congratulated Chris. "Hey, you're famous. The paramedics at the scene said that patient wouldn't have made it if you hadn't started CPR. And they said you were a big help because you knew what the rhythm was and what to do. Good job."

Introduction

Ventricular rhythms originate in one or more irritable foci in the ventricular tissue below the conduction system pathway. Without the benefit of this pathway to speed the impulses through the tissue, the impulses trudge very slowly, cell by cell, through the ventricle, producing a wide QRS complex that measures >0.12 seconds. The impulse does sometimes travel backward to depolarize the atria, but the resultant P wave is usually lost in the mammoth QRS complex. Slow ventricular rhythms are the heart's last gasp as a pacemaker, kicking in when the higher pacemakers can't. Rapid ventricular arrhythmias can result in drastically decreased cardiac output, cardiovascular collapse, and death. See Figures 10–1 and 10–2.

In Figure 10–1, a single ventricular focus sends its impulse out, depolarizing the ventricles and providing the QRS complex. The impulse then heads backwards toward the atria to depolarize them, resulting in a P wave that may or may not be seen.

In Figure 10–2, multiple ventricular foci are firing off, each depolarizing its own little piece of ventricular territory. Rather than a QRS, which implies coordinated ventricular depolarization, this scenario results in a waveform that resembles static—no QRS in sight. This is a lethal rhythm unless properly treated.

The Word on Ventricular Rhythms

Ventricular rhythms, the most lethal of all the rhythms, command great respect from health care personnel. They can result from escape or usurpation and can have a heart rate varying from 0 to more than 250 beats per minute. Although some ventricular rhythms can be well tolerated, many will cause symptoms of decreased cardiac output or—even worse—cardiac standstill.

Most ventricular rhythms respond well to medications. Unfortunately, some of the medications used to treat ventricular rhythms can *cause* them in some circumstances. Some ventricular rhythms can be treated only by electric shock to the heart. And others, despite aggressive treatment, are usually fatal.

Some ventricular rhythms have no QRS at all; others have wide, bizarre QRS complexes. *Depending on the lead being monitored and the ventricle propagating the ventricular beats, the QRS may be positive or negative.* The best lead(s) to use for identification of ventricular rhythms is V$_1$ or MCL1; with these leads, it's possible to tell from which ventricle the rhythm/beats originated. This can be very important. *Left-ventricular premature ventricular complexes (PVCs) have an upward deflection in* V$_1$/MCL1. *Right-ventricular PVCs have a downward deflection in* V$_1$/MCL1. If the rhythm or beat in question meets *any* of the criteria that follow, it is ventricular in origin:

■ Wide QRS (>0.12 secs) without preceding P wave *or*
■ No QRS at all (*or* can't be sure if there are QRS complexes) *or*
■ Premature, wide QRS beat without preceding P wave, interrupting another rhythm

Let's look at these rhythms in detail now.

FIGURE 10–1

Conduction of a single ventricular focus.

Premature Ventricular Complexes (PVCs)

Premature ventricular complexes (PVCs) are premature beats that originate in irritable ventricular tissue before the next sinus beat is due.

Rate	Can occur at any rate
Regularity	Regular but interrupted
P waves	Usually not seen on PVCs
Intervals	PR not applicable QRS interval >0.12 secs; QRS wide and bizarre in shape
T wave	Slopes off in the opposite direction to the QRS. If the QRS points upward, for example, the T wave will point downward.
Cause	The big three causes are heart disease, **hypokalemia** (low blood potassium level), and hypoxia. Other causes include low blood magnesium level, stimulants, caffeine, stress, or anxiety. All these factors can cause the ventricle to become irritable and fire early beats.
Adverse effects	Occasional PVCs are of no concern. Frequent PVCs (6 or more per minute) or PVCs that are close to or land on the downstroke of the previous beat's T wave (called **R-on-T phenomenon**) can progress to lethal arrhythmias such as ventricular tachycardia or ventricular fibrillation. Multifocal PVCs

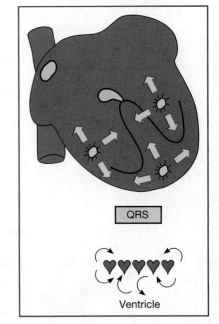

FIGURE 10–2

Conduction of multiple ventricular foci.

(those with differing shapes) are also cause for concern, since they mean that there are multiple irritable areas.

Treatment   Occasional PVCs don't require treatment. They can occur in normal, healthy individuals. If PVCs are more frequent, treat the cause. For example, if the potassium level is low, give supplemental potassium. Start oxygen. Amiodarone, an antiarrhythmic medication used to treat both atrial and ventricular arrhythmias, may be used to treat PVCs. For frequent PVCs during a slow bradycardia, however, do not treat with antiarrhythmics; treat with atropine instead. Bradycardic rhythm PVCs are the heart's attempt to increase the heart rate by providing another beat from *somewhere*. Giving antiarrhythmics could knock out the PVCs, leaving a slower heart rate. Atropine would speed up the underlying rhythm and the PVCs should go away on their own. See Figure 10–3.

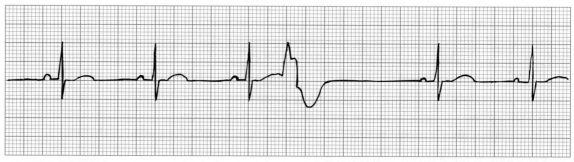

FIGURE 10–3

PVC (example of R-on-T PVC).

Figure 10–3 shows QRS complexes, all except the fourth beat having the same shape. The fourth beat has a wide QRS complex. Regularity is regular but interrupted by the premature beat. Heart rate is 60. There are matching upright P waves on all beats except the fourth beat, which has no P wave at all. PR interval is 0.16 on the sinus beats, no PR interval on the PVC. QRS interval is 0.08 on the sinus beats, 0.14 on the PVC. Interpretation: sinus rhythm with one PVC. This is an example of an R-on-T PVC, as you'll note the PVC lands on the downstroke of the previous beat's T wave. This is a potentially disastrous occurrence. This patient will need treatment to prevent lethal arrhythmias.

PVCs that come from a single focus all look alike. They're called **unifocal** PVCs. PVCs from different foci look different. They're called **multifocal** PVCs. See Figure 10–4.

Note in Figure 10–4 that A's PVCs are shaped the same—they're unifocal. B's PVCs are shaped differently—they're multifocal.

Two consecutive PVCs are called a **couplet.** Couplets can be either unifocal or multifocal. See Figure 10–5.

PVCs can be regular at times. If every other beat is a PVC, it's called ventricular **bigeminy.** If every third beat is a PVC, it's called ventricular **trigeminy.** If every fourth beat is a PVC, it's ventricular **quadrigeminy,** and so on. See Figure 10–6.

In Figure 10–6, note that every third beat is a PVC. This is ventricular trigeminy.

PVCs usually have a pause, called a **complete compensatory pause,** following them. This allows the regular rhythm to resume right on time as if the PVC had never happened. A complete compensatory pause measures two R-R cycles from the beat preceding the PVC to the beat following the PVC. See Figure 10–7.

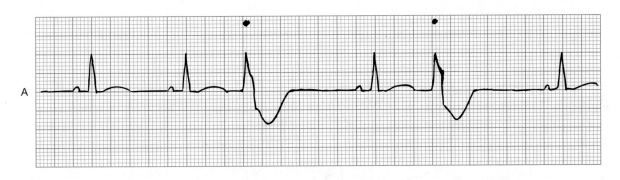

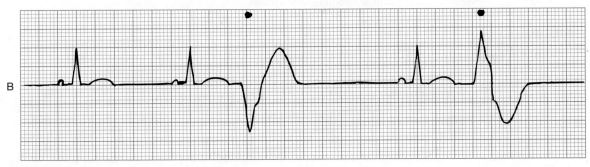

FIGURE 10–4

(A) Unifocal PVCs; (B) Multifocal PVCs.

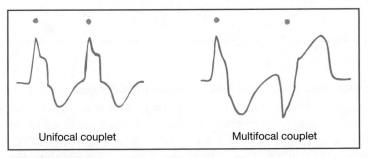

Unifocal couplet   Multifocal couplet

FIGURE 10–5

Unifocal and multifocal couplets.

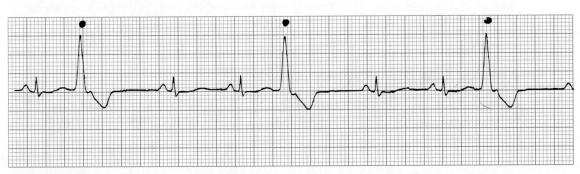

FIGURE 10–6

Ventricular trigeminy.

Sometimes a sinus impulse arrives to depolarize the ventricle at the same time a premature ventricular impulse was starting to depolarize the same tissue. The resultant QRS complex is intermediate in shape and size between the sinus beat and the PVC. Imagine the sinus beat as the mother and the PVC as the father. **Fusion beats**, as these beats are called, are their offspring. Just as in humans, where some children look more like their mother and

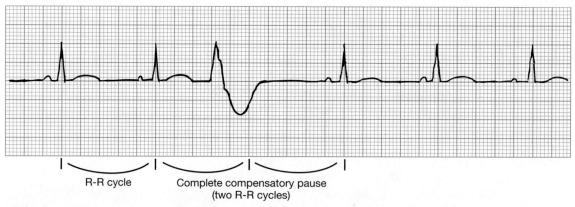

R-R cycle   Complete compensatory pause
(two R-R cycles)

FIGURE 10–7

Complete compensatory pause.

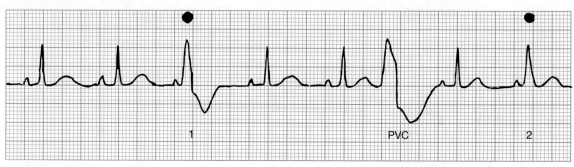

1   PVC   2

FIGURE 10–8

Fusion beats.

others resemble their father, some fusion beats will look more like the sinus beat (just a little wider and/or taller or deeper), and others will look more like the PVC (but narrower). See Figure 10–8. Here the dotted QRS complexes represent fusion beats. Note the shape of the sinus beats and the PVC. Look at fusion beat 1. It looks more like a narrowed PVC, doesn't it? The ventricle obviously contributed more to its shape than the sinus node did. Now look at fusion beat 2. It looks more like the sinus beats, but with a thicker R wave. Its shape was contributed mostly by the sinus beat with a little contribution from the ventricle. Note on both fusion beats that a P wave precedes the QRS. This is not always the case. If there is a P wave, the PR interval will be shorter than on the surrounding sinus beats. Fusion beats are caused by the same factors that cause PVCs and are treated the same way.

Agonal Rhythm (Dying Heart)

Agonal rhythm is an irregular rhythm in which the severely impaired heart is only able to "cough out" an occasional beat from its only remaining pacemaker, the ventricle. The higher pacemakers have all failed.

Rate	<20, although an occasional beat might come in at a slightly higher rate
Regularity	Irregular
P waves	None
Intervals	PR not applicable QRS interval >0.12 secs; QRS wide and bizarre
T wave	Slopes off in the opposite direction to the QRS

Cause	The patient is dying, usually from profound cardiac or other damage or from hypoxia.
Adverse effects	Profound shock, unconsciousness; death if untreated. Agonal rhythm usually does not provide a pulse—and even if it does, the cardiac output it produces will be incompatible with life.
Treatment	CPR, epinephrine and/or vasopressin, atropine, oxygen

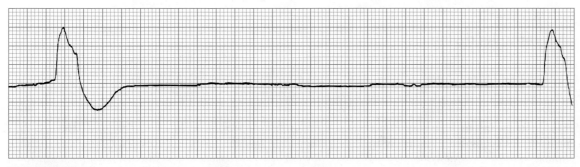

FIGURE 10–9

Agonal rhythm.

Figure 10–9 shows two QRS complexes, both the same shape, wide and bizarre. Regularity is indeterminate on this strip because there are only 2 QRS complexes. (Three are needed to determine regularity.) Heart rate is about 12. There are no P waves, therefore no PR interval. QRS interval is 0.28, extremely wide. Interpretation: agonal rhythm.

Idioventricular Rhythm (IVR)

Idioventricular rhythm (IVR) is a rhythm originating in the ventricle at its inherent rate. Higher pacemakers have failed, so the ventricle escapes to save the patient's life.

Rate	20 to 40
Regularity	Regular
P waves	None
Intervals	PR not applicable QRS interval >0.12 secs; QRS wide and bizarre
T wave	Slopes off in the opposite direction to the QRS
Cause	Usually implies massive cardiac or other damage, hypoxia
Adverse effects	Decreased cardiac output, cardiovascular collapse. IVR may or may not result in a pulse.
Treatment	Atropine, epinephrine, pacemaker, oxygen, dopamine. If the patient is pulseless, do CPR.

Figure 10–10 shows QRS complexes, all wide and bizarre. Regularity is regular. Heart rate is 37. There are no P waves, therefore no PR interval. QRS interval is 0.20, extremely wide. Interpretation: idioventricular rhythm.

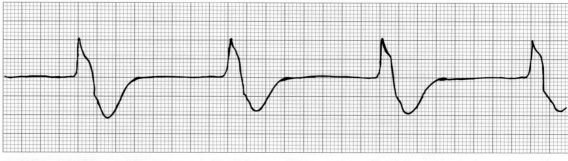

FIGURE 10–10

Idioventricular rhythm.

---

chapter CHECKUP

We're about halfway through this chapter. To evaluate your understanding of the material thus far, answer the following questions. If you have trouble with them, review the material again before continuing.

Mr. Kirk has a slow regular rhythm with a narrow QRS complex, matching upright P waves in Lead II, and a heart rate of 40. He's now having very frequent PVCs. He complains of feeling faint and you note his blood pressure has dropped alarmingly. You call for help. A coworker, having seen the rhythm, brings in amiodarone in case the physician orders it.

1. Is this the right medication for this situation? Why or why not?
2. If not, what medication would be indicated?

Accelerated Idioventricular Rhythm (AIVR)

Accelerated idioventricular rhythm (AIVR) is a rhythm originating in the ventricle, with a heart rate faster than the ventricle's normal rate. It can result from escape or usurpation.

Rate	40 to 100
Regularity	Usually regular, but can be a little irregular at times
P waves	Usually not seen
Intervals	No PR interval since no P waves QRS interval >0.12 secs; QRS wide and bizarre
T wave	Slopes off in the opposite direction to the QRS
Cause	Very common after an MI. Can be caused by the same factors that cause PVCs. AIVR is also common after administration of thrombolytic (clot-dissolving) medications, and in that context it was once considered a **reperfusion** arrhythmia, implying the heart muscle was once again getting blood flow after the clot was dissolved. Current studies, however, have shown that AIVR occurs just as often without reperfusion as with it, so it's no longer considered a sign of reperfusion.
Adverse effects	Usually no ill effects because the heart rate is close to normal
Treatment	Could be treated with atropine if the patient is symptomatic. Consider starting oxygen. Usually no treatment is necessary as AIVR tends to be a self-limiting rhythm.

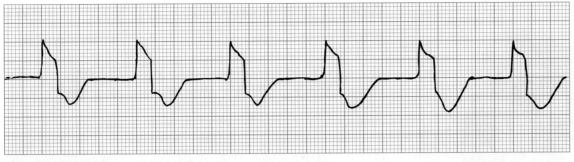

FIGURE 10–11

Accelerated idioventricular rhythm (AIVR).

Figure 10–11 shows QRS complexes, all wide and bizarre. Regularity is regular. Heart rate is 60. There are no P waves and thus no PR interval. QRS interval is about 0.18, very wide. Interpretation: accelerated idioventricular rhythm.

Ventricular Tachycardia (V-tach)

In *ventricular tachycardia* (V-tach), an irritable ventricular focus has usurped the sinus node to become the pacemaker and is firing very rapidly.

Rate	>100
Regularity	Usually regular, but can be a little irregular at times
P waves	Usually none seen, but dissociated from the QRS if present
Intervals	Variable PR if even present QRS >0.12 secs; QRS wide and bizarre
T wave	Slopes off in the opposite direction to the QRS
Cause	Same as PVCs
Adverse effects	This rhythm may be tolerated for short bursts, but prolonged runs of V-tach can cause profound shock, unconsciousness, and death if untreated.
Treatment	Amiodarone or lidocaine intravenously *if the patient is stable.* Electric shock to the heart (cardioversion or defibrillation) is indicated if the patient is unstable or pulseless. Also treat the cause (low potassium, magnesium, or oxygen levels, etc.). CPR is indicated if the patient is pulseless.

Figure 10–12 shows QRS complexes, all wide and bizarre. Regularity is regular. Heart rate is 214. P waves are absent. PR interval is not applicable. QRS interval is 0.13. Interpretation: ventricular tachycardia.

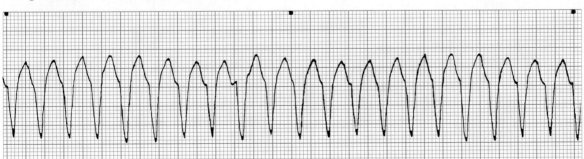

FIGURE 10–12

Ventricular tachycardia.

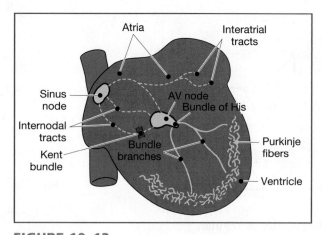

FIGURE 10–13

The bypass tract in WPW.

Wolff-Parkinson-White Syndrome (WPW)

Before we move on from V-tach, it's important to note a condition that can produce supraventricular tachycardias (particularly atrial fibrillation) with wide QRS complexes that mimic V-tach. This condition is **Wolff-Parkinson-White Syndrome (WPW)**, a syndrome in which there is an accessory conductive pathway between the atrium and ventricle. This accessory pathway, called the **Kent bundle**, allows some impulses to bypass the AV node and arrive at the ventricle earlier than if they'd gone through the AV node. For this reason, WPW is known as a **pre-excitation syndrome**. The ventricle is excited (depolarized) earlier than usual. WPW is recognized by a short PR interval and a **delta wave**, a slurred or slanted upstroke to the R wave of the QRS complex. This delta wave makes the QRS wider than normal. See Figures 10–13 and 10–14.

Since atrial fib with WPW can result in a wide QRS complex, it is often initially confused with V-tach—until the irregularity of the rhythm makes it clear that it's atrial fib. (Remember V-tach is usually regular.) *The problem lies not with thinking the rhythm is V-tach, but with realizing it's not.* Say you have a 24-year-old patient in your emergency department. He has come in because of episodes of "palpitations" and is now in what looks like V-tach. His blood pressure is OK so far, but he does admit to feeling light-headed, not a surprise since his heart rate is more than 200. You notify the physician, who declares the rhythm is V-tach. Since the patient is not unstable (yet), the physician elects not to do electric shock, but rather tells you to get amiodarone ready. As you prepare to inject the amiodarone into the IV, the physician, who had been examining the rhythm strip, stops you. "Wait, that's not V-tach; it's atrial fib with a wide QRS. Let's give a beta-blocker instead." So you toss the amiodarone, get out the beta blocker medication, inject it into the IV line, and watch in horror as your patient's heart rate shoots up to 280 and deteriorates into V-fib—cardiac arrest. What happened? Beta blockers are appropriate treatment for atrial fib, right?

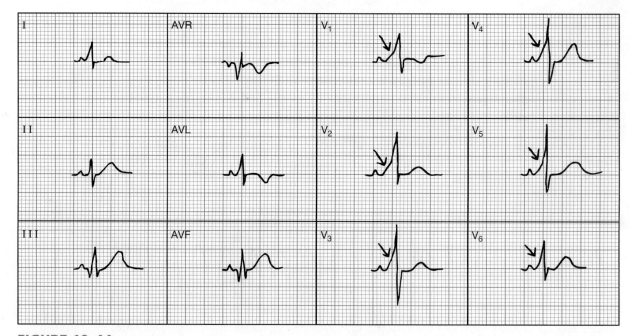

FIGURE 10–14

The delta wave and short PR interval in WPW. The arrow points out the delta wave.

Didn't we learn that in Chapter 8? Yes, but *here the problem is not the atrial fib—it's the WPW. We must treat rhythms with WPW only with medications that do not slow AV conduction.* Medications that slow AV node conduction, such as beta blockers, calcium channel blockers, or digitalis, can actually speed up the heart rate with WPW, since *once those meds slow down the AV node conduction, the accessory pathway is the path of least resistance and the impulses will blast down the Kent bundle.* This results in a much faster heart rate than before. As you can see, with the incorrect treatment, a bad situation can become life-threatening. Amiodarone and electrical cardioversion or defibrillation, routine treatments for V-tach, are also effective treatment for supraventricular tachycardias with WPW. So had our physician continued to think the rhythm was V-tach, he would have properly treated the rhythm. *It is important to recognize WPW so you'll know which medications* not *to give.*

WPW is a condition most often seen in males, although it is still rare. *It is most easily recognized on a routine 12-lead EKG when the heart rate is not tachycardic. The delta wave is more noticeable then.* Treatment includes ablation (destruction) of the accessory pathway.

Torsades de Pointes

Torsades de pointes (pronounced *tor-sahd de point*) is a French term meaning "twisting of the points." It's a form of **polymorphic** (multiple-shaped) ventricular tachycardia that is recognized primarily by its classic shape—it oscillates around an axis, with the QRS complexes pointing up, then becoming smaller, then rotating around until they point down. Torsades is not usually well tolerated in longer bursts and often deteriorates into ventricular fibrillation.

Rate	>200
Regularity	May be regular or irregular
P waves	None seen
Intervals	PR not applicable QRS >0.12 secs, often hard to measure; QRS wide and bizarre *QT interval on a pre-torsades strip will be prolonged.*
T wave	Opposite the QRS, but may not be seen due to the rapidity of the rhythm
Cause	Can be caused by antiarrhythmic medications such as quinidine, procainamide, or amiodarone, which cause an increased QT interval. Otherwise it is caused by the same factors that cause V-tach.
Adverse effects	May be tolerated for short runs, but usually results in cardiac arrest if sustained
Treatment	Intravenous magnesium is the usual treatment. Electrical cardioversion or defibrillation may be needed. Start oxygen.

Figure 10–15 shows QRS complexes, not all the same shape. Some point downward, some point upward, and others are very small. Regularity is regular. Heart rate is about 375. P waves are absent; therefore no PR interval. QRS interval is 0.16. Interpretation: torsades de pointes. The big clue here is the oscillating character of the QRS complexes—bigger, then smaller, then bigger again, and so on. That's classic for torsades.

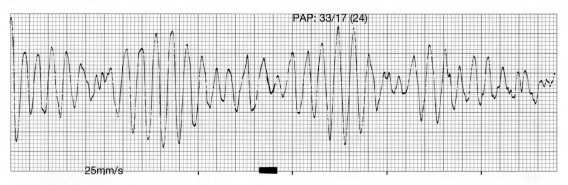

PAP: 33/17 (24)

25mm/s

FIGURE 10–15

Torsades de pointes.

Ventricular Fibrillation (V-fib)

In *ventricular fibrillation* (V-fib), hundreds of impulses in the ventricle are firing, each depolarizing its own little piece of territory. As a result, the ventricles wiggle instead of contract. The heart's electrical system is in chaos, and the resultant rhythm looks like static.

Rate	Cannot be counted
Regularity	None detectable
P waves	None
Intervals	No PR interval since no P waves No QRS interval since no QRS complexes—just a wavy or spiked baseline
T wave	None
Cause	Same as V-tach; also can be caused by drowning, drug overdoses, accidental electric shock
Adverse effects	Profound cardiovascular collapse. There is no cardiac output whatsoever. There is no pulse, no breathing, nothing. The patient is functionally dead. New onset V-fib has coarse fibrillatory waves. These waves get progressively finer the longer it lasts.
Treatment	Immediate defibrillation (electric shock to the heart), epinephrine, CPR, amiodarone, lidocaine, oxygen. The rhythm will not be converted with just medications. Defibrillation must be done. The medications make the defibrillation more successful and can prevent recurrences of V-fib.

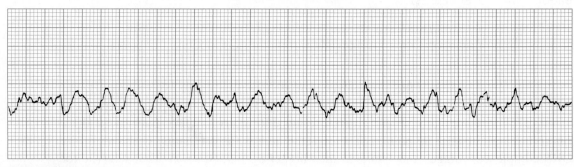

FIGURE 10–16

Ventricular fibrillation.

Figure 10–16 shows no identifiable QRS complexes—just a wavy, spiked baseline resembling static. Regularity is not determinable. Heart rate is not measurable since there are no QRS complexes. P waves are not present. PR and QRS intervals cannot be measured. Interpretation: ventricular fibrillation.

Asystole

Asystole is flat-line EKG. Every one of the heart's pacemakers has failed.

Rate	Zero
Regularity	None
P waves	None
Intervals	No PR interval since no P waves; no QRS interval since no QRS
T wave	None
Cause	Profound cardiac or other body system damage; profound hypoxia. Even with vigorous resuscitative efforts, this is usually a terminal rhythm.
Adverse effects	Death if untreated
Treatment	Atropine to reverse any vagal influence, epinephrine and/or vasopressin, CPR, oxygen. There is rarely a need to utilize a pacemaker. Depending on the situation, it may be appropriate to forgo resuscitative efforts.

Figure 10–17 shows no QRS complexes, only a flat line. There is no regularity. Heart rate is zero. There are no P waves, no PR interval, and no QRS interval. Interpretation: asystole.

There is another kind of asystole in which there are no QRS complexes but there are still P waves. This is called **P wave asystole** or **ventricular asystole**. The still-functioning sinus node fires its impulses, but they do not cause ventricular depolarization either because the ventricle is too damaged to respond to the stimulus or because there is a complete block in conduction of the impulse to the ventricle. Since the atria depolarize but the ventricles don't, there is no QRS after the Ps. Eventually the sinus impulses will slow and stop, since there is no cardiac output to feed blood to the sinus node. Remember—*if there is no QRS complex, there is no cardiac output.* Treatment is the same as for asystole.

Quick Tip

Do not use electrical shock to treat asystole—it will only result in more asystole. Shocking is used to recoordinate the heart's electrical activity. *In asystole, there is no electrical activity to recoordinate.* (Exception: If it's debated whether the rhythm may actually be a very fine V-fib instead of asystole, a trial defibrillation may be done.)

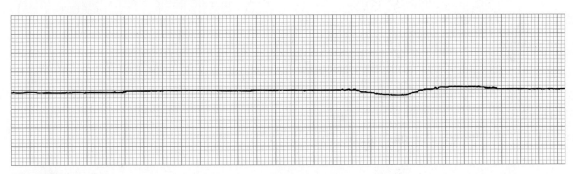

FIGURE 10–17

Asystole.

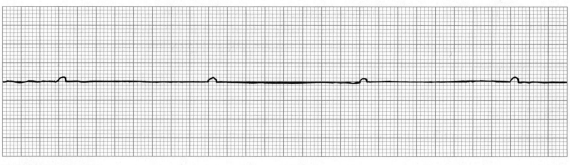

FIGURE 10–18

P wave asystole.

Figure 10–18 shows no QRS complexes. Regularity is not applicable. Heart rate is zero. P waves are present, regular, with an atrial rate of 37. There is no PR interval or QRS interval. Interpretation: P wave asystole.

Pacemaker Rhythm

Pacemakers are electronic devices that can be implanted into or attached to the patient to send out an electrical impulse to cause the heart to depolarize. Pacemakers are used when the heart is temporarily or permanently unable to generate or transmit its own impulses, or when it does so too slowly to provide a reasonable cardiac output. They can be used to pace the atria, the ventricles, or both.

When the pacemaker sends out its signal, a vertical spike is recorded on the EKG paper. Ventricular pacing provides a spike followed by a wide QRS. Atrial pacing has a spike followed by a P wave. Dual-chamber pacing (both atrium and ventricle) has a spike before both the P and the QRS. See Figure 10–19.

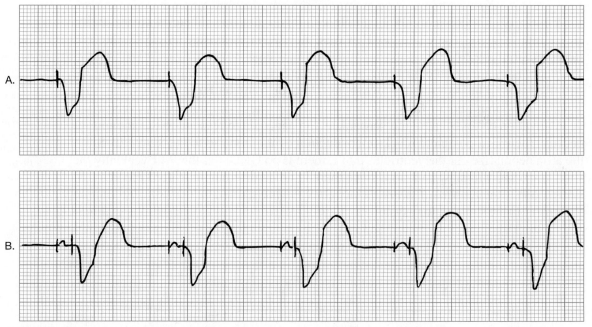

FIGURE 10–19

Pacemakers: (A) Ventricular pacing; (B) Dual-chamber pacing.

In Figure 10–19A, there are QRS complexes, all wide, all shaped the same. Each QRS is preceded by a pacemaker spike. Regularity is regular. Heart rate is 50. There are no P waves, therefore no PR interval. QRS interval is 0.24 secs. Interpretation: ventricular pacing.

In Figure 10–19B, there are QRS complexes, all wide, all shaped the same. Regularity is regular. Heart rate is 50. There are matching P waves, each preceded by a pacemaker spike. PR interval is not measured in paced rhythms. The **AV interval** (the interval between atrial and ventricular pacing spikes) is 0.16 secs and should be constant as this interval is preset when the pacemaker is implanted. QRS interval is 0.24 secs. Interpretation: dual-chamber pacing (also called AV pacing).

For in-depth information on pacemakers, see Chapter 16.

Practice Strips: Ventricular Rhythms

The first 10 strips are single-lead strips; the last 15 are double-lead strips.

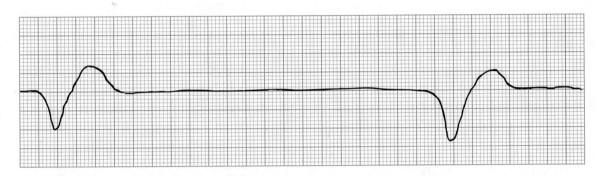

1. QRS complexes _____ Regularity _____ Heart rate _____

P waves _____

PR interval _____ QRS interval _____

Interpretation (name of rhythm) _____

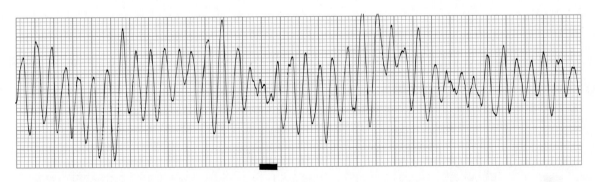

2. QRS complexes _____ Regularity _____ Heart rate _____

P waves _____

PR interval _____ QRS interval _____

Interpretation _____

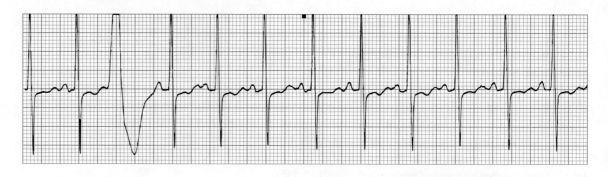

3. QRS complexes _____ Regularity _____ Heart rate _____

P waves _____

PR interval _____ QRS interval _____

Interpretation _____

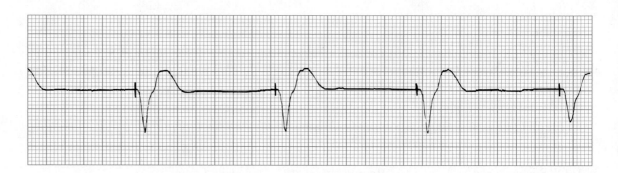

4. QRS complexes _____ Regularity _____ Heart rate _____

P waves _____

PR interval _____ QRS interval _____

Interpretation _____

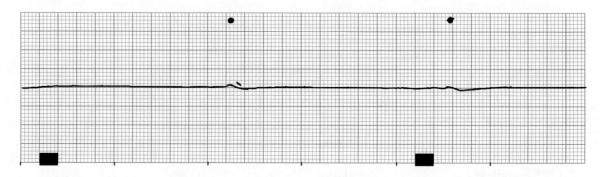

5. QRS complexes _____ Regularity _____ Heart rate _____

P waves _____

PR interval _____ QRS interval _____

Interpretation _____

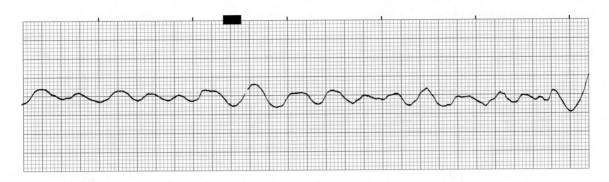

6. QRS complexes _____ Regularity _____ Heart rate _____

P waves _____

PR interval _____ QRS interval _____

Interpretation _____

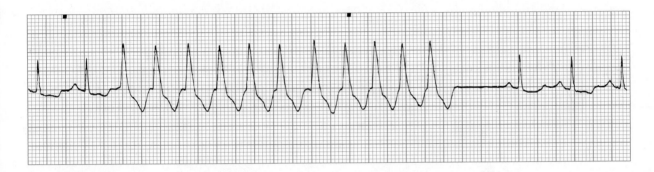

7. QRS complexes _____ Regularity _____ Heart rate _____

P waves _____

PR interval _____ QRS interval _____

Interpretation _____

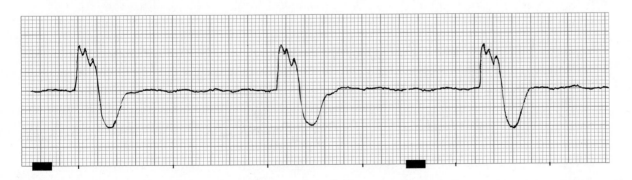

8. QRS complexes _____ Regularity _____ Heart rate _____

P waves _____

PR interval _____ QRS interval _____

Interpretation _____

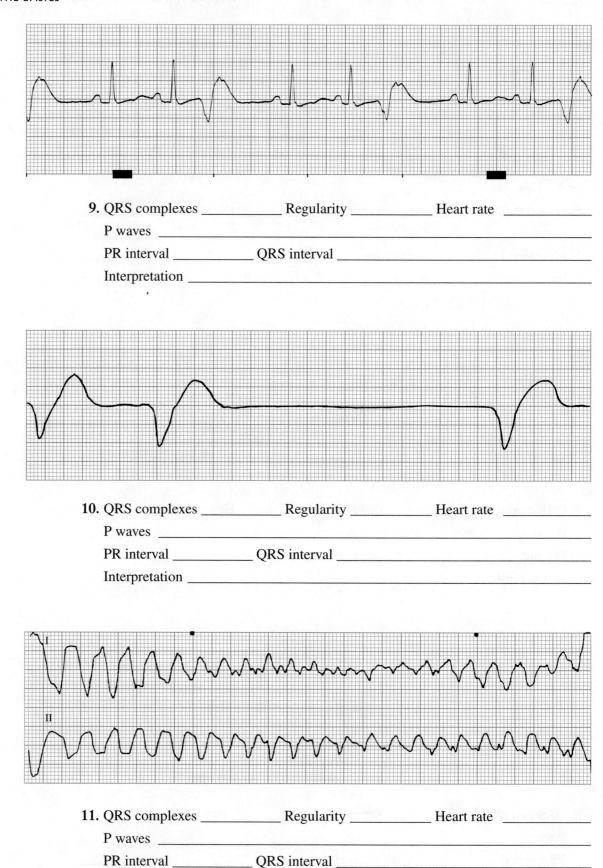

9. QRS complexes _____ Regularity _____ Heart rate _____

P waves _____

PR interval _____ QRS interval _____

Interpretation _____

10. QRS complexes _____ Regularity _____ Heart rate _____

P waves _____

PR interval _____ QRS interval _____

Interpretation _____

11. QRS complexes _____ Regularity _____ Heart rate _____

P waves _____

PR interval _____ QRS interval _____

Interpretation _____

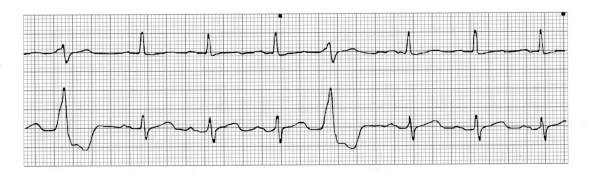

12. QRS complexes _____ Regularity _____ Heart rate _____

P waves _____

PR interval _____ QRS interval _____

Interpretation _____

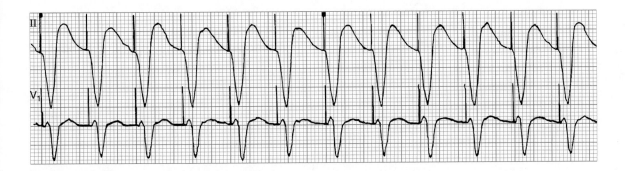

13. QRS complexes _____ Regularity _____ Heart rate _____

P waves _____

PR interval _____ QRS interval _____

Interpretation _____

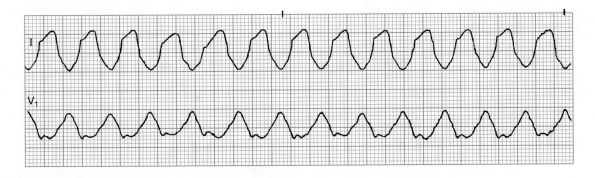

14. QRS complexes _____ Regularity _____ Heart rate _____

P waves _____

PR interval _____ QRS interval _____

Interpretation _____

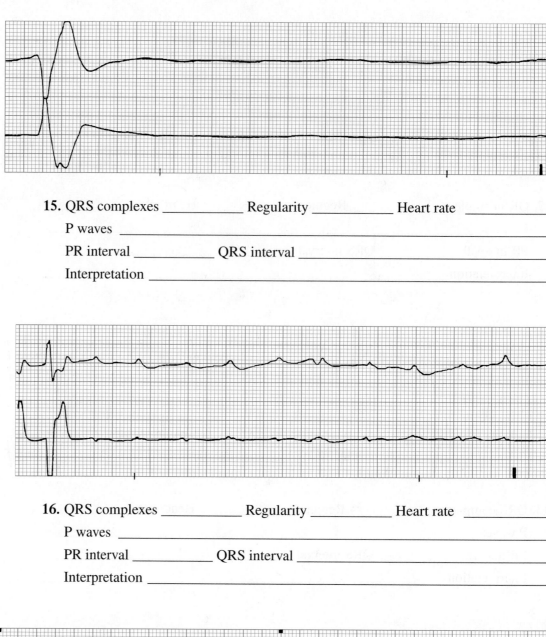

15. QRS complexes _____ Regularity _____ Heart rate _____

P waves _____

PR interval _____ QRS interval _____

Interpretation _____

16. QRS complexes _____ Regularity _____ Heart rate _____

P waves _____

PR interval _____ QRS interval _____

Interpretation _____

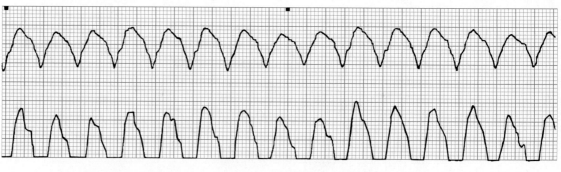

17. QRS complexes _____ Regularity _____ Heart rate _____

P waves _____

PR interval _____ QRS interval _____

Interpretation _____

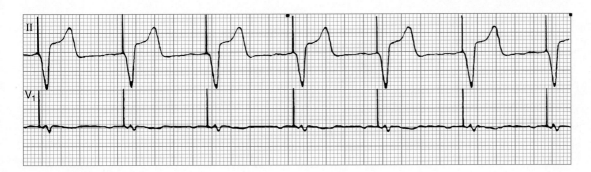

18. QRS complexes _____ Regularity _____ Heart rate _____

    P waves _____

    PR interval _____ QRS interval _____

    Interpretation _____

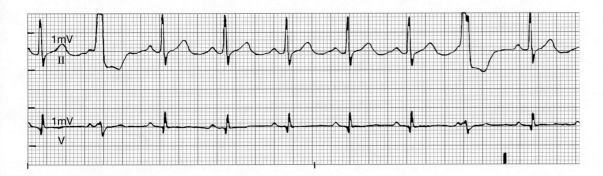

19. QRS complexes _____ Regularity _____ Heart rate _____

    P waves _____

    PR interval _____ QRS interval _____

    Interpretation _____

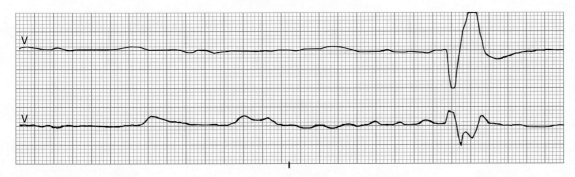

20. QRS complexes _____ Regularity _____ Heart rate _____

    P waves _____

    PR interval _____ QRS interval _____

    Interpretation _____

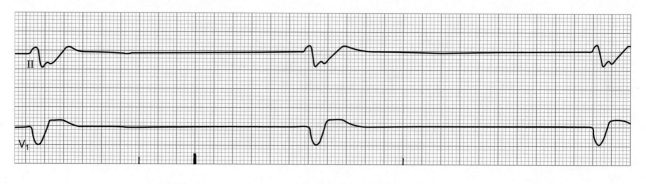

21. QRS complexes _____ Regularity _____ Heart rate _____

P waves _____

PR interval _____ QRS interval _____

Interpretation _____

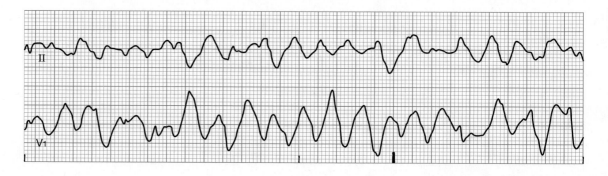

22. QRS complexes _____ Regularity _____ Heart rate _____

P waves _____

PR interval _____ QRS interval _____

Interpretation _____

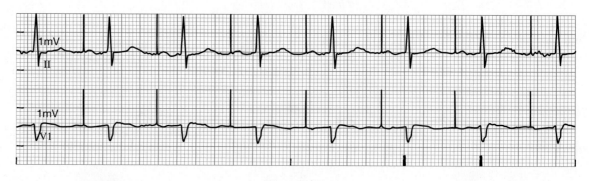

23. QRS complexes _____ Regularity _____ Heart rate _____

P waves _____

PR interval _____ QRS interval _____

Interpretation _____

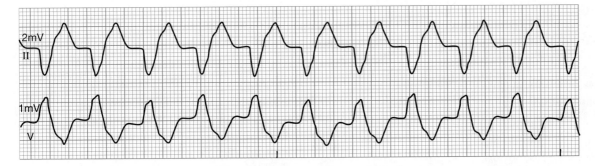

24. QRS complexes _____ Regularity _____ Heart rate _____

P waves _____

PR interval _____ QRS interval _____

Interpretation _____

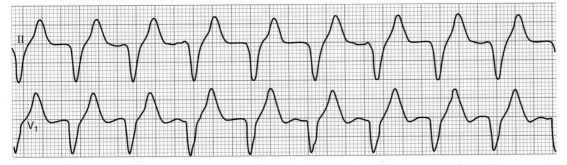

25. QRS complexes _____ Regularity _____ Heart rate _____

P waves _____

PR interval _____ QRS interval _____

Interpretation _____

chapter ten notes TO SUM IT ALL UP . . .

- **Ventricular rhythms**—Originate in an irritable focus in the ventricle—travel cell by cell through the tissue. Ventricular rhythm impulses do not travel through the bundle branches. QRS complex is wide and bizarre in appearance.
- **In ventricular rhythms, QRS may be positive or negative depending on the lead being monitored and the ventricle originating the rhythm.** In V_1 or MCL1, PVCs from left ventricle will have a positive QRS. PVCs from right ventricle will have negative QRS.
- **PVCs:**
  - *Heart rate*—Can occur at any rate
  - *Regularity*—Regular but interrupted by a premature beat
  - *P waves*—None
  - *Intervals*—PR—not applicable; QRS >0.12 secs.
  - *T wave*—Opposite the QRS
  - *Causes*—Heart disease, hypokalemia, hypoxia, low magnesium level, stress, caffeine, anxiety
  - *Adverse effects*—Can lead to worsening arrhythmias such as V-tach or V-fib
  - *Treatment*—Treat the cause; oxygen, amiodarone. Treat bradycardia PVCs with atropine.
- **Unifocal PVCs**—Have same shape. Multifocal PVCs—have differing shapes.

- **R-on-T PVCs**—Land on the T wave of the preceding beat—are more dangerous than PVCs that land after the T wave—can cause V-tach or V-fib.
- **Couplets**—Paired PVCs; can be unifocal or multifocal
- **Fusion beats**—Combination of sinus beat and PVC
- **Agonal rhythm:**
  - *Heart rate*—<20
  - *Regularity*—Irregular
  - *P waves*—None
  - *Intervals*—PR—not applicable; QRS >0.12 secs
  - *T wave*—Opposite the QRS
  - *Causes*—Dying patient
  - *Adverse effects*—Shock, unconsciousness, death if untreated
  - *Treatment*—CPR, epinephrine or vasopressin, atropine, oxygen
- **Idioventricular rhythm:**
  - *Heart rate*—20–40
  - *Regularity*—Regular
  - *P waves*—None
  - *Intervals*—PR—not applicable; QRS >0.12 secs
  - *T wave*—Opposite the QRS
  - *Causes*—Hypoxia, massive heart or other organ damage

- *Adverse effects*—Decreased cardiac output, cardiovascular collapse
- *Treatment*—Oxygen, atropine, epinephrine and/or vasopressin, pacemaker if indicated, dopamine infusion, CPR if pulseless or cardiac output ineffective

■ **Accelerated idioventricular rhythm:**
- *Heart rate*—40–100
- *Regularity*—Usually regular
- *P waves*—Usually none
- *Intervals*—PR—not applicable; QRS >0.12 secs
- *T wave*—Opposite the QRS
- *Causes*—MI
- *Adverse effects*—Usually none—could have decreased cardiac output at slower heart rates
- *Treatment*—Oxygen, atropine if symptoms from slow heart rate

■ **Ventricular tachycardia:**
- *Heart rate*—>100
- *Regularity*—Usually regular
- *P waves*—Usually none; if present will be dissociated from QRS
- *Intervals*—PR—not applicable; QRS >0.12 secs
- *T waves*—Opposite the QRS
- *Causes*—Same as PVCs
- *Adverse effects*—Decreased cardiac output, shock, unconsciousness, death
- *Treatment*—Amiodarone or lidocaine if stable; electrical cardioversion if unstable; defibrillation if pulseless

■ **Wolff-Parkinson-White Syndrome**—Pre-excitation syndrome characterized by a short PR interval and a delta wave—can result in supraventricular tachycardias that resemble V-tach. Treatment can involve cardioversion, defibrillation, or *medications that* do not *slow AV conduction.*

■ **Torsades de pointes:**
- *Heart rate*—>200
- *Regularity*—Regular or irregular
- *P waves*—None

- *Intervals*—PR—none; QRS >0.12 secs
- *T wave*—Opposite the QRS; T waves hard to see because of fast rate
- *Causes*—Antiarrhythmic medications such as amiodarone, quinidine, procainamide; otherwise causes same as for V-tach
- *Adverse effects*—Cardiac arrest if sustained
- *Treatment*—Oxygen, IV magnesium, cardioversion or defibrillation

■ **Ventricular fibrillation:**
- *Heart rate*—Cannot count
- *Regularity*—Cannot determine
- *P waves*—None
- *Intervals*—Not applicable
- *T waves*—None
- *Causes*—Same as V-tach plus drowning, accidental electric shock, drug overdoses
- *Adverse effects*—Cardiac arrest; death if untreated
- *Treatment*—Defibrillation, CPR, oxygen, amiodarone or lidocaine, epinephrine and/or vasopressin

■ **Asystole:**
- *Heart rate*—Zero
- *Regularity*—Not applicable
- *P waves*—None unless it's P wave asystole/ventricular asystole
- *Intervals*—Not applicable
- *T wave*—None
- *Causes*—Profound hypoxia or heart or other damage
- *Adverse effects*—Death if untreated
- *Treatment*—CPR, atropine, epinephrine and/or vasopressin, oxygen. Find and treat the cause. Consider termination of resuscitative efforts.

■ **Pacemakers**—Devices that are attached to or implanted into a patient—stimulate the atria, ventricles, or both to depolarize when the patient's own conduction system is too slow or unable to do it.
- *Atrial pacing*—Pacer spike then P wave
- *Ventricular pacing*—Pacer spike then QRS complex

Practice Quiz

1. The three main causes of PVCs are _____ _____ _____

2. The rhythm that has no QRS complexes but instead has a wavy, static-looking baseline is _____ _____

3. Appropriate treatment for PVCs interrupting a sinus bradycardia with a heart rate of 32 would be _____

4. *Torsades de pointes* is a French term that means _____

5. How does asystole differ from P wave asystole? _____ _____

6. Your patient has a ventricular rhythm with a heart rate of 39, but no pulse. What treatment would be appropriate? _____ _____

7. True or false: Asystole is treated with electric shock to the heart.

8. The treatment of choice for ventricular fibrillation is _____ _____

9. True or false: Pacemakers can pace the atrium, the ventricle, or both.

10. True or false: Antiarrhythmics should be given to treat agonal rhythm.

Putting It All Together—Critical Thinking Exercises

These exercises may consist of diagrams to label, scenarios to analyze, brain-stumping questions to ponder, or other challenging exercises to boost your understanding of the chapter material.

Let's play with ventricular rhythms a bit. The following scenario will provide you with information about a fictional patient and ask you to analyze the situation, answer questions, and decide on appropriate actions.

Mr. Winston, age 45, arrives in your ER complaining of intermittent dizziness. He feels he has come close to passing out a few times in the past 24 hours. Other than a past medical history of diet-controlled diabetes, he's been healthy. See his initial rhythm strip in the ER, Figure 10–20. Vital signs are stable. Mr. Winston denies feeling dizzy at this time.

1. What is this rhythm? _____

2. Does this rhythm require emergency treatment?

   _____

   _____

3. Name three factors that can cause this rhythm.

   _____

   _____

Lab tests reveal Mr. Winston's potassium level to be 1.9, extremely low. The physician orders potassium to be given intravenously. Half an hour later, an alarm sounds and the following rhythm strip prints out. See Figure 10–21.

4. What is this rhythm? _____

5. Does this rhythm require emergency treatment?

   _____

6. Mr. Winston has no breathing and no pulse. What intervention must be employed to terminate this rhythm?

   _____

After successful intervention, Mr. Winston returns to sinus rhythm and has no more problems. After an uneventful course in the intensive care unit, Mr. Winston goes home taking amiodarone.

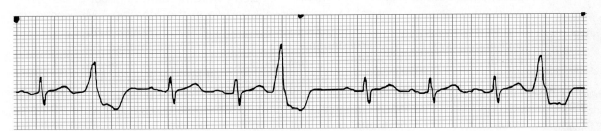

FIGURE 10–20

Mr. Winston's initial strip.

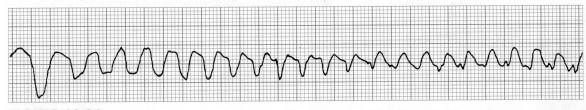

FIGURE 10-21

Rhythm causing alarm.

AV Blocks

CHAPTER 11 OBJECTIVES

Upon completion of this chapter, the student will be able to:

- State the criteria, causes, adverse effects, and treatment for each type of AV block.
- State whether the block is at the AV node or the bundle branches.
- Identify each type of AV block on a variety of strips.

What It's All About

Mr. Pomeroux, age 54, was having a heart attack. He'd just finished watching his beloved New Orleans Saints win the Super Bowl when he began to notice left-sided chest pain. His wife dragged him from in front of the TV and brought him to the emergency room where his heart rate was discovered to be 42. The doctor said it was third-degree AV block, whatever that was. Mr. Pomeroux didn't care much for hospitals and especially didn't care for this doctor who looked younger than his 15-year-old daughter telling him what to do. "We need to get you to the cath lab and put in a pacemaker," the doctor had told him. "No, I don't want no darned pacemaker. I don't need no pacemaker. I want to go home. I'll be fine in the morning." Mr. Pomeroux signed himself out of the emergency room against medical advice and against the protestations of his wife and daughter. He insisted on driving himself home, his wife and daughter cringing beside him. A few hours later, Mr. Pomeroux was rushed back to the ER by ambulance, this time extremely dizzy and in third-degree AV block with a heart rate of 27 and a wide QRS. ER nurses Glenn and Ron started oxygen and attached transcutaneous pacemaker patches to Mr. Pomeroux's chest while ER nurse Paul started an IV line and gave him atropine. The heart rate improved with the pacemaker, but the atropine did no good. Mr. Pomeroux was taken immediately to the cardiac cath lab and a pacemaker was inserted. He woke up in the ICU. Although still not happy to be in the hospital, he expressed gratitude that his family had called 911 to get him back to the hospital. "I almost died of stubbornness," he declared.

Introduction

With **AV blocks** (atrioventricular), the sinus node fires its impulses as usual, but there is a problem down the line—a partial or complete interruption in the transmission of these impulses to the ventricles. The site of the block is the AV node or the bundle branches. See Figures 11–1 and 11–2.

In Figure 11–1, the sinus node sends its impulse through the atria and a P wave is written on the EKG. The impulse travels to the AV node where there is a block in conduction. The impulse dies out here. In Figure 11–2, the impulse travels as far as the bundle branches, where it is stopped by a block. In either case, the impulse can just end there, with a P wave and no QRS (since it never made it to the ventricle), or a lower pacemaker can escape to provide stimulus to the ventricle, thus providing a QRS.

Degrees of AV Block

There are 3 degrees of block, varying in severity from benign to life threatening. See Table 11–1.

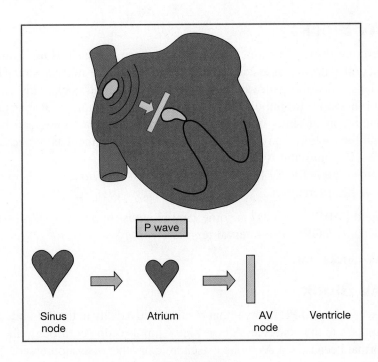

FIGURE 11–1

Block at the AV node.

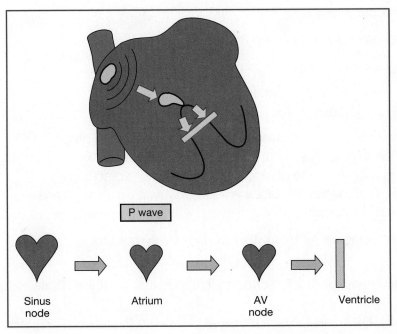

FIGURE 11–2

Block at the bundle branches.

TABLE 11–1   Degrees of AV Block

Kind of AV Block	Site of Block	Feature	Clinical Importance
First degree	AV node	Delay in impulse transmission from sinus node to ventricles.	No clinical danger—no symptoms
Second degree	AV node or bundle branches	Some impulses from sinus node get through; some don't.	Can progress to higher degree of block—can cause decreased cardiac output
Third degree	AV node or bundle branches	None of the impulses get through to the ventricles. A lower pacemaker assumes control.	Can be life-threatening, causing severe symptoms

The Word on AV Blocks

In AV blocks, the underlying rhythm is sinus. The impulse is born in the sinus node and starts down the conduction pathway as usual. Thus, the P waves are normal sinus P waves. Farther down the conduction pathway, however, there is a roadblock. This can result in either a simple delay in impulse transmission or a complete or partial interruption in the conduction of sinus impulses to the ventricle. Heart rates can be normal or very slow, and symptoms may be present or absent. Treatment is aimed at increasing the heart rate and improving AV conduction.

There are two possible criteria for AV blocks. *If either of these criteria is met, there is an AV block.* Let's look at the criteria:

- PR interval prolonged (>0.20 seconds) in some kind of sinus rhythm *or*
- Some Ps not followed by a QRS; P-P interval regular

Let's look at the AV blocks now.

First-Degree AV Block

First-degree AV block is a prolonged PR interval that results from a delay in the AV node's conduction of sinus impulses to the ventricle. All the sinus impulses do get through; they just take longer than normal because the AV node is ischemic or otherwise suppressed.

Rate	Can occur at any rate
Regularity	Depends on the underlying rhythm.
P waves	Upright, matching; one P to each QRS
Intervals	PR prolonged (>0.20 secs), constant QRS <0.12 secs
Cause	AV node ischemia, digitalis toxicity or a side effect of other medications such as beta-blockers or calcium channel blockers. This is a benign type of block, but be alert for worsening AV block. *First-degree AV block is seen only with rhythms originating in the sinus node.*
Adverse effects	The first-degree AV block itself causes no symptoms.
Treatment	Remove any medication causing it. Otherwise, treat the cause.

Figure 11–3 shows QRS complexes, all shaped the same. Regularity is regular. Heart rate is 62. P waves are upright, matching, one to each QRS. PR interval is 0.28. QRS interval is 0.08. Interpretation: sinus rhythm with a first-degree AV block.

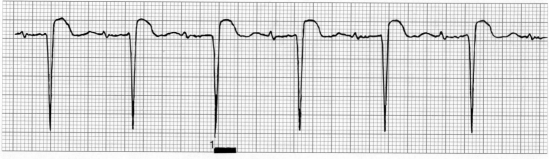

FIGURE 11–3

First-degree AV block.

Mobitz I Second-Degree AV Block (Wenckebach)

Usually a transient block, *Wenckebach* usually lasts only a few days. It occurs when the AV node becomes progressively weaker and less able to conduct the sinus impulses until finally it is unable to send the impulse down to the ventricle at all. As a result, the PR intervals grow progressively longer until there is a P wave that has no QRS behind it.

Rate	Atrial rate usually 60 to 100; ventricular rate less than the atrial rate due to nonconducted beats.
Regularity	Usually irregular, but can look regular but interrupted at times. A hallmark of Wenckebach is groups of beats, then a pause.
P waves	Normal sinus P waves. All Ps except the blocked P are followed by a QRS. P-P interval is regular. There may be P waves that are hidden in the QRS complex or the T wave. Find two consecutive P waves and then march out where the rest of the P waves are, keeping in mind they will all have the same P-P interval, so they'll all be the same distance apart.
Intervals	PR gradually prolongs until a QRS is dropped. QRS <0.12 secs
Cause	Myocardial infarction (MI), digitalis toxicity, medication side effects
Adverse effects	Usually no ill effects. Watch for worsening block.
Treatment	Prepare for transcutaneous pacing if signs of decreased cardiac output exist. Administer atropine if a pacemaker is not immediately available and the patient is symptomatic. Most patients with Wenckebach require nothing more than cautious observation.

Figure 11–4 shows QRS complexes, all shaped the same. Regularity is irregular. Heart rate is 50 to 83, with a mean rate of 70. P waves are matching, upright, some not followed by a QRS. Some Ps are at the end of the T waves. P-P interval is regular. Atrial rate is 83. PR interval varies from 0.04 to 0.28. Note the relatively short PR of the first beat on the strip. Compare this to the third beat. The PR interval prolongs from beat to beat until the fourth P wave does not conduct through to the ventricle at all. We know it doesn't get through to the ventricle because that P wave is not followed by a QRS complex. The cycle then repeats, with prolonging PR intervals, until the eighth P wave is not conducted. QRS interval is 0.10. Interpretation: Mobitz I second-degree AV block (Wenckebach).

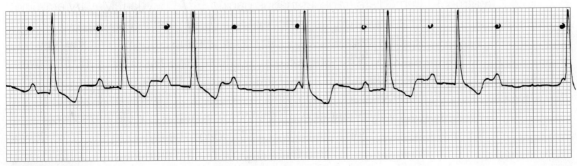

FIGURE 11–4

Wenckebach.

We're about halfway through this chapter. To evaluate your understanding of the material thus far, answer the following questions. If you have trouble with them, review the material again before continuing.

Mrs. Uhura had a heart attack yesterday. Today the nurse notices her rhythm has changed. Her PR intervals are prolonging and then a QRS is dropped. This is happening in cycles. Her blood pressure is fine and she has no symptoms.

1. What is this new rhythm?
2. Is this an emergency?
3. What treatment, if any, is required?

Mobitz II Second-Degree AV Block

Mobitz II is a block caused by an intermittent block at the AV node or the bundle branches, preventing some sinus impulses from getting to the ventricles. *With AV node block, the resultant QRS complexes will be narrow. With block at the bundle branches, the QRS will be wide.* Usually, *Mobitz II* patients already have a bundle branch block, meaning that one of their bundle branches does not let impulses through. They are therefore dependent on the other bundle branch to conduct the impulses through to the ventricles. If that other bundle branch becomes suddenly blocked, then none of the sinus impulses can get through. Sinus P waves therefore conduct through to the ventricles when the one bundle branch is open, but they don't get through at all when both bundle branches are blocked. When the impulses do get through, they do so with an unchanging PR interval every time. Bottom line: *Mobitz II second-degree AV block looks like a sinus rhythm with all P waves in place, but with some QRS-Ts removed.*

Rate	Atrial rate usually 60 to 100; ventricular rate less than atrial rate due to dropped beats.
Regularity	May be regular, irregular, or regular but interrupted.
P waves	Normal sinus P waves. All Ps except the blocked Ps have a QRS behind them. P-P interval is regular. Some P waves may be hidden inside QRS complexes or T waves.
Intervals	PR constant on the conducted beats. QRS <0.12 secs if the block is at the AV node; ≥0.12 secs if the block is at the bundle branches.
Cause	MI, conduction system lesion, medication side effect, hypoxia.
Adverse effects	Since the heart rate can be very slow, the patient may have signs of decreased cardiac output. Mobitz II can progress to third-degree block if untreated.
Treatment	Immediate transcutaneous pacing. Start oxygen. May try atropine or an epinephrine or dopamine infusion first if a pacemaker is not readily available. Depending on where the block is, atropine may not work. Atropine speeds up the rate of sinus node firing and improves AV node conduction. If the block is at the AV node, atropine will improve conduction, and the impulse will travel on down the pathway unimpeded. If the block is at the bundle branches, however, the impulse will blast through the AV node and head down the pathway only to find that both bundle branches are still blocked. Atropine has no effect on the bundle branches. So bottom line: *With Mobitz II and narrow QRS (<0.12 secs), atropine should work. With wide QRS (≥0.12 secs), epinephrine may be a better choice.*

look 2:1 ?

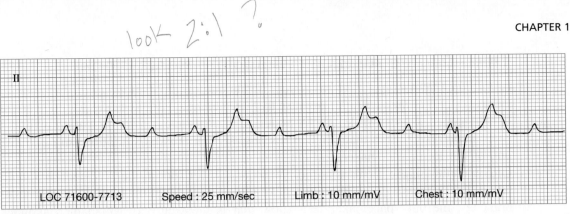

LOC 71600-7713   Speed : 25 mm/sec   Limb : 10 mm/mV   Chest : 10 mm/mV

FIGURE 11–5

Mobitz II second-degree AV block.

Figure 11–5 shows QRS complexes, all the same shape. Regularity is regular. Heart rate is 44. P waves are upright, matching, some not followed by a QRS. P-P interval is regular. Atrial rate is 137. PR interval is constant at 0.12. QRS interval is 0.12. Interpretation: Mobitz II second-degree AV block and a wide QRS, indicating a likely bundle branch block.

2:1 AV Block

2:1 AV block is a type of second-degree block in which there are two P waves to each QRS complex. The first P wave in each pair of P waves is blocked. 2:1 AV block can be caused by either Wenckebach or Mobitz II.

Rate	Atrial rate 60 to 100; ventricular rate half the atrial rate
Regularity	Regular
P waves	Normal sinus P waves; two Ps to each QRS; P-P interval regular
Intervals	PR constant on the conducted beats
	QRS <0.12 secs if the block is at the AV node; ≥0.12 secs if the block is at the bundle branches
Cause	Same as Wenckebach or Mobitz II
Adverse effects	Decreased cardiac output if the heart rate is too slow.
Treatment	Transcutaneous pacing if the patient has symptoms of decreased cardiac output. May try atropine or an epinephrine or dopamine infusion first if a pacemaker is not readily available. Start oxygen.

Figure 11–6 shows QRS complexes, all the same shape. Regularity is regular. Heart rate is 37. Atrial rate is 75. P waves are upright and matching, two to each QRS. P-P interval is regular. PR interval is 0.16. QRS interval is 0.08. Interpretation: 2:1 AV block.

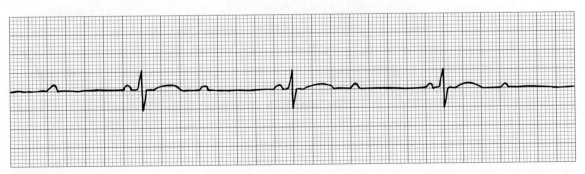

FIGURE 11–6

2:1 AV block.

Third-Degree AV Block (Complete Heart Block)

In *third-degree AV block,* the sinus node sends out its impulses as usual, *but none of them ever gets to the ventricles* because there is a complete block at the AV node or the bundle branches. Meanwhile, the AV node and the ventricle are waiting patiently for the sinus impulses to reach them. When it's obvious that the sinus impulse isn't coming, one of the lower pacemakers escapes and assumes pacemaking control to provide a QRS complex. If the block is at the AV node, a lower spot in the AV junction should take over as pacemaker and provide a heart rate of 40 to 60. If the block is at the bundle branches, the only pacemaker left below that is the ventricle, which then assumes control with a heart rate of 20 to 40. Even though the lower pacemaker has assumed control of providing the QRS complex, the sinus node is unaware of that, so it continues firing out its impulses as usual, providing P waves.

Rate	Atrial rate usually 60 to 100; ventricular rate usually 20 to 60.
Regularity	Regular
P waves	Normal sinus P waves; P-P interval is regular; P waves may be hidden inside QRS complexes or T waves. P waves are not associated with any of the QRS complexes, even though there may at times appear to be a relationship. This is called **AV dissociation**, and it is a hallmark of third-degree block. AV dissociation means that the sinus node is firing at its normal rate, and the lower pacemaker is firing at its slower rate, and the two have nothing to do with each other. AV dissociation results in independent beating of the atria and the ventricles.
	Imagine the lower pacemaker that controls the ventricles as an old man jogging around a circular racetrack at 2 miles per hour. The sinus node is an 18-year-old boy sprinting at 4 miles per hour. Since the boy is going faster than the old man, he will periodically catch up with him and then pass him. An onlooker might see the boy at the split second he's side by side with the old man and assume they are together and that there is a relationship between the two. There isn't, of course. Their being side by side was just coincidence, just as it's coincidence that a sinus P wave might land right in front of a QRS in third-degree AV block and make it seem as though there is a relationship there.
Intervals	PR varies. QRS narrow (<0.12 secs) or wide (>0.12 secs) depending on the location of the block. If the block is at the AV node, the AV junction should become the pacemaker and the QRS will be narrow. If the block is at the bundle branches, the ventricle will become the pacemaker, with a wide QRS.
Cause	MI, conduction system lesion, medication side effects, hypoxia.
Adverse effects	Signs of low cardiac output may occur if the heart rate is slow enough.
Treatment	Transcutaneous pacing is indicated if the patient is symptomatic. Atropine, epinephrine, or dopamine can be given until a more permanent transvenous pacemaker can be inserted if needed. Start oxygen.

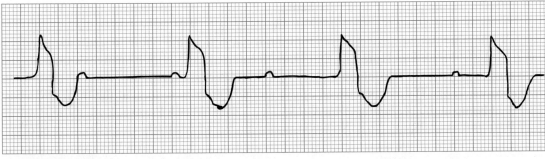

FIGURE 11–7

Third-degree AV block.

Figure 11–7 shows QRS complexes, all shaped the same. Regularity is regular. Heart rate is 37. P waves are upright and matching. Atrial rate is 60. P-P interval is regular. One P wave is hidden in the ST segment of the third QRS complex. PR interval varies. QRS interval is 0.20. Interpretation: third-degree AV block with a ventricular escape rhythm. Since the QRS is wide, we know the ventricle is the pacemaker. If the AV junction had been the pacemaker, the QRS would have been narrow and the heart rate a bit faster.

Before we get started on our practice strips, let's look at an algorithm (flow chart) to help identify second- and third-degree AV blocks. (First-degree AV blocks are easier to identify because there are no dropped beats). See Figure 11–8. It includes the algorithm and a practice example.

> **Quick Tip**
>
> Here's a quick way to differentiate the AV blocks:
>
> First-degree AV block—no dropped QRS, PR interval >0.20 secs.
>
> Wenckebach—gradually prolonging PR intervals until a QRS is dropped.
>
> Mobitz II second-degree AV block—PR intervals constant, some QRS complexes dropped.
>
> 2:1 AV block—2 P waves to every QRS.
>
> Third-degree AV block—PR intervals vary, some QRS complexes dropped, R-R interval constant.

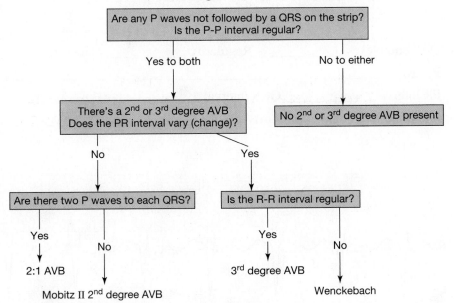

2nd and 3rd Degree AV Block Algorithm

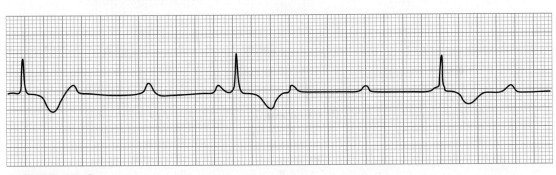

FIGURE 11–8

Second- and third-degree AV block algorithm.

On the practice example, are there any P waves not followed by a QRS? Yes, lots of them. Is the P-P interval regular? Yes, the Ps are all about the same distance apart from one another. We've answered yes to both, so we follow the arrow. There's a second- or third-degree AV block present. Does the PR interval vary (does it change throughout the strip)? For this we look at the P wave right in front of the QRS. Yes, it varies quite a bit. See where the P wave is in front of the second QRS? Now look at the third QRS. See that hump at the beginning of the QRS? That's the start of a P wave. Both those P waves have different PR intervals. So we've again answered yes to the question, so we follow the yes arrow (if we'd answered no we would follow the no arrow). Is the R-R interval regular? Yes, the QRS complexes are evenly spaced. We follow the yes arrow and it takes us to the answer—third-degree AV block.

Now practice some strips on your own. Use the algorithm if you wish, but be sure to do it without as well, to be sure you know the criteria.

Practice Strips: AV Blocks

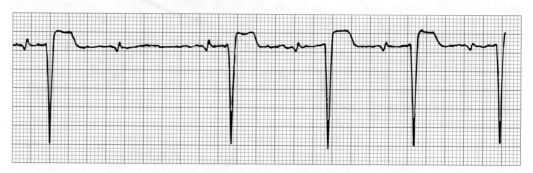

1. QRS complexes _____ Regularity _Reg w/ interrupt_ Heart rate _60 w/interrupt_

   P waves _____

   PR interval _0.28_____ QRS interval _____

   Interpretation (name of rhythm) _Mobitz I 2nd° Wenckebach_

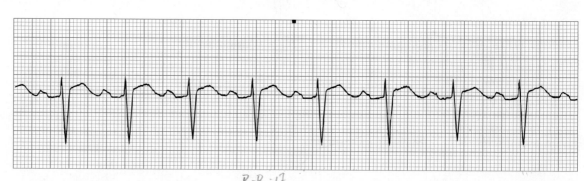

P R int 0.12-0.2

QRS < 0.12

R-R: 17

2. QRS complexes _____ Regularity _Regular_____ Heart rate _84___

   P waves _regular upright_____

   .12-.2   PR interval _0.28____ QRS interval _0.12_____

   Interpretation _____Sinus Rhythm w/ 1st degree block_____

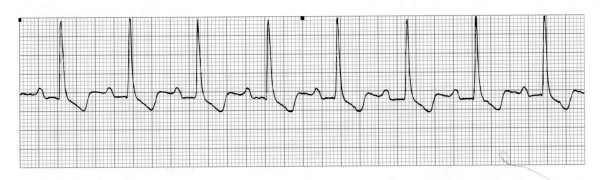

3. QRS complexes _yes_ Regularity _Reg_ Heart rate _84 bpm_

P waves _____

PR interval _0.24_ QRS interval _0.12_

Interpretation _Sinus Rhythm w/ 1st deg. AV Block_

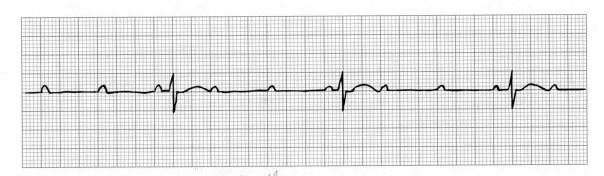

4. QRS complexes _Present, all shaped same_ Regularity _____ Heart rate _____

P waves _upright, matching, 3 p's to every QRS_

PR interval _0.20_ QRS interval _0.08_

Interpretation _Mobitz I 2nd Degree AV Block (Wenckebach)_

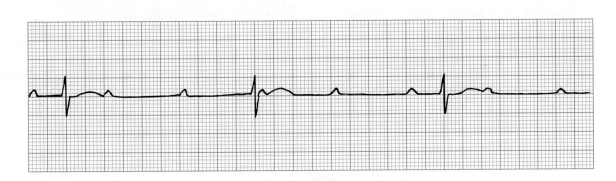

5. QRS complexes _____ Regularity _____ Heart rate _____

P waves _____

PR interval _____ QRS interval _____

Interpretation _3rd Degree AV Block w/ a Junctional Escape Rhythm_

b/c QRS is < 0.12

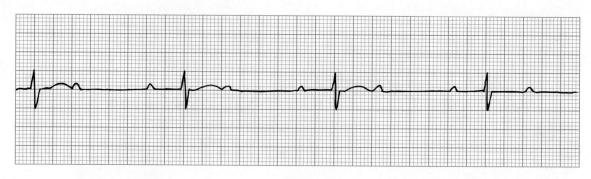

6. QRS complexes _____ Regularity __Regular__ Heart rate __38bpm__

   P waves __Regular, upright, 2:1 QRS__

   PR interval _____ QRS interval __0.08__

   Interpretation __2:1 AV Block__

give range for irregular HR

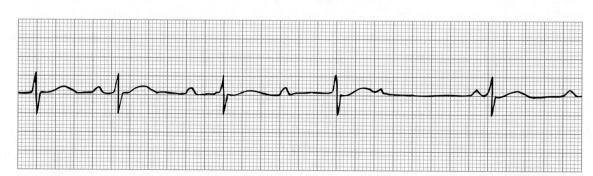

7. QRS complexes __present__ Regularity __irregular__ Heart rate __37-68__

   P waves __upright, regular, increasing PRi__

   PR interval __increases__ QRS interval __0.08__

   Interpretation __Mobitz I 2nd deg. Block Wenckebach__

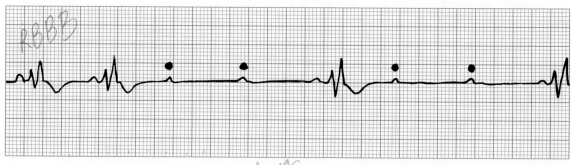

RBBB

8. QRS complexes __present, some missing__ Regularity __irregular__ Heart rate __25-75__

   P waves __upright, regular, not all followed by QRS__

   PR interval _____ QRS interval _____

   Interpretation __Mobitz II 2nd Deg Bloc__

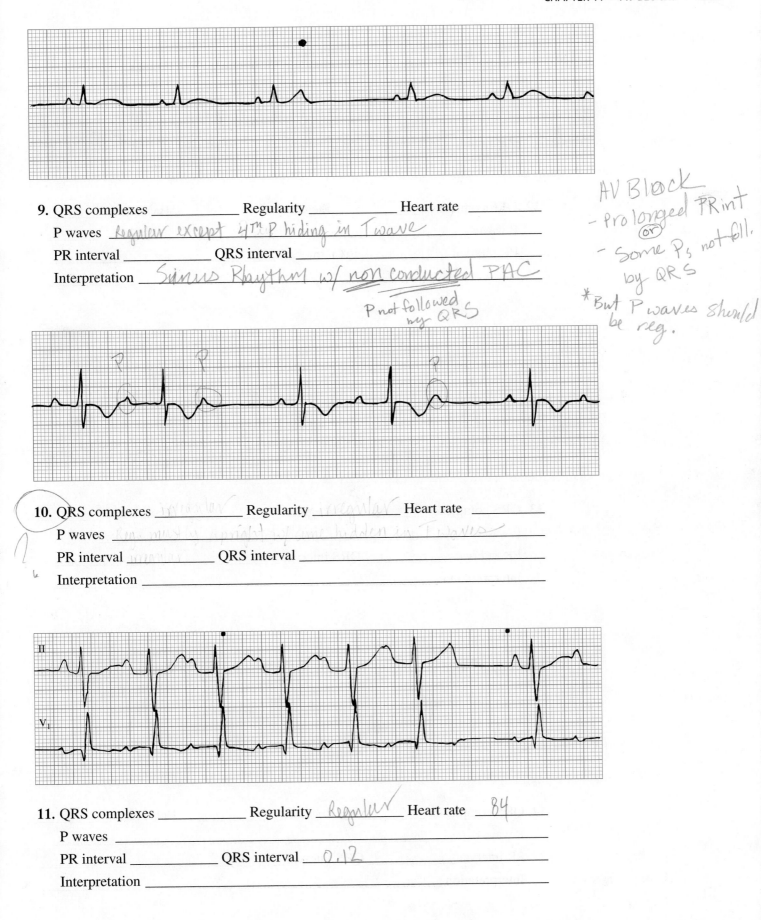

9. QRS complexes _____ Regularity _____ Heart rate _____

P waves _Regular except 4th P hiding in T wave_

PR interval _____ QRS interval _____

Interpretation _Sinus Rhythm w/ non conducted PAC_

P not followed by QRS

AV Block
- Prolonged PR int
(or)
- Some Ps not foll. by QRS
* But P waves should be reg.

10. QRS complexes _irregular_ Regularity _irregular_ Heart rate _____

P waves _Reg mostly upright of some hidden in T waves_

PR interval _irregular_ QRS interval _____

Interpretation _____

11. QRS complexes _____ Regularity _Regular_ Heart rate _84_

P waves _____

PR interval _____ QRS interval _0.12_

Interpretation _____

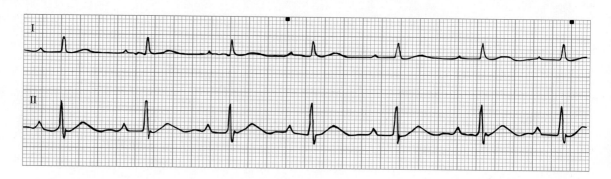

12. QRS complexes _____ Regularity _____ Heart rate _____

P waves _____

PR interval _____ QRS interval _____

Interpretation _____

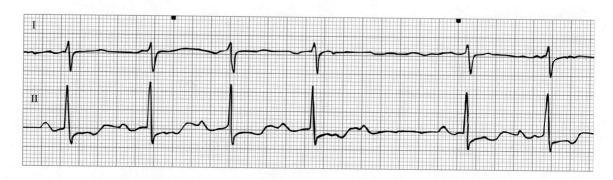

13. QRS complexes _____ Regularity _____ Heart rate _____

P waves _____

PR interval _____ QRS interval _____

Interpretation _____

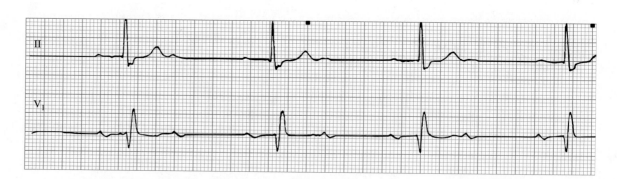

14. QRS complexes _____ Regularity _____ Heart rate _____

P waves _____

PR interval _____ QRS interval _____

Interpretation _____

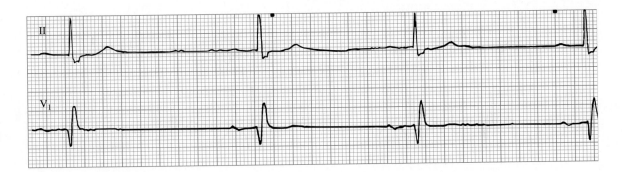

15. QRS complexes _____ Regularity _____ Heart rate _____

P waves _____

PR interval _____ QRS interval _____

Interpretation _____

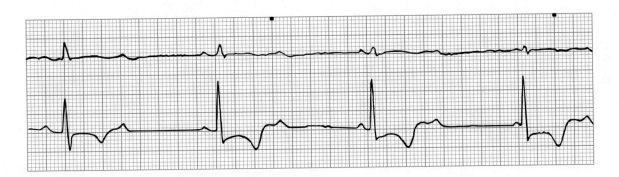

16. QRS complexes _____ Regularity _____ Heart rate _____

P waves _____

PR interval _____ QRS interval _____

Interpretation _____

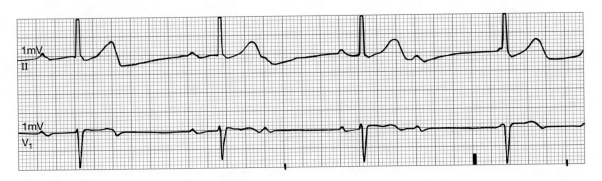

17. QRS complexes _____ Regularity _____ Heart rate _____

P waves _____

PR interval _____ QRS interval _____

Interpretation _____

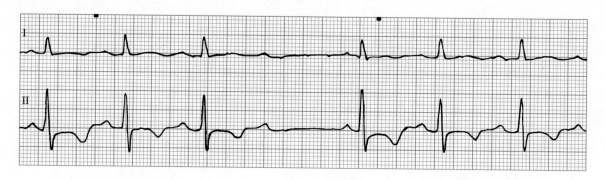

18. QRS complexes _____ Regularity _____ Heart rate _____

P waves _____

PR interval _____ QRS interval _____

Interpretation _____

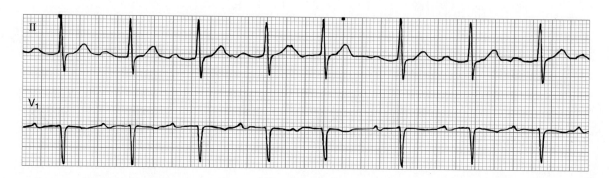

19. QRS complexes _____ Regularity _____ Heart rate _____

P waves _____

PR interval _____ QRS interval _____

Interpretation _____

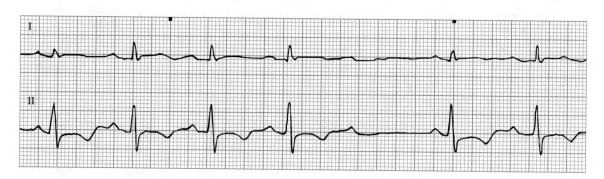

20. QRS complexes _____ Regularity _____ Heart rate _____

P waves _____

PR interval _____ QRS interval _____

Interpretation _____

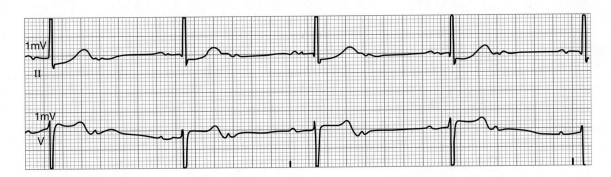

21. QRS complexes _____ Regularity _____ Heart rate _____

    P waves _____

    PR interval _____ QRS interval _____

    Interpretation _____

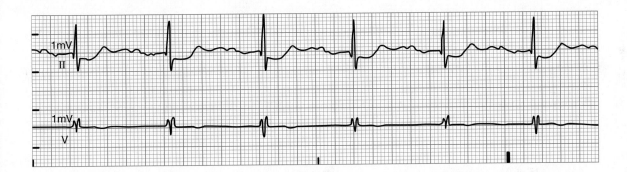

22. QRS complexes _____ Regularity _____ Heart rate _____

    P waves _____

    PR interval _____ QRS interval _____

    Interpretation _____

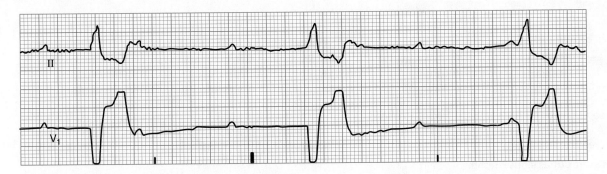

23. QRS complexes _____ Regularity _____ Heart rate _____

    P waves _____

    PR interval _____ QRS interval _____

    Interpretation _____

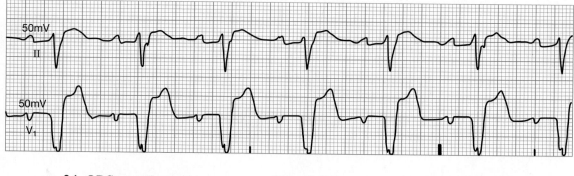

24. QRS complexes _____ Regularity _____ Heart rate _____

P waves _____

PR interval _____ QRS interval _____

Interpretation _____

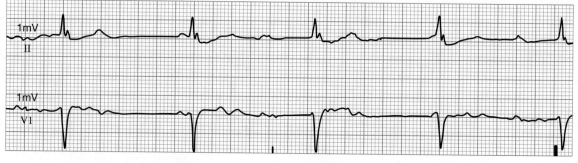

25. QRS complexes _____ Regularity _____ Heart rate _____

P waves _____

PR interval _____ QRS interval _____

Interpretation _____

chapter eleven notes TO SUM IT ALL UP . . .

- **Three degrees of AV blocks:**
  - *First degree*—Delay in impulse transmission between atria and ventricles. All impulses do make it through.
  - *Second degree*—Some impulses get through to ventricles; some don't.
  - *Third degree*—No impulses make it through from atria to ventricles. A lower pacemaker has to escape to provide stimulus to ventricles.

- **All AV blocks start out as sinus rhythms.** Therefore all P waves are sinus Ps.

- **The block can occur in the AV node or the bundle branches.**

- **First-degree AV block:**
  - *Heart rate*—Can occur at any rate
  - *Regularity*—Depends on underlying rhythm
  - *P waves*—Sinus Ps; one P per QRS
  - *Intervals*—PR >0.20 secs; QRS <0.12 secs
  - *Causes*—AV node ischemia, digitalis toxicity, other medication side effects
  - *Adverse effects*—None
  - *Treatment*—Treat the cause

- **Mobitz I second-degree AV block (Wenckebach):**
  - *Heart rate*—Atrial rate 60–100; ventricular rate slower than atrial due to dropped beats

- *Regularity*—Irregular or regular but interrupted in appearance
- *P waves*—Sinus P waves; some not followed by a QRS
- *Intervals*—PR varies, gradually prolonging until a QRS is dropped; QRS <0.12 secs
- *Causes*—MI, digitalis toxicity, medication side effects
- *Adverse effects*—Usually none since heart rate is usually good
- *Treatment*—Usually none needed; watch for worsening block; oxygen, atropine, pacemaker if symptomatic from low heart rate

■ **Mobitz II second-degree AV block:**
- *Heart rate*—Atrial rate 60–100; ventricular rate slower due to dropped beats
- *Regularity*—Regular, irregular, or regular but interrupted in appearance
- *P waves*—Sinus Ps; some Ps not followed by a QRS
- *Intervals*—PR 0.12–0.20 secs constant on the conducted beats. QRS <0.12 secs if the block is at the AV node; >0.12 secs if the block is at the bundle branches
- *Causes*—MI, conduction system lesion, medications, hypoxia
- *Adverse effects*—Decreased cardiac output
- *Treatment*—Oxygen, pacemaker; atropine, epinephrine or dopamine infusions can be used while awaiting pacemaker arrival.

■ **2:1 AV block:**
- *Heart rate*—Atrial rate 60–100; ventricular rate half of atrial rate
- *Regularity*—Regular
- *P waves*—Sinus Ps; every other P not followed by a QRS
- *Intervals*—PR 0.12–0.20 secs constant on conducted beats. QRS <0.12 secs if the block is at the AV node; ≥0.12 secs if the block is at the bundle branches.
- *Causes*—Same as Wenckebach or Mobitz II
- *Adverse effects*—Decreased cardiac output if heart rate too slow
- *Treatment*—Oxygen, pacemaker, atropine, epinephrine or dopamine infusion

■ **Third-degree AV block:**
- *Heart rate*—Atrial rate 60–100; ventricular rate much slower due to dropped beats
- *Regularity*—Regular
- *P waves*—Sinus Ps; some not followed by a QRS
- *Intervals*—PR varies. QRS <0.12 secs if the block is at the AV node; >0.12 secs if the block is at the bundle branches.
- *Causes*—MI, conduction system lesion, medication side effects, hypoxia
- *Adverse effects*—Decreased cardiac output
- *Treatment*—Pacemaker, oxygen. May use atropine, epinephrine or dopamine infusion while awaiting pacemaker arrival.

Practice Quiz

1. Name the two typical locations of the block in AV blocks. _____
_____

2. True or false: People with a first-degree AV block need a pacemaker inserted.

3. Wenckebach is another name for which kind of block? _____
_____

4. AV dissociation is a hallmark of which kind of AV block? _____
_____
_____

5. True or false: Atropine is effective in all types of AV blocks, whether the block is at the AV node or the bundle branches.

6. The AV block that merely results in a prolonged PR interval is _____
_____

7. What is atropine's mode of action? _____
_____

8. The most dangerous type of AV block is _____

9. The least dangerous type of AV block is _____

10. True or false: All AV blocks require atropine or epinephrine to increase the heart rate.

Putting It All Together—Critical Thinking Exercises

These exercises may consist of diagrams to label, scenarios to analyze, brain-stumping questions to ponder, or other challenging exercises to boost your understanding of the chapter material.

Let's play with AV blocks a bit. The following scenario will provide you with information about a fictional patient and will ask you to analyze the situation, answer questions, and decide on appropriate actions.

Ms. Watson, age 89, presents to her physician's office complaining of feeling weak and tired for the past 3 days. She has a history of atrial fibrillation and has been taking digoxin for years. She also takes insulin for diabetes and beta-blockers for high blood pressure. Vital signs are stable and within normal limits. Suspecting that Ms. Watson's atrial fib has again gotten out of control, the nurse records the rhythm strip below. See Figure 11–9.

1. What is the rhythm and heart rate? _____

_____

2. Does this rhythm require emergency treatment?

_____

Suddenly, Ms. Watson says "I feel funny," and the nurse helps her lie back on the examining table. Vital signs are still within normal limits, but her BP has dropped some. Her repeat rhythm strip is seen in Figure 11–10.

3. What has happened? _____

4. Which of Ms. Watson's medications could be responsible for this rhythm? _____

_____

The physician admits Ms. Watson to the telemetry floor and orders a digoxin level, which comes back elevated. Further questioning of Ms. Watson reveals that she'd doubled up on her digoxin the past three days because she thought it would help her feel better.

5. Given this latest information, what treatment is appropriate for this rhythm? _____

_____

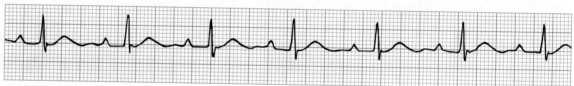

FIGURE 11–9

Ms. Watson's initial strip.

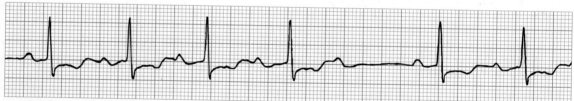

FIGURE 11–10

Ms. Watson's "funny" strip.

Rhythm Practice Strips

CHAPTER 12 OBJECTIVES

Upon completion of this chapter, the student will be able to:

- Correctly identify the rhythms.
- Identify any weak areas for further study.

What It's All About

"So what's up with Mr. Cohen's rhythm there? He looks like he's in third-degree AV block," asked Chianti of her colleague Josiah on the cardiovascular floor. "Yeah, I know; I was just looking at that. I think it's third-degree block also. I've got a call in to Dr. Howell—I'm just waiting for her to call me back. Mr. Cohen's heart rate is 42 and he's a bit pale and complaining of very mild dizziness, but his blood pressure is holding within his normal limits so far. I've already got the transcutaneous pacemaker out on standby just in case we need it," answered Josiah. "I'll get out the atropine," Chianti offered. Dr. Howell came in, looked at the rhythm strip, and agreed with the nurses that the rhythm was third-degree AV block. She called the cath lab team in to do an emergency transvenous pacemaker and ordered atropine to be given intravenously in the meantime. The next morning, with his new pacemaker working well, Mr. Cohen stated he hadn't felt so good in years. "Dr. Howell thinks maybe I've had heart block off and on for awhile," he told Chianti and Josiah.

Introduction

This chapter focuses on the interpretation of rhythm strips utilizing the five steps you learned in Chapter 6 and the rhythm descriptions in Chapters 7 through 11. Additionally, two other analysis tools are included here to help you analyze rhythms: *Rhythm summary sheets* present a summary of all the rhythm criteria along with a pictorial review, so you can turn to this section for a quick comparison of criteria. And the *rhythm regularity summary* points out the type of regularity of each rhythm. For example, if you know the rhythm is irregular but aren't sure what rhythm it is, you can turn to this summary to determine which rhythms are irregular and which are not.

Rhythm Summary Sheets

Rhythm Summary: Sinus Rhythms

	Rate	Regularity	P Wave	PR Interval	QRS Interval	Cause	Adverse Effects	Treatment
Sinus rhythm	60–100	Regular	Upright in Lead II; one per QRS; uniform shape	0.12–0.20; constant	<0.12	Normal	None	None
Sinus bradycardia	<60	Regular	Upright in Lead II; one per QRS; uniform shape	0.12–0.20; constant	<0.12	MI, vagal stimulation, hypoxia	None necessarily; maybe decreased cardiac output	Atropine if symptoms; consider O_2
Sinus tachycardia	101–160	Regular	Upright in Lead II; one per QRS; uniform shape	0.12–0.20; constant	<0.12	SNS stimulation, MI, hypoxia, pulmonary embolus, CHF, thyroid storm, fever, vagal inhibition	Maybe none; maybe decreased cardiac output	Treat the cause; consider O_2 and beta blockers
Sinus arrhythmia	Varies-↑ with inspiration, ↓ with expiration	Irregular; R-R varies by ≥0.16 secs	Upright in Lead II; one per QRS; uniform shape	0.12–0.20; constant	<0.12	The breathing pattern	Usually none	Atropine if HR slow and symptoms
Sinus arrest	Can occur at any rate	Regular but interrupted	Normal before the pause; may be different or absent after	Normal before pause; may be different or absent after	<0.12 unless ventricular escape beat present	Sinus node ischemia, hypoxia, digitalis toxicity, excessive vagal tone, medication side effects	Maybe none; maybe decreased cardiac output; lower pacemaker may take over after pause	Consider O_2; atropine or pacemaker if symptoms
Sinus exit block	Can occur at any rate	Regular but interrupted	Normal before and after the pause; all shaped the same	0.12–0.20	<0.12	Medication side effects, excessive vagal tone, hypoxia	Same as sinus arrest; pause is a multiple of R-R; sinus resumes after pause	Consider O_2; atropine or pacemaker if symptoms

Sinus Rhythms Pictorial Review

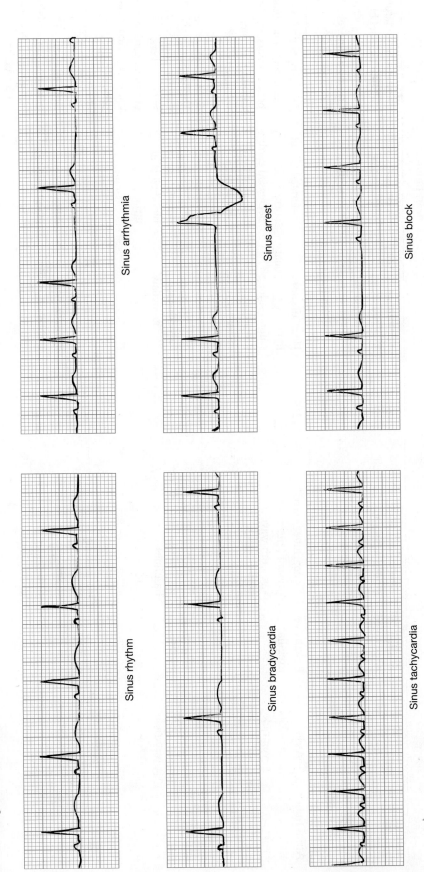

Sinus arrhythmia

Sinus arrest

Sinus block

Sinus rhythm

Sinus bradycardia

Sinus tachycardia

Rhythm Summary: Atrial Rhythms

	Rate	Regularity	P Wave	QRS Interval	Cause	Adverse Effects	Treatment
Wandering atrial pacemaker (WAP)	Mean rate <100	Irregular	At least 3 different shapes; sometimes no P at all on some beats	<0.12	MI, medication side effects, hypoxia, vagal stimulation	Usually no ill effects	Usually none; atropine or pacemaker if HR slow and symptoms
Multifocal atrial tachycardia	Mean rate >100	Irregular	Same as WAP	<0.12	COPD	Decreased cardiac output at higher heart rates	Beta blockers or calcium channel blockers
PACs _premature atrial complexes_	Can occur at any rate	Regular but interrupted	Shaped differently from sinus Ps; often hidden in preceding T wave	<0.12; QRS absent after nonconducted PAC	Stimulants, caffeine, hypoxia, heart disease, or normal	None if occasional; can be a sign of early heart failure	Remove the causes; consider O_2, digitalis, calcium channel blockers
Paroxysmal atrial tachycardia (PAT)	161–250 once in atrial tach	Regular but interrupted	Shaped differently from sinus Ps but same as each other	<0.12	Stimulants, caffeine, hypoxia, heart disease, or normal	Decreased cardiac output; some people tolerate OK for a while	Digitalis, amiodarone, calcium channel blockers, beta blockers, sedation, O_2, adenosine, electrical cardioversion
Atrial flutter	Atria: 251–350; ventricle: varies	Regular or irregular	None; flutter waves present (zigzag or sawtooth waves)	<0.12	Heart disease, hypoxia, pulmonary embolus, lung disease, valve disease, thyroid storm	Tolerated OK at normal rate; decreased cardiac output at faster or slower rates	Digitalis, amiodarone, calcium channel blockers, beta blockers; consider O_2, carotid massage, electrical cardioversion
Atrial fib	Atria: 350–700; ventricle: varies	Irregularly irregular	None; fibrillatory waves present (waviness of the baseline)	<0.12	MI, lung disease, valve disease, thyrotoxicosis	Decreased cardiac output; can cause blood clots in atria	Digitalis, amiodarone, calcium channel blockers, beta blockers; consider O_2; electrical cardioversion; consider anticoagulation to prevent clots
SVT _supraventricular tachycardia_	≥130	Regular	May be present but hard to see	<0.12	Stimulants, caffeine, hypoxia, heart disease, or normal	Decreased cardiac output; some people tolerate OK for a while	Digitalis, amiodarone, calcium channel blockers, beta blockers, sedation, O_2, adenosine, electrical cardioversion

Atrial Rhythms Pictorial Review

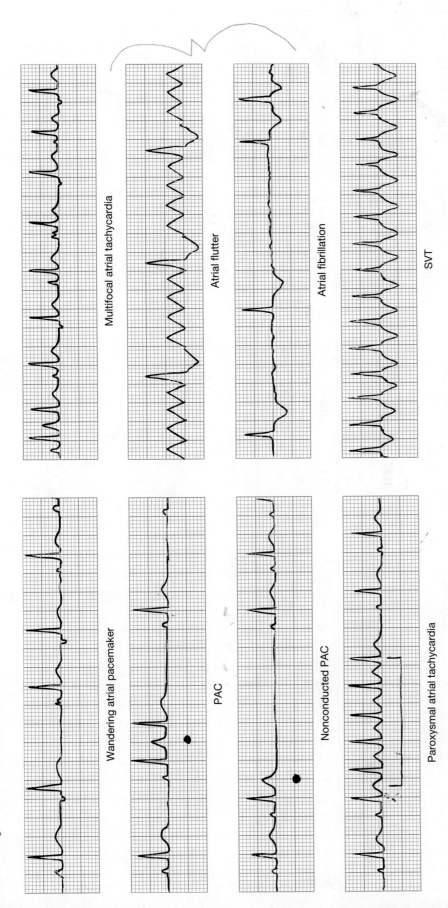

Multifocal atrial tachycardia

Atrial flutter

Atrial fibrillation

SVT

Wandering atrial pacemaker

PAC

Nonconducted PAC

Paroxysmal atrial tachycardia

Rhythm Summary: Junctional Rhythms

	Rate	Regularity	P Wave	QRS	Cause	Adverse Effects	Treatment
PJCs	Can occur at any rate	Regular but interrupted	Inverted before or after QRS or hidden inside QRS	<0.12	Stimulants, caffeine, hypoxia, heart disease, or normal	Usually no ill effects	Usually none required
Junctional bradycardia	<40	Regular	Inverted before or after QRS or hidden inside QRS	<0.12	Vagal stimulation, hypoxia, sinus node ischemia, MI	Decreased cardiac output	Pacemaker or atropine if symptoms; hold medications that can slow the HR; start O_2
Junctional rhythm	40–60	Regular	Inverted before or after QRS or hidden inside QRS	<0.12	Vagal stimulation, hypoxia, sinus node ischemia, MI	Well tolerated if HR closer to 50–60; decreased cardiac output possible	Pacemaker or atropine if symptoms; hold medications that can slow the HR; start O_2
Accelerated junctional	60–100	Regular	Inverted before or after QRS or hidden inside QRS	<0.12	Heart disease, stimulant drugs, caffeine	Usually no ill effects	Usually none needed
Junctional tach	>100	Regular	Inverted before or after QRS or hidden inside QRS	<0.12	Digitalis toxicity, heart disease, stimulants, SNS stimulation	Decreased cardiac output at faster heart rates	Beta-blockers, calcium channel blockers, adenosine; consider O_2 and electrical cardioversion

Junctional Rhythms Pictorial Review

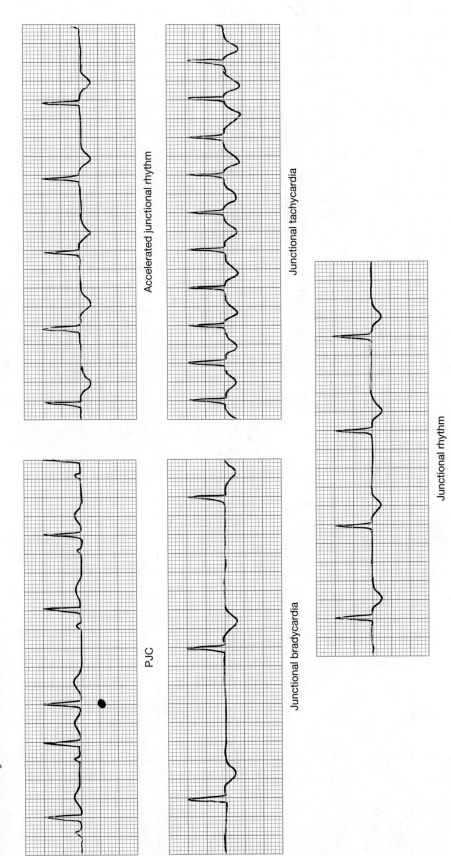

Accelerated junctional rhythm

Junctional tachycardia

PJC

Junctional bradycardia

Junctional rhythm

Rhythm Summary: Ventricular Rhythms

	Rate	Regularity	P Wave	QRS	Cause	Adverse Effects	Treatment
PVCs	Can occur at any rate	Regular but interrupted	Usually none	>0.12; wide and bizarre in shape	Hypoxia, MI, hypokalemia, low magnesium, caffeine, stimulants, stress	Occasional are no problem; can lead to lethal arrhythmias if frequent or after an MI	Amiodarone, O_2, lidocaine; atropine for bradycardic PVCs
Agonal rhythm	<20	Irregular	None	>0.12; wide and bizarre in shape	Profound cardiac or other damage, profound hypoxia	Shock, unconsciousness, death if untreated	CPR, atropine, epinephrine, dopamine, O_2
Idioventricular rhythm	20–40	Regular	None	>0.12; wide and bizarre in shape	Massive cardiac or other damage hypoxia	↓ CO	Atropine, epinephrine, dopamine, O_2, pacemaker
AIVR	40–100	Usually regular—can be irregular at times	Dissociated if even present	>0.12; wide and bizarre in shape	Most often seen during MI	Usually well tolerated	Atropine, epinephrine, dopamine if HR low and symptoms
V-tach	100–250	Usually regular—can be irregular at times	Dissociated if even present	>0.12; wide and bizarre in shape	Hypoxia, MI, hypokalemia, low magnesium, caffeine, stimulants, stress	May be tolerated OK for short bursts; can cause shock, unconsciousness, and death if untreated	Amiodarone, lidocaine, O_2, cardioversion or defib; CPR if no pulse
Torsades de pointes	>200	Regular or irregular	None seen	>0.12; QRS oscillates around an axis	Medications such as quinidine or pro-cainamide; hypoxia, MI, hypokalemia, low magnesium, caffeine, stimulants, stress	Circulatory collapse if sustained; tolerated OK for short bursts	IV magnesium, overdrive pacing, cardioversion or defib, O_2
V-fib	Cannot be counted	None detectable	None	None; just a wavy baseline that looks like static	Hypoxia, MI, hypokalemia, low magnesium, caffeine, stimulants, stress	Cardiovascular collapse; no pulse, breathing, zero cardiac output	Defibrillation, lidocaine, amiodarone, epinephrine, O_2, CPR
Asystole	Zero	None	None	None	Profound cardiac or other damage, hypoxia	Death if untreated	Atropine, epinephrine, CPR, O_2
P wave asystole	Zero	Ps regular	Sinus Ps	None	Profound cardiac or other damage, hypoxia	Death if untreated	Same as asystole

174

Ventricular Rhythms Pictorial Review

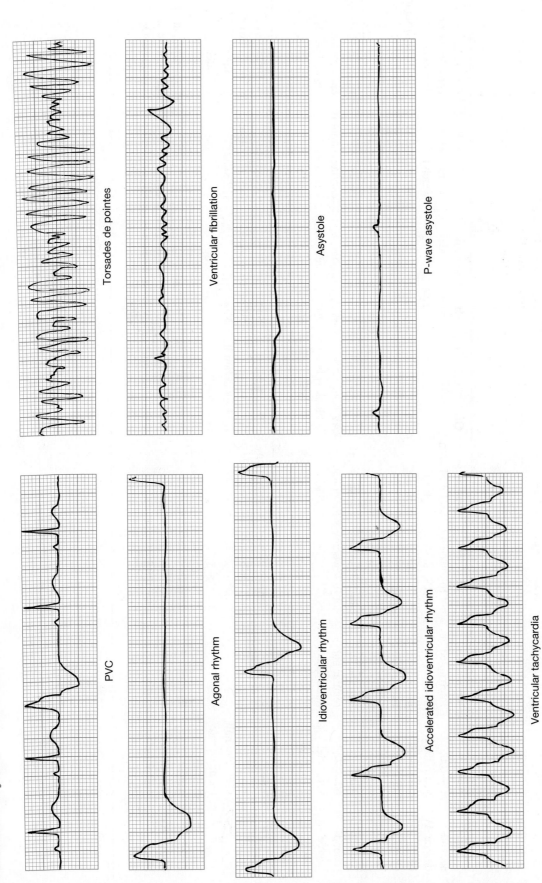

Torsades de pointes

Ventricular fibrillation

Asystole

P-wave asystole

PVC

Agonal rhythm

Idioventricular rhythm

Accelerated idioventricular rhythm

Ventricular tachycardia

Rhythm Summary: AV Blocks

	Rate	Regularity	P Wave	PR Interval	QRS Interval	Cause	Adverse Effects	Treatment
First-degree AV block	Can occur at any rate	Depends on underlying rhythm	Normal; one per QRS; all shaped the same	>0.20; constant	<0.12	AV node ischemia, prolonged bundle branch depolarization time, digitalis toxicity, other medication side effects	Usually no ill effects	Remove the cause
Mobitz I second-degree AV block (Wencke-bach)	Atria: 60–100; ventricle: less than atrial rate	Regular but interrupted or irregular; groups of beats, then a pause	Normal; one not followed by a QRS; all shaped the same	Gradually prolongs until a QRS is dropped	QRS <0.12	MI, digitalis toxicity, medication side effects	Usually well tolerated, but watch for worsening AV block	Pacemaker, atropine, epinephrine or dopamine if symptoms from low HR
Mobitz II second-degree AV block	Atria: 60–100; ventricle: less than atrial rate	Regular, regular but interrupted, or irregular	Normal; some not followed by a QRS	Constant on the conducted beats	<0.12 if block at AV node; ≥0.12 if block at bundle branches	MI, conduction system lesion, hypoxia, medication side effects	Decreased cardiac output if HR slow	Pacemaker, atropine, epinephrine or dopamine, O$_2$
2:1 AVB	Atria: 60–100; ventricle: half the atrial rate	Regular	Normal; 2 Ps to each QRS	Constant on the conducted beats	<0.12 if block at AV node; ≥0.12 if block at bundle branches	Same as Wenckebach and Mobitz II	Decreased cardiac output if HR slow	Pacemaker, atropine, epinephrine or dopamine, consider O$_2$
Third-degree AV block	Atria: 60–100; ventricle: 20–60	Regular	Normal; dissociated from QRS	Varies	<0.12 if AV node is the pacemaker; >0.12 if ventricle is the pacemaker	MI, conduction system lesion, hypoxia, medication side effect	Decreased cardiac output if HR slow	Pacemaker, atropine, epinephrine or dopamine, O$_2$

< 0.12s

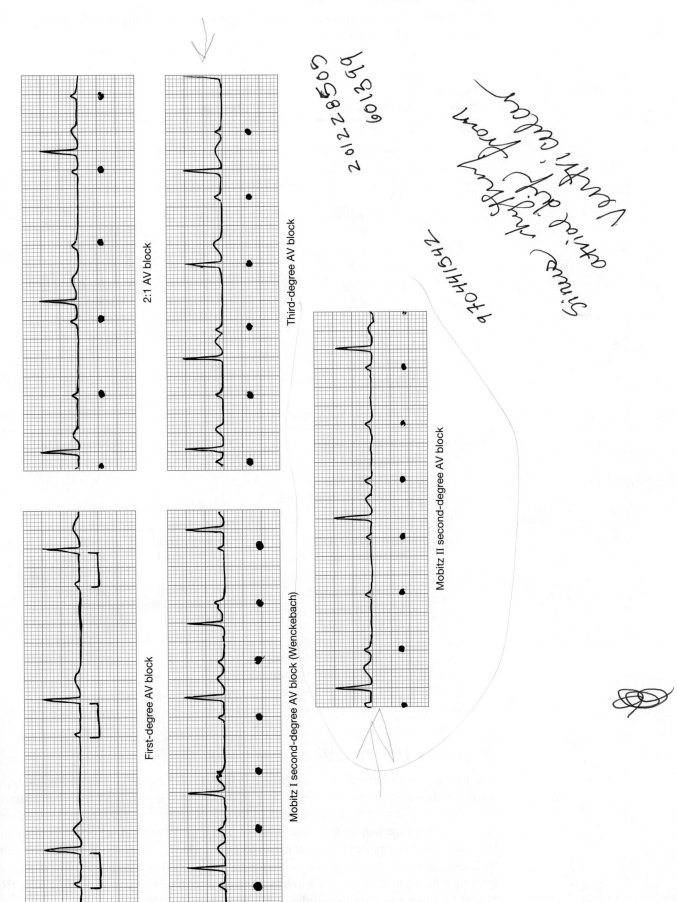

First-degree AV block

2:1 AV block

Mobitz I second-degree AV block (Wenckebach)

Third-degree AV block

Mobitz II second-degree AV block

Rhythm Regularity Summary

The following table points out the type of regularity of each rhythm. *Only rhythms with QRS complexes are shown here.*

Origin of Rhythm	Regular	Regular But Interrupted	Irregular
Sinus	• Sinus rhythm • Sinus bradycardia • Sinus tachycardia	• Sinus arrest • Sinus exit block	• Sinus arrhythmia
Atrial	• SVT • Atrial tachycardia (nonparoxysmal) • Atrial flutter (if the conduction ratio is constant)	• PACs • Paroxysmal atrial tachycardia	• Wandering atrial pacemaker • Multifocal atrial tachycardia • Atrial fibrillation • Atrial flutter (if the conduction ratio varies)
Junctional	• Junctional bradycardia • Junctional rhythm • Accelerated junctional rhythm • Junctional tachycardia	• PJCs	• None
Ventricular	• Idioventricular rhythm • Accelerated idioventricular rhythm • Ventricular tachycardia • Paced rhythm	• PVCs • Paced beats	• Agonal rhythm • Torsades de pointes
AV blocks	• First-degree AV block (if the underlying rhythm is regular) • 2:1 AV block • Mobitz II second-degree AV block (if the conduction ratio is constant and it does not interrupt another rhythm) • Third-degree AV block	• Mobitz II second-degree AV block (if it interrupts another rhythm) • Wenckebach	• First-degree AV block (if the underlying rhythm is irregular) • Wenckebach • Mobitz II second-degree AV block (if the conduction ratio varies)

Rhythms for Practice

OK, let's get down to work. Some rhythms in this chapter are on single-lead strips; others are on double-lead strips. Remember that on double-lead strips, both leads represent the same rhythm, just seen in different leads. Thus the heart rate, interval measurements, and other interpretation will be the same whether you assess the top lead or the bottom lead. Use either lead you prefer to do your interpretation. On the intervals, allow plus or minus 0.02 secs for your answer. (If the answer for a PR interval is listed as 0.16, for example, anywhere between 0.14 to 0.18 would still be correct. Intervals can vary just a little from beat to beat in a normally functioning nervous system).

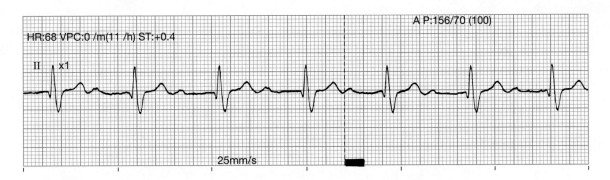

1. QRS complexes_____ Regularity_____ Heart rate_____

   P waves_____

   PR interval_____ QRS interval_____

   Interpretation_____

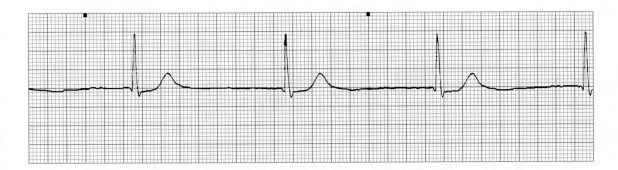

2. QRS complexes_____ Regularity_____ Heart rate_____

   P waves_____

   PR interval_____ QRS interval_____

   Interpretation_____

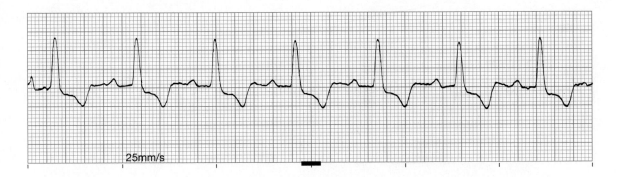

3. QRS complexes_____ Regularity_____ Heart rate_____

   P waves_____

   PR interval_____ QRS interval_____

   Interpretation_____

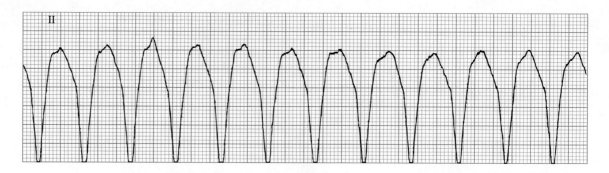

4. QRS complexes_____ Regularity_____ Heart rate_____

P waves_____

PR interval_____ QRS interval_____

Interpretation_____

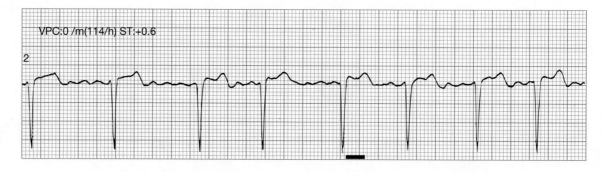

5. QRS complexes_____ Regularity_____ Heart rate_____

P waves_____

PR interval_____ QRS interval_____

Interpretation_____

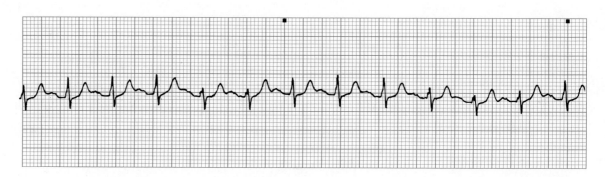

6. QRS complexes_____ Regularity_____ Heart rate_____

P waves_____

PR interval_____ QRS interval_____

Interpretation_____

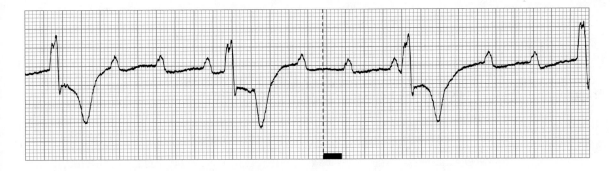

7. QRS complexes_____ Regularity_____ Heart rate_____

   P waves_____

   PR interval_____ QRS interval_____

   Interpretation_____

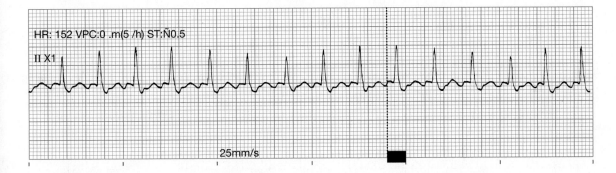
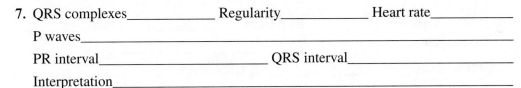

HR: 152 VPC:0 .m(5 /h) ST:Ñ0.5

II X1

25mm/s

8. QRS complexes_____ Regularity_____ Heart rate_____

   P waves_____

   PR interval_____ QRS interval_____

   Interpretation_____

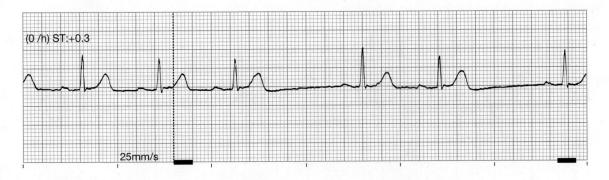
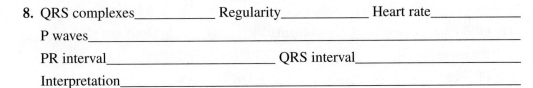

(0 /h) ST:+0.3

25mm/s

9. QRS complexes_____ Regularity_____ Heart rate_____

   P waves_____

   PR interval_____ QRS interval_____

   Interpretation_____

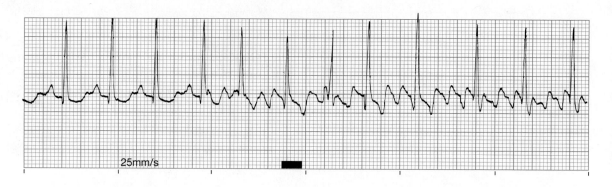

10. QRS complexes_____ Regularity_____ Heart rate_____

P waves_____

PR interval_____ QRS interval_____

Interpretation_____

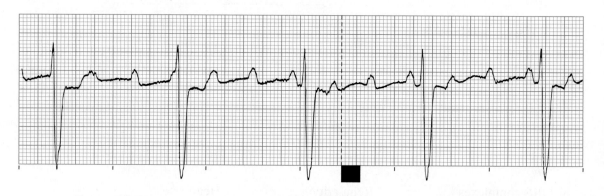

11. QRS complexes_____ Regularity_____ Heart rate_____

P waves_____

PR interval_____ QRS interval_____

Interpretation_____

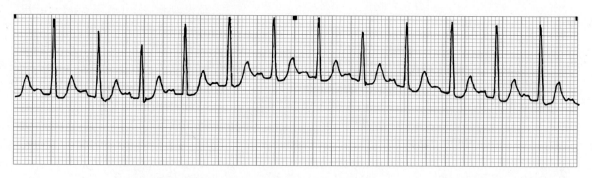

12. QRS complexes_____ Regularity_____ Heart rate_____

P waves_____

PR interval_____ QRS interval_____

Interpretation_____

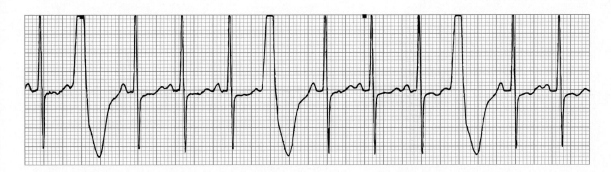

13. QRS complexes_____ Regularity_____ Heart rate_____

P waves_____

PR interval_____ QRS interval_____

Interpretation_____

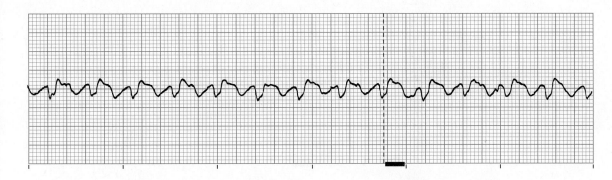

14. QRS complexes_____ Regularity_____ Heart rate_____

P waves_____

PR interval_____ QRS interval_____

Interpretation_____

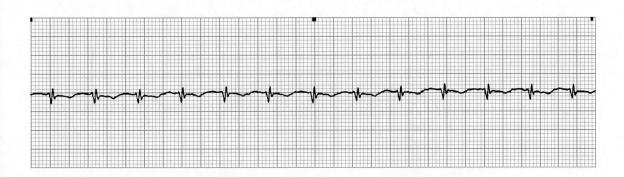

15. QRS complexes_____ Regularity_____ Heart rate_____

P waves_____

PR interval_____ QRS interval_____

Interpretation_____

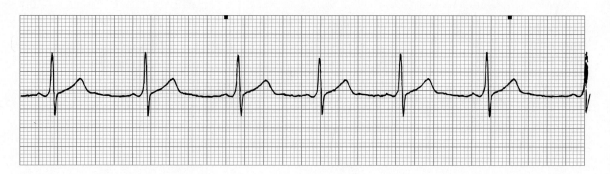

16. QRS complexes_____ Regularity_____ Heart rate_____

P waves_____

PR interval_____ QRS interval_____

Interpretation_____

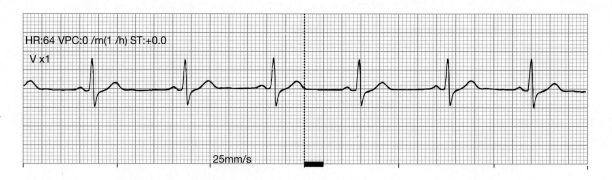

17. QRS complexes_____ Regularity_____ Heart rate_____

P waves_____

PR interval_____ QRS interval_____

Interpretation_____

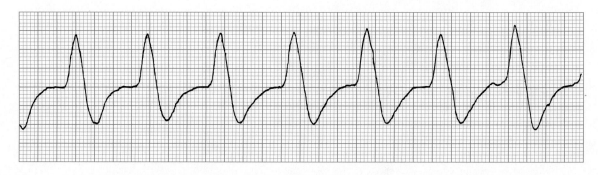

18. QRS complexes_____ Regularity_____ Heart rate_____

P waves_____

PR interval_____ QRS interval_____

Interpretation_____

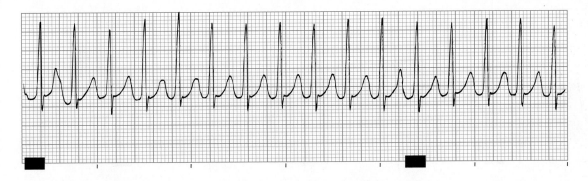

19. QRS complexes_____ Regularity_____ Heart rate_____

P waves_____

PR interval_____ QRS interval_____

Interpretation_____

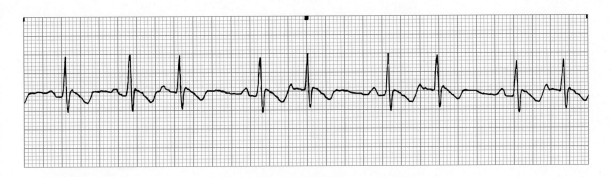

20. QRS complexes_____ Regularity_____ Heart rate_____

P waves_____

PR interval_____ QRS interval_____

Interpretation_____

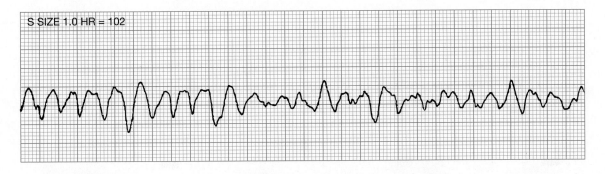

S SIZE 1.0 HR = 102

21. QRS complexes_____ Regularity_____ Heart rate_____

P waves_____

PR interval_____ QRS interval_____

Interpretation_____

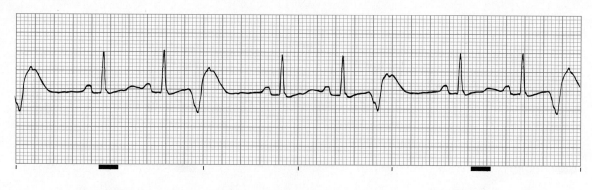

22. QRS complexes_____ Regularity_____ Heart rate_____

P waves_____

PR interval_____ QRS interval_____

Interpretation_____

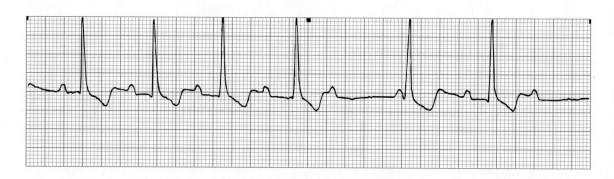

23. QRS complexes_____ Regularity_____ Heart rate_____

P waves_____

PR interval_____ QRS interval_____

Interpretation_____

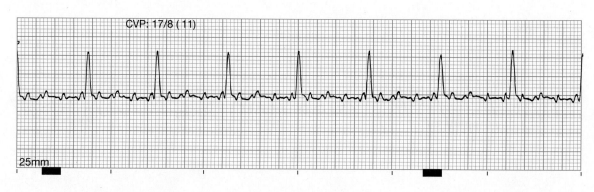

CVP: 17/8 (11)

25mm

24. QRS complexes_____ Regularity_____ Heart rate_____

P waves_____

PR interval_____ QRS interval_____

Interpretation_____

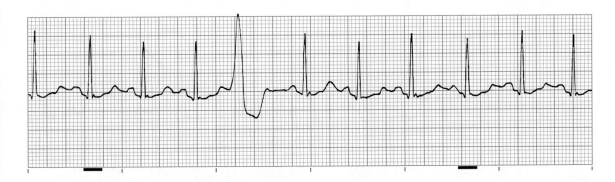

25. QRS complexes_____ Regularity_____ Heart rate_____

P waves_____

PR interval_____ QRS interval_____

Interpretation_____

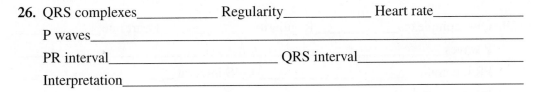

26. QRS complexes_____ Regularity_____ Heart rate_____

P waves_____

PR interval_____ QRS interval_____

Interpretation_____

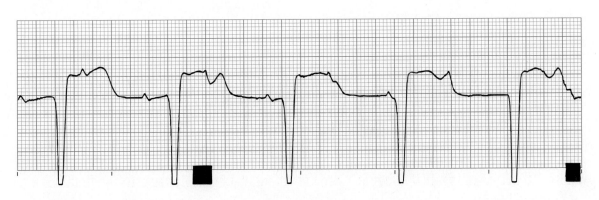

27. QRS complexes_____ Regularity_____ Heart rate_____

P waves_____

PR interval_____ QRS interval_____

Interpretation_____

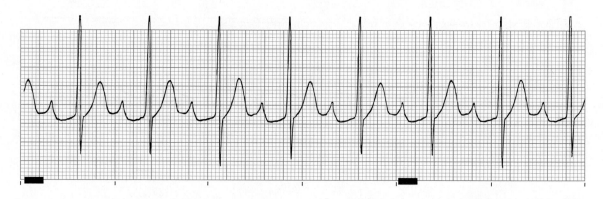

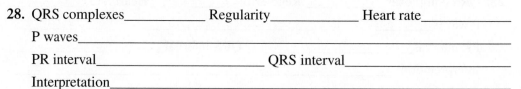

28. QRS complexes_____ Regularity_____ Heart rate_____

P waves_____

PR interval_____ QRS interval_____

Interpretation_____

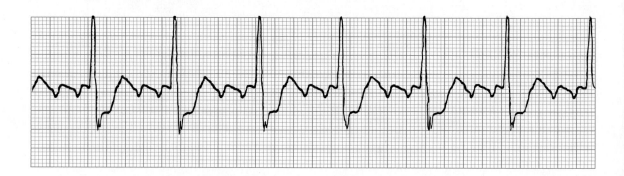

29. QRS complexes_____ Regularity_____ Heart rate_____

P waves_____

PR interval_____ QRS interval_____

Interpretation_____

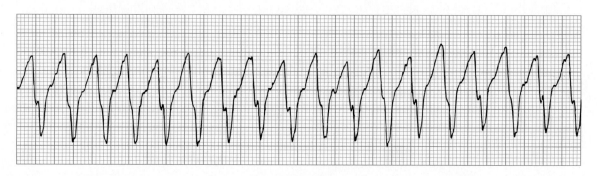

30. QRS complexes_____ Regularity_____ Heart rate_____

P waves_____

PR interval_____ QRS interval_____

Interpretation_____

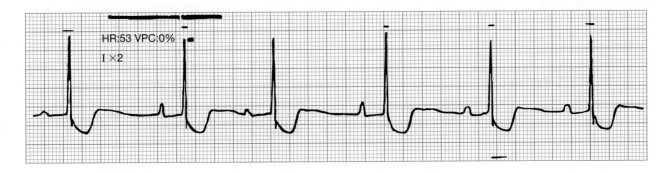

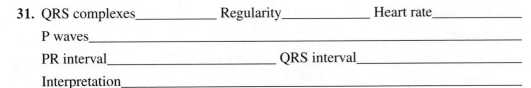

31. QRS complexes_____ Regularity_____ Heart rate_____

P waves_____

PR interval_____ QRS interval_____

Interpretation_____

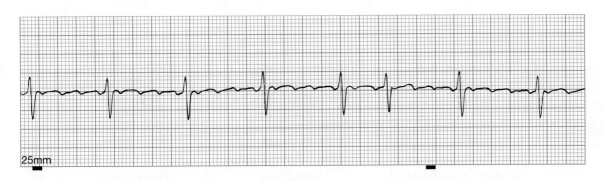

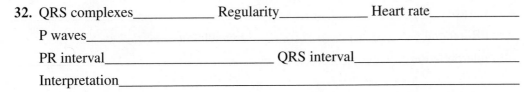

32. QRS complexes_____ Regularity_____ Heart rate_____

P waves_____

PR interval_____ QRS interval_____

Interpretation_____

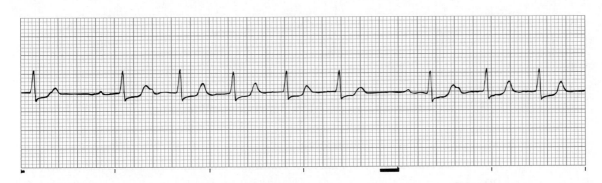

33. QRS complexes_____ Regularity_____ Heart rate_____

P waves_____

PR interval_____ QRS interval_____

Interpretation_____

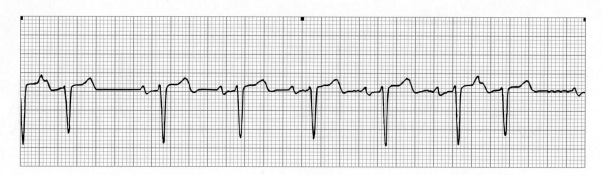

34. QRS complexes_____ Regularity_____ Heart rate_____

P waves_____

PR interval_____ QRS interval_____

Interpretation_____

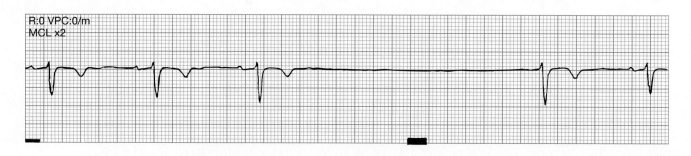

35. QRS complexes_____ Regularity_____ Heart rate_____

P waves_____

PR interval_____ QRS interval_____

Interpretation_____

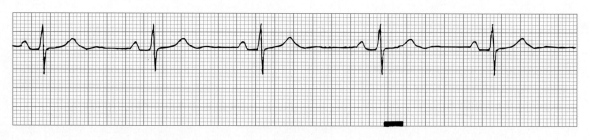

36. QRS complexes_____ Regularity_____ Heart rate_____

P waves_____

PR interval_____ QRS interval_____

Interpretation_____

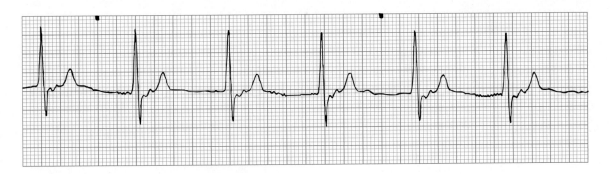

37. QRS complexes_____ Regularity_____ Heart rate_____

P waves_____

PR interval_____ QRS interval_____

Interpretation_____

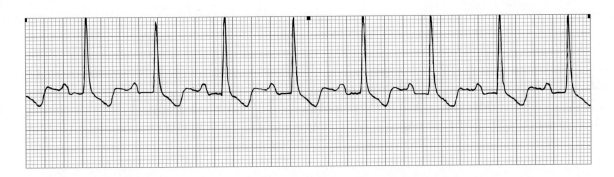

38. QRS complexes_____ Regularity_____ Heart rate_____

P waves_____

PR interval_____ QRS interval_____

Interpretation_____

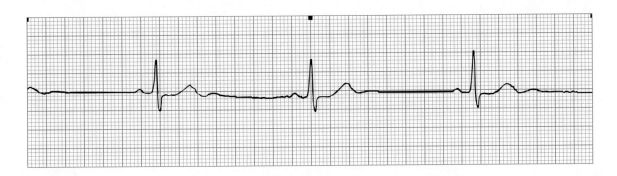

39. QRS complexes_____ Regularity_____ Heart rate_____

P waves_____

PR interval_____ QRS interval_____

Interpretation_____

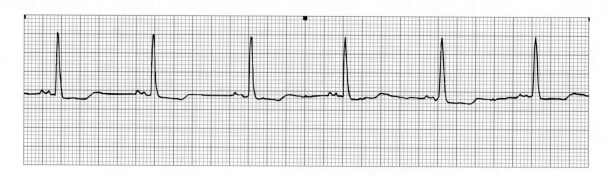

40. QRS complexes_____ Regularity_____ Heart rate_____

P waves_____

PR interval_____ QRS interval_____

Interpretation_____

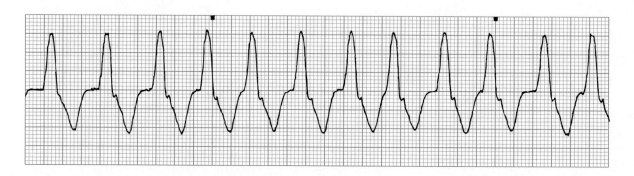

41. QRS complexes_____ Regularity_____ Heart rate_____

P waves_____

PR interval_____ QRS interval_____

Interpretation_____

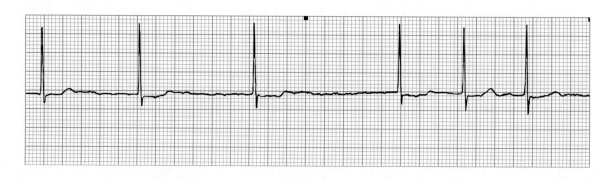

42. QRS complexes_____ Regularity_____ Heart rate_____

P waves_____

PR interval_____ QRS interval_____

Interpretation_____

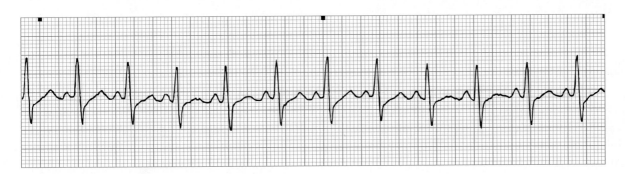

43. QRS complexes_____ Regularity_____ Heart rate_____

P waves_____

PR interval_____ QRS interval_____

Interpretation_____

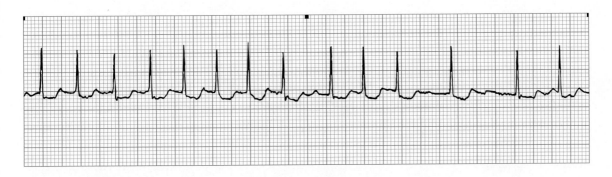

44. QRS complexes_____ Regularity_____ Heart rate_____

P waves_____

PR interval_____ QRS interval_____

Interpretation_____

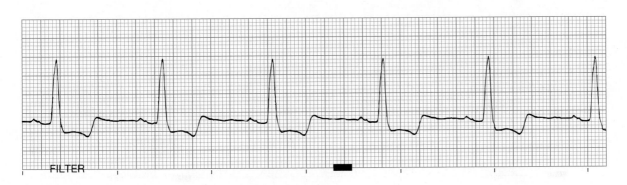

FILTER

45. QRS complexes_____ Regularity_____ Heart rate_____

P waves_____

PR interval_____ QRS interval_____

Interpretation_____

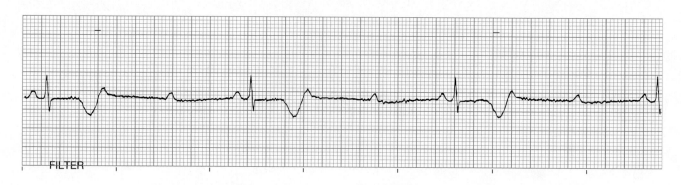

FILTER

46. QRS complexes_____ Regularity_____ Heart rate_____

P waves_____

PR interval_____ QRS interval_____

Interpretation_____

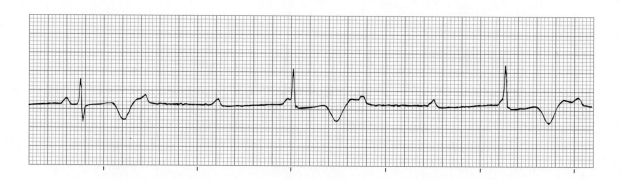

47. QRS complexes_____ Regularity_____ Heart rate_____

P waves_____

PR interval_____ QRS interval_____

Interpretation_____

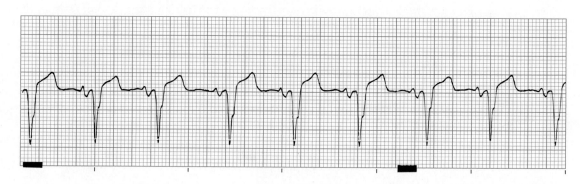

48. QRS complexes_____ Regularity_____ Heart rate_____

P waves_____

PR interval_____ QRS interval_____

Interpretation_____

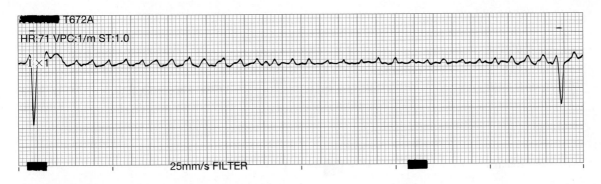

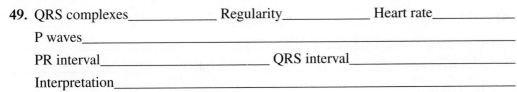

49. QRS complexes_____ Regularity_____ Heart rate_____

P waves_____

PR interval_____ QRS interval_____

Interpretation_____

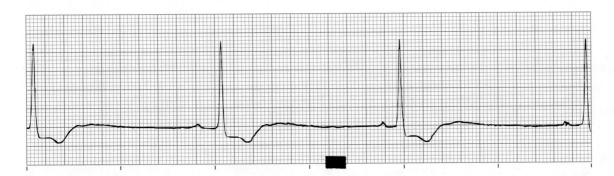

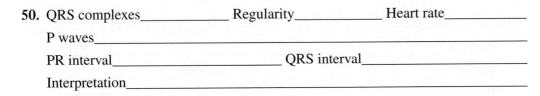

50. QRS complexes_____ Regularity_____ Heart rate_____

P waves_____

PR interval_____ QRS interval_____

Interpretation_____

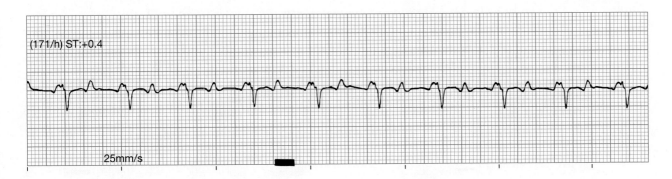

51. QRS complexes_____ Regularity_____ Heart rate_____

P waves_____

PR interval_____ QRS interval_____

Interpretation_____

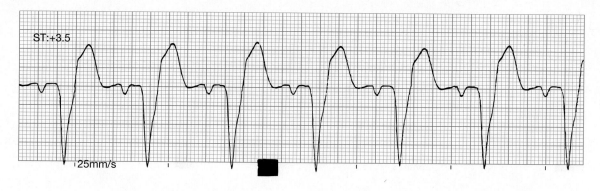

ST:+3.5

25mm/s

52. QRS complexes_____ Regularity_____ Heart rate_____

P waves_____

PR interval_____ QRS interval_____

Interpretation_____

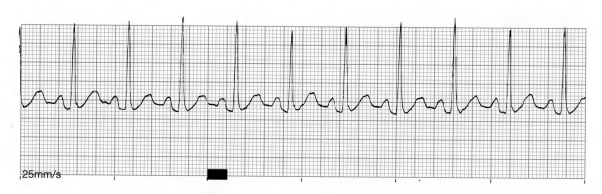

25mm/s

53. QRS complexes_____ Regularity_____ Heart rate_____

P waves_____

PR interval_____ QRS interval_____

Interpretation_____

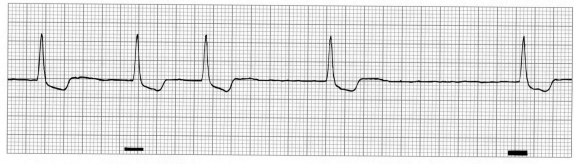

54. QRS complexes_____ Regularity_____ Heart rate_____

P waves_____

PR interval_____ QRS interval_____

Interpretation_____

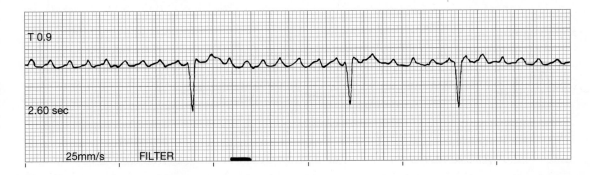

55. QRS complexes_____ Regularity_____ Heart rate_____

P waves_____

PR interval_____ QRS interval_____

Interpretation_____

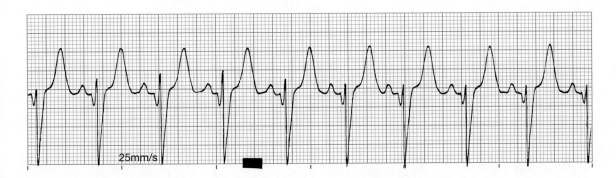

56. QRS complexes_____ Regularity_____ Heart rate_____

P waves_____

PR interval_____ QRS interval_____

Interpretation_____

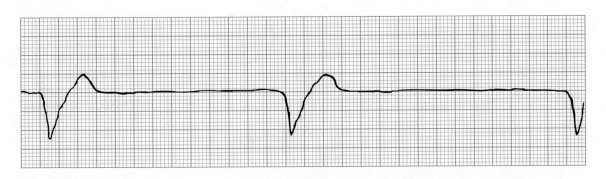

57. QRS complexes_____ Regularity_____ Heart rate_____

P waves_____

PR interval_____ QRS interval_____

Interpretation_____

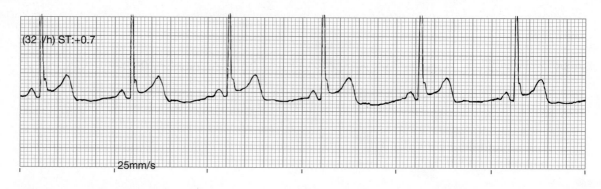

(32 /h) ST:+0.7

25mm/s

58. QRS complexes_____ Regularity_____ Heart rate_____

P waves_____

PR interval_____ QRS interval_____

Interpretation_____

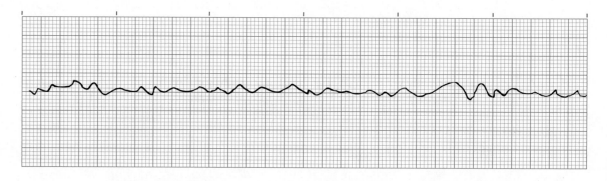

59. QRS complexes_____ Regularity_____ Heart rate_____

P waves_____

PR interval_____ QRS interval_____

Interpretation_____

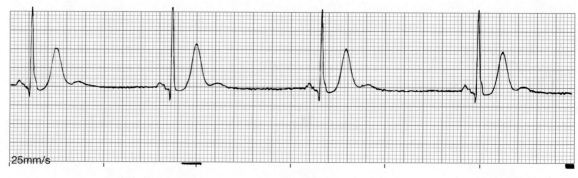

25mm/s

60. QRS complexes_____ Regularity_____ Heart rate_____

P waves_____

PR interval_____ QRS interval_____

Interpretation_____

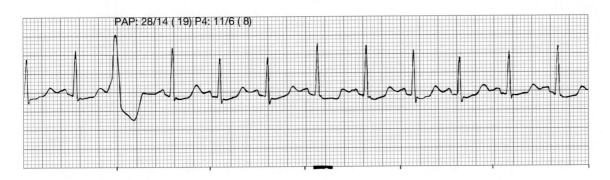

PAP: 28/14 (19) P4: 11/6 (8)

61. QRS complexes_____ Regularity_____ Heart rate_____

P waves_____

PR interval_____ QRS interval_____

Interpretation_____

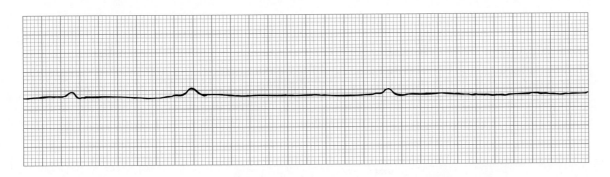

62. QRS complexes_____ Regularity_____ Heart rate_____

P waves_____

PR interval_____ QRS interval_____

Interpretation_____

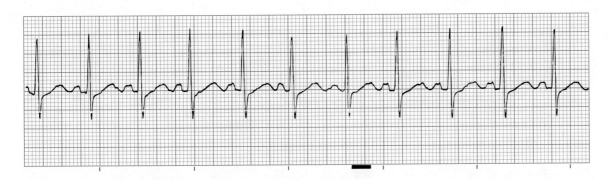

63. QRS complexes_____ Regularity_____ Heart rate_____

P waves_____

PR interval_____ QRS interval_____

Interpretation_____

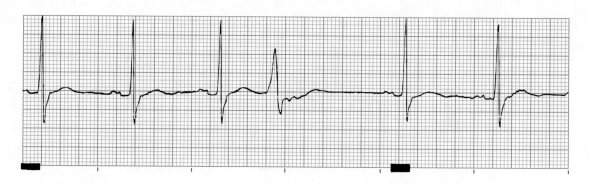

64. QRS complexes_____ Regularity_____ Heart rate_____

P waves_____

PR interval_____ QRS interval_____

Interpretation_____

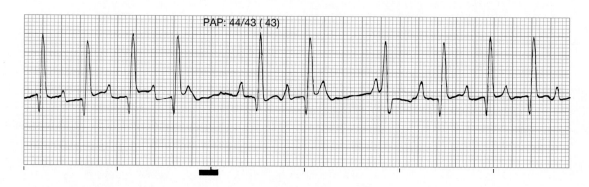

65. QRS complexes_____ Regularity_____ Heart rate_____

P waves_____

PR interval_____ QRS interval_____

Interpretation_____

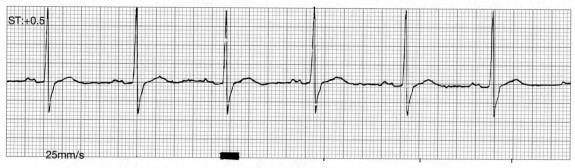

66. QRS complexes_____ Regularity_____ Heart rate_____

P waves_____

PR interval_____ QRS interval_____

Interpretation_____

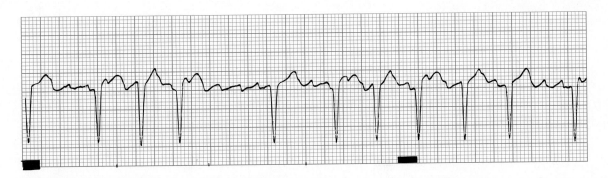

67. QRS complexes_____ Regularity_____ Heart rate_____

P waves_____

PR interval_____ QRS interval_____

Interpretation_____

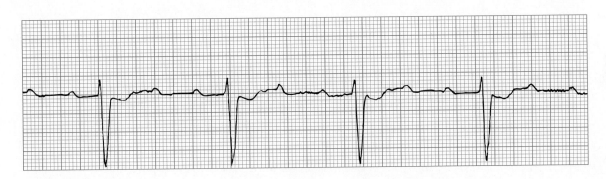

68. QRS complexes_____ Regularity_____ Heart rate_____

P waves_____

PR interval_____ QRS interval_____

Interpretation_____

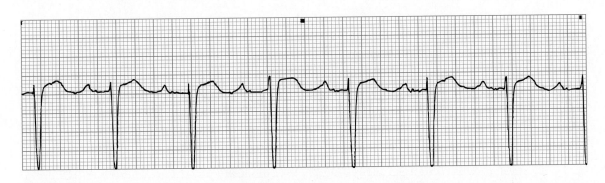

69. QRS complexes_____ Regularity_____ Heart rate_____

P waves_____

PR interval_____ QRS interval_____

Interpretation_____

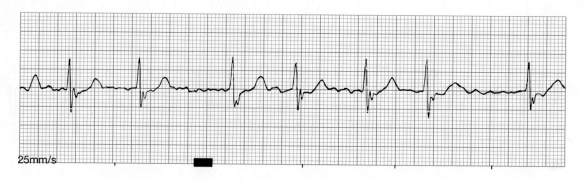

25mm/s

70. QRS complexes_____ Regularity_____ Heart rate_____

P waves_____

PR interval_____ QRS interval_____

Interpretation_____

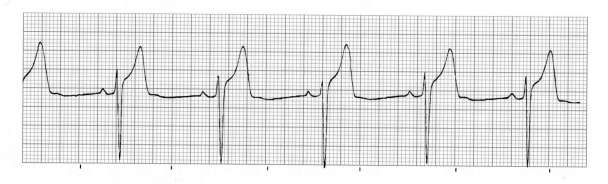

71. QRS complexes_____ Regularity_____ Heart rate_____

P waves_____

PR interval_____ QRS interval_____

Interpretation_____

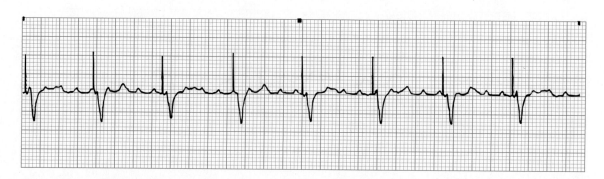

72. QRS complexes_____ Regularity_____ Heart rate_____

P waves_____

PR interval_____ QRS interval_____

Interpretation_____

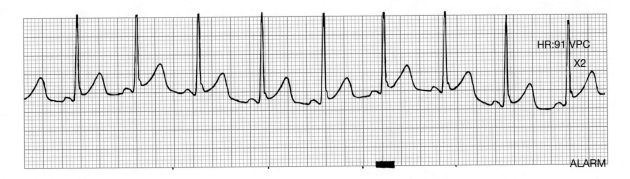

73. QRS complexes_____ Regularity_____ Heart rate_____

P waves_____

PR interval_____ QRS interval_____

Interpretation_____

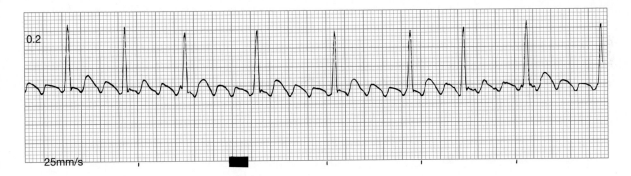

74. QRS complexes_____ Regularity_____ Heart rate_____

P waves_____

PR interval_____ QRS interval_____

Interpretation_____

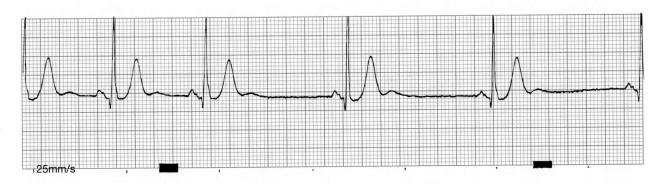

75. QRS complexes_____ Regularity_____ Heart rate_____

P waves_____

PR interval_____ QRS interval_____

Interpretation_____

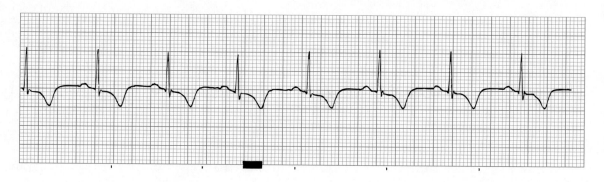

76. QRS complexes_____ Regularity_____ Heart rate_____

P waves_____

PR interval_____ QRS interval_____

Interpretation_____

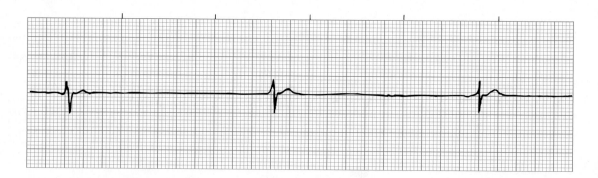

77. QRS complexes_____ Regularity_____ Heart rate_____

P waves_____

PR interval_____ QRS interval_____

Interpretation_____

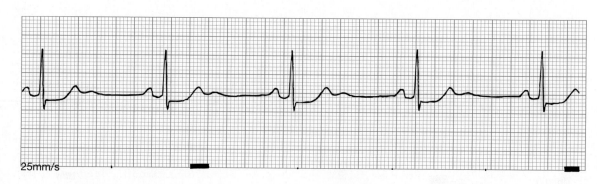

25mm/s

78. QRS complexes_____ Regularity_____ Heart rate_____

P waves_____

PR interval_____ QRS interval_____

Interpretation_____

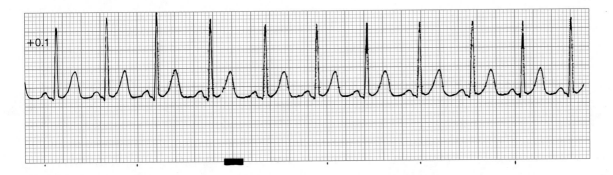

79. QRS complexes_____ Regularity_____ Heart rate_____

P waves_____

PR interval_____ QRS interval_____

Interpretation_____

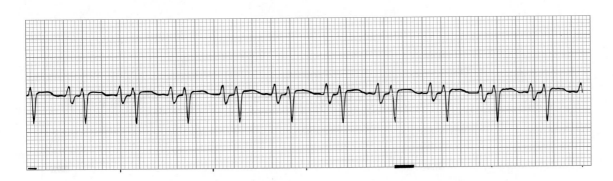

80. QRS complexes_____ Regularity_____ Heart rate_____

P waves_____

PR interval_____ QRS interval_____

Interpretation_____

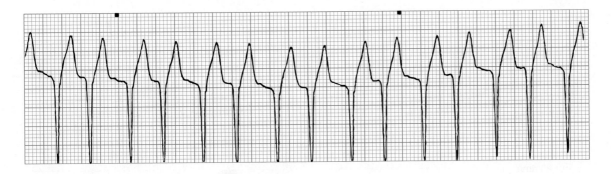

81. QRS complexes_____ Regularity_____ Heart rate_____

P waves_____

PR interval_____ QRS interval_____

Interpretation_____

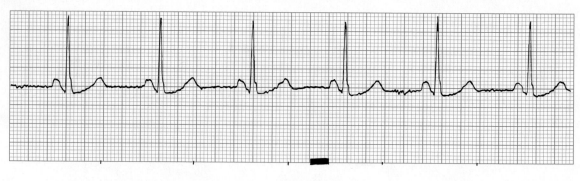

82. QRS complexes_____ Regularity_____ Heart rate_____

   P waves_____

   PR interval_____ QRS interval_____

   Interpretation_____

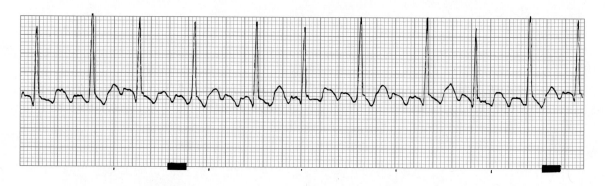

83. QRS complexes_____ Regularity_____ Heart rate_____

   P waves_____

   PR interval_____ QRS interval_____

   Interpretation_____

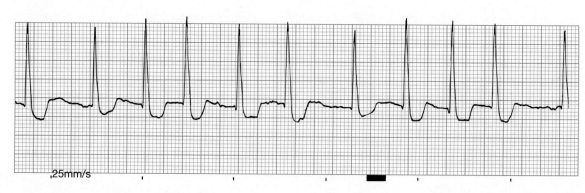

,25mm/s

84. QRS complexes_____ Regularity_____ Heart rate_____

   P waves_____

   PR interval_____ QRS interval_____

   Interpretation_____

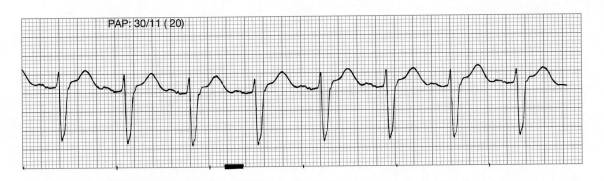

PAP: 30/11 (20)

85. QRS complexes_____ Regularity_____ Heart rate_____

P waves_____

PR interval_____ QRS interval_____

Interpretation_____

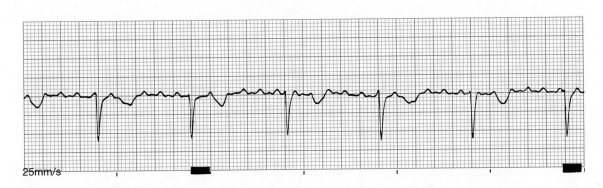

25mm/s

86. QRS complexes_____ Regularity_____ Heart rate_____

P waves_____

PR interval_____ QRS interval_____

Interpretation_____

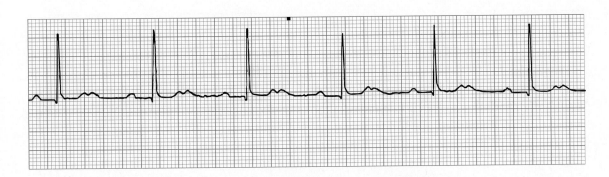

87. QRS complexes_____ Regularity_____ Heart rate_____

P waves_____

PR interval_____ QRS interval_____

Interpretation_____

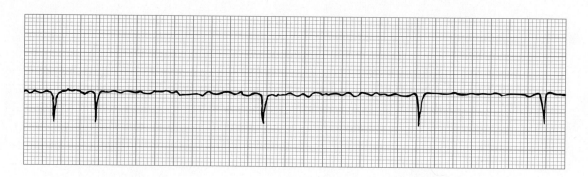

88. QRS complexes_____ Regularity_____ Heart rate_____

P waves_____

PR interval_____ QRS interval_____

Interpretation_____

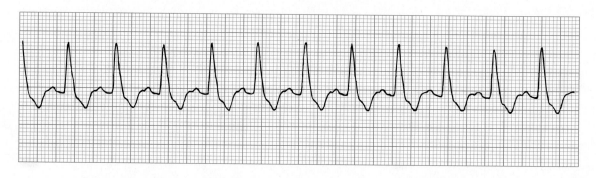

89. QRS complexes_____ Regularity_____ Heart rate_____

P waves_____

PR interval_____ QRS interval_____

Interpretation_____

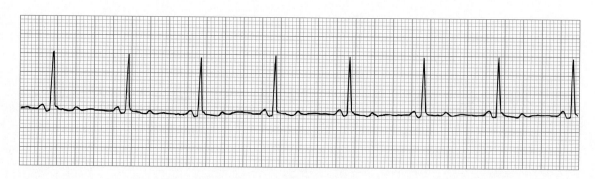

90. QRS complexes_____ Regularity_____ Heart rate_____

P waves_____

PR interval_____ QRS interval_____

Interpretation_____

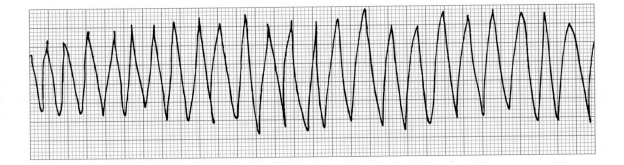

91. QRS complexes_____ Regularity_____ Heart rate_____

P waves_____

PR interval_____ QRS interval_____

Interpretation_____

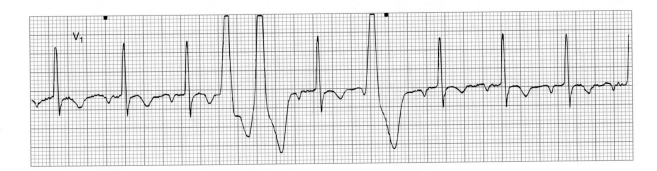

92. QRS complexes_____ Regularity_____ Heart rate_____

P waves_____

PR interval_____ QRS interval_____

Interpretation_____

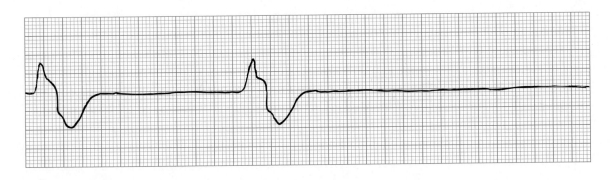

93. QRS complexes_____ Regularity_____ Heart rate_____

P waves_____

PR interval_____ QRS interval_____

Interpretation_____

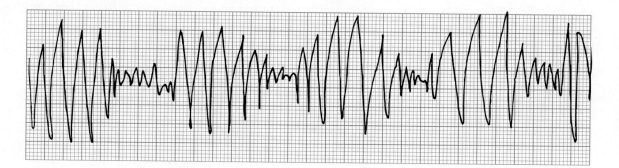

94. QRS complexes_____ Regularity_____ Heart rate_____
    P waves_____
    PR interval_____ QRS interval_____
    Interpretation_____

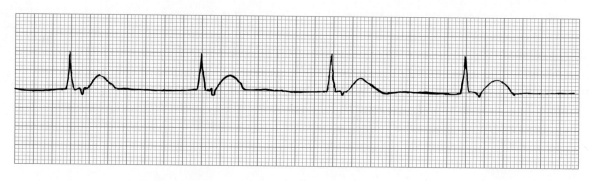

95. QRS complexes_____ Regularity_____ Heart rate_____
    P waves_____
    PR interval_____ QRS interval_____
    Interpretation_____

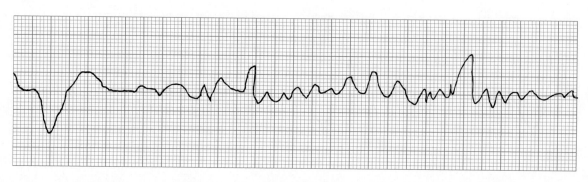

96. QRS complexes_____ Regularity_____ Heart rate_____
    P waves_____
    PR interval_____ QRS interval_____
    Interpretation_____

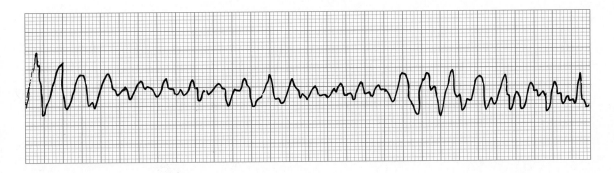

97. QRS complexes_____ Regularity_____ Heart rate_____

P waves_____

PR interval_____ QRS interval_____

Interpretation_____

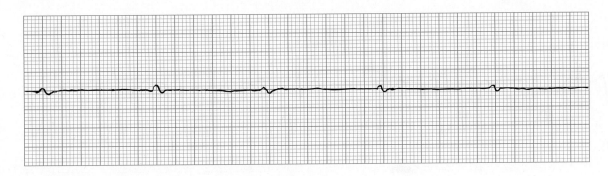

98. QRS complexes_____ Regularity_____ Heart rate_____

P waves_____

PR interval_____ QRS interval_____

Interpretation_____

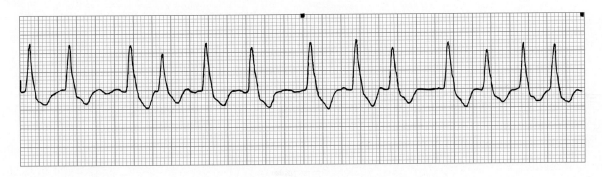

99. QRS complexes_____ Regularity_____ Heart rate_____

P waves_____

PR interval_____ QRS interval_____

Interpretation_____

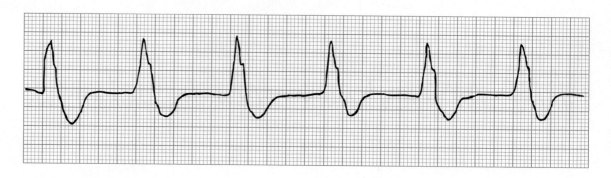

100. QRS complexes_____ Regularity_____ Heart rate_____

P waves_____

PR interval_____ QRS interval_____

Interpretation_____

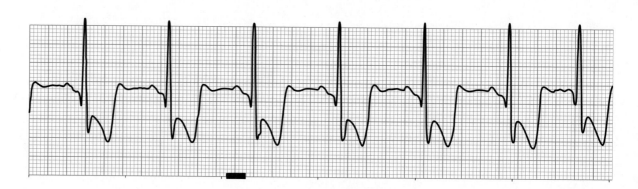

101. QRS complexes_____ Regularity_____ Heart rate_____

P waves_____

PR interval_____ QRS interval_____

Interpretation_____

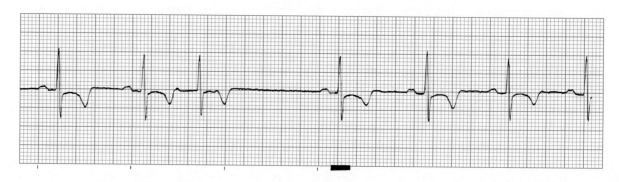

102. QRS complexes_____ Regularity_____ Heart rate _____

P waves_____

PR interval_____ QRS interval_____

Interpretation_____

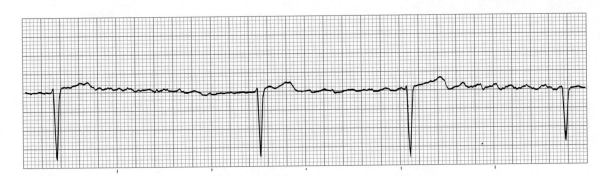

103. QRS complexes_____ Regularity_____ Heart rate_____

P waves_____

PR interval_____ QRS interval_____

Interpretation_____

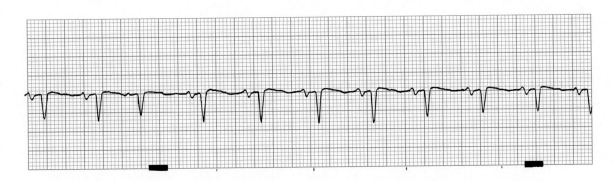

104. QRS complexes_____ Regularity_____ Heart rate_____

P waves_____

PR interval_____ QRS interval_____

Interpretation_____

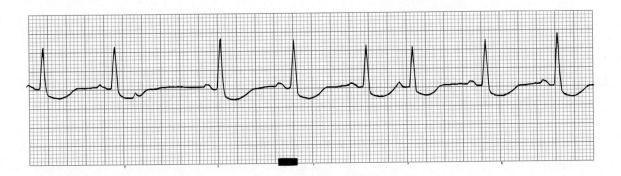

105. QRS complexes_____ Regularity_____ Heart rate_____

P waves_____

PR interval_____ QRS interval_____

Interpretation_____

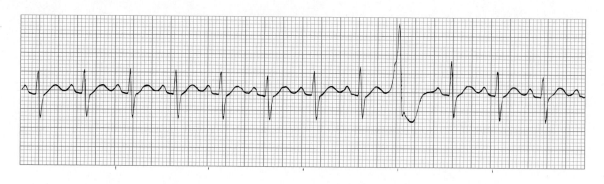

106. QRS complexes_____ Regularity_____ Heart rate_____

P waves_____

PR interval_____ QRS interval_____

Interpretation_____

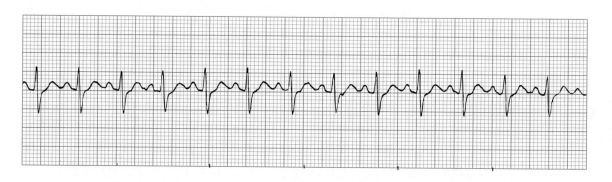

107. QRS complexes_____ Regularity_____ Heart rate_____

P waves_____

PR interval_____ QRS interval_____

Interpretation_____

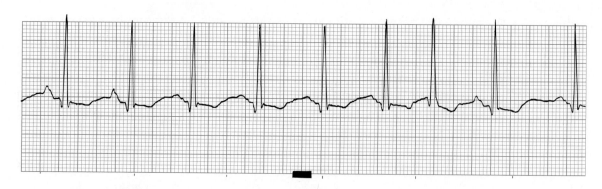

108. QRS complexes_____ Regularity_____ Heart rate_____

P waves_____

PR interval_____ QRS interval_____

Interpretation_____

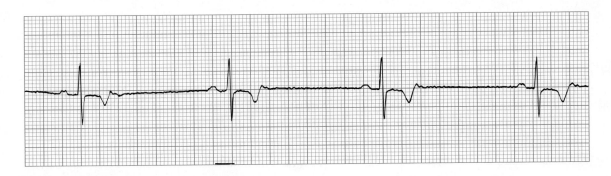

109. QRS complexes_____ Regularity_____ Heart rate_____

P waves_____

PR interval_____ QRS interval_____

Interpretation_____

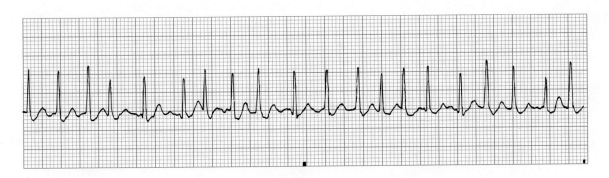

110. QRS complexes_____ Regularity_____ Heart rate_____

P waves_____

PR interval_____ QRS interval_____

Interpretation_____

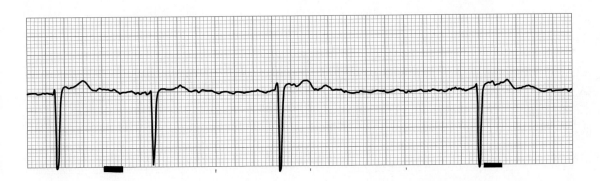

111. QRS complexes_____ Regularity_____ Heart rate_____

P waves_____

PR interval_____ QRS interval_____

Interpretation_____

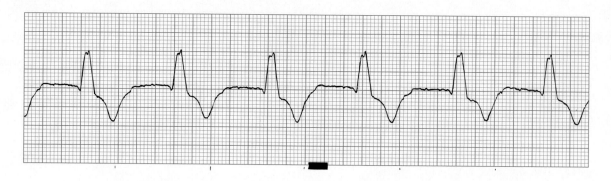

112. QRS complexes_____ Regularity_____ Heart rate_____

P waves_____

PR interval_____ QRS interval_____

Interpretation_____

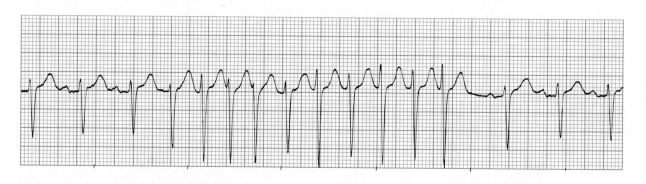

113. QRS complexes_____ Regularity_____ Heart rate_____

P waves_____

PR interval_____ QRS interval_____

Interpretation_____

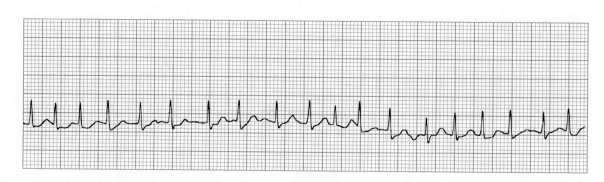

114. QRS complexes_____ Regularity_____ Heart rate_____

P waves_____

PR interval_____ QRS interval_____

Interpretation_____

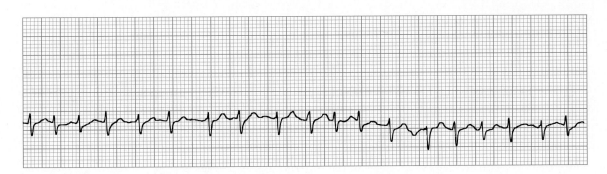

115. QRS complexes_____ Regularity_____ Heart rate_____

P waves_____

PR interval_____ QRS interval_____

Interpretation_____

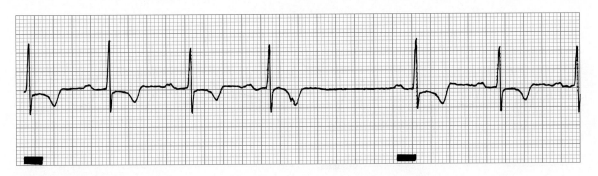

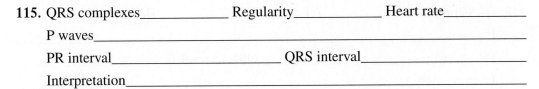

116. QRS complexes_____ Regularity_____ Heart rate_____

P waves_____

PR interval_____ QRS interval_____

Interpretation_____

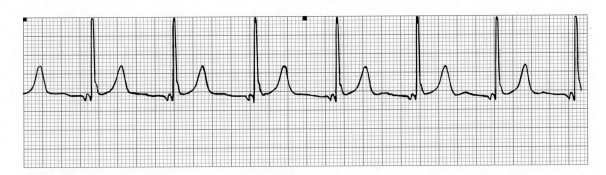

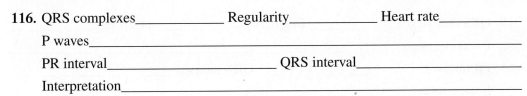

117. QRS complexes_____ Regularity_____ Heart rate_____

P waves_____

PR interval_____ QRS interval_____

Interpretation_____

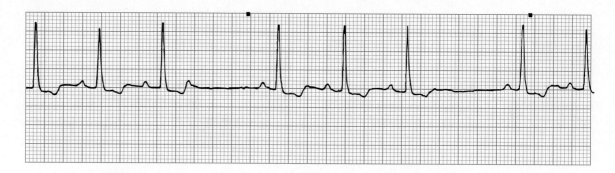

118. QRS complexes_____ Regularity_____ Heart rate_____

P waves_____

PR interval_____ QRS interval_____

Interpretation_____

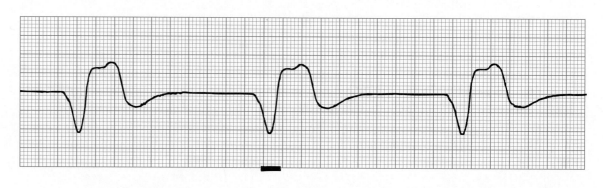

119. QRS complexes_____ Regularity_____ Heart rate_____

P waves_____

PR interval_____ QRS interval_____

Interpretation_____

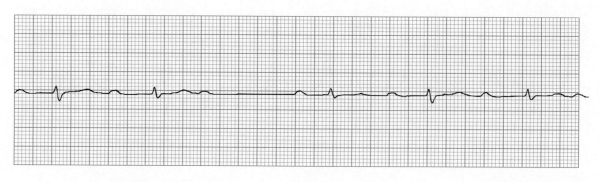

120. QRS complexes_____ Regularity_____ Heart rate_____

P waves_____

PR interval_____ QRS interval_____

Interpretation_____

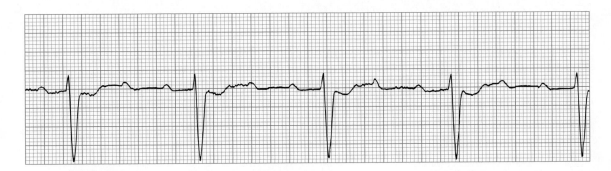

121. QRS complexes_____ Regularity_____ Heart rate_____

P waves_____

PR interval_____ QRS interval_____

Interpretation_____

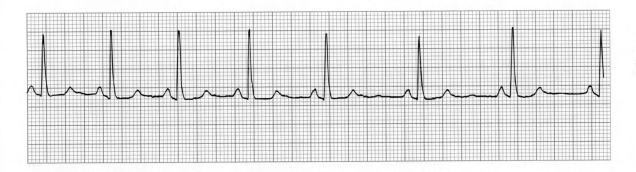

122. QRS complexes_____ Regularity_____ Heart rate_____

P waves_____

PR interval_____ QRS interval_____

Interpretation_____

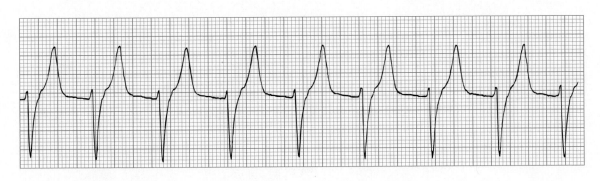

123. QRS complexes_____ Regularity_____ Heart rate_____

P waves_____

PR interval_____ QRS interval_____

Interpretation_____

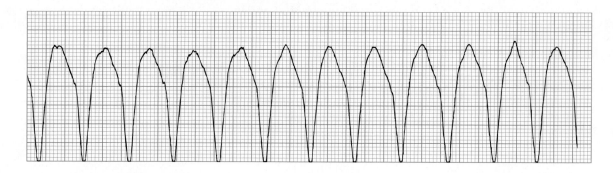

124. QRS complexes_____ Regularity_____ Heart rate_____

P waves_____

PR interval_____ QRS interval_____

Interpretation_____

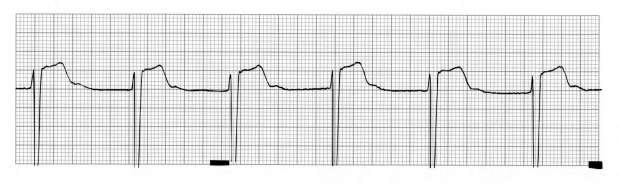

125. QRS complexes_____ Regularity_____ Heart rate_____

P waves_____

PR interval_____ QRS interval_____

Interpretation_____

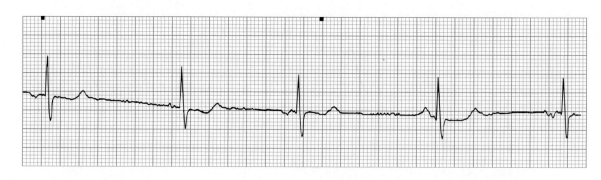

126. QRS complexes_____ Regularity_____ Heart rate_____

P waves_____

PR interval_____ QRS interval_____

Interpretation_____

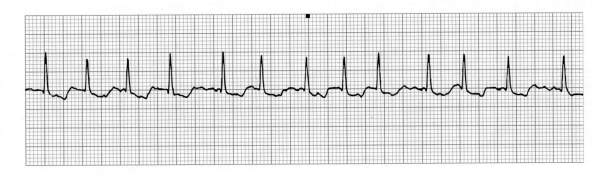

127. QRS complexes_____ Regularity_____ Heart rate_____

P waves_____

PR interval_____ QRS interval_____

Interpretation_____

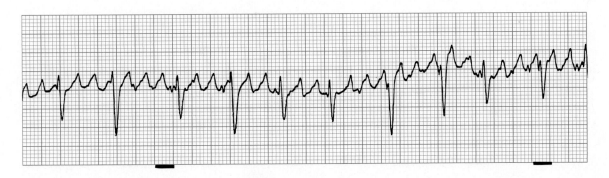

128. QRS complexes_____ Regularity_____ Heart rate_____

P waves_____

PR interval_____ QRS interval_____

Interpretation_____

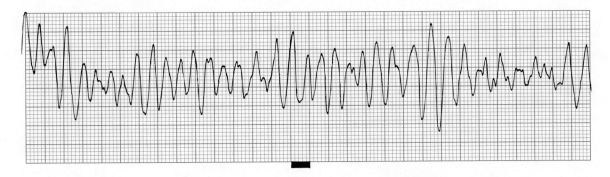

129. QRS complexes_____ Regularity_____ Heart rate_____

P waves_____

PR interval_____ QRS interval_____

Interpretation_____

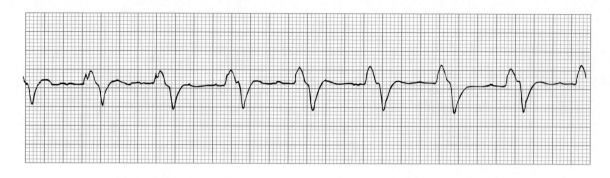

130. QRS complexes_____ Regularity_____ Heart rate_____

P waves_____

PR interval_____ QRS interval_____

Interpretation_____

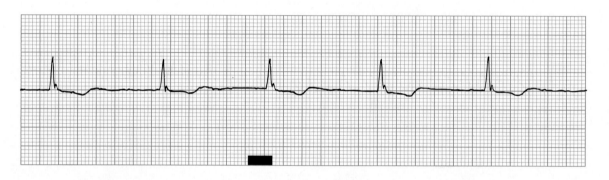

131. QRS complexes_____ Regularity_____ Heart rate_____

P waves_____

PR interval_____ QRS interval_____

Interpretation_____

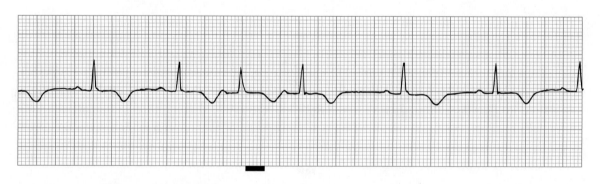

132. QRS complexes_____ Regularity_____ Heart rate_____

P waves_____

PR interval_____ QRS interval_____

Interpretation_____

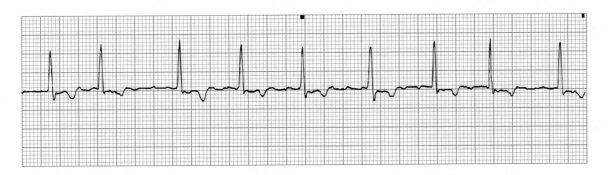

133. QRS complexes_____ Regularity_____ Heart rate_____

P waves_____

PR interval_____ QRS interval_____

Interpretation_____

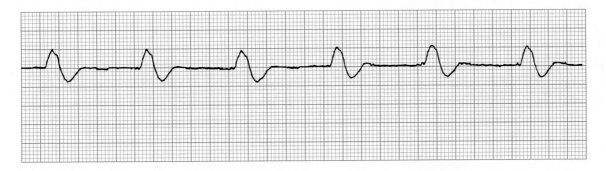

134. QRS complexes_____ Regularity_____ Heart rate_____

P waves_____

PR interval_____ QRS interval_____

Interpretation_____

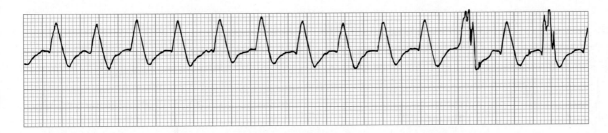

135. QRS complexes_____ Regularity_____ Heart rate_____

P waves_____

PR interval_____ QRS interval_____

Interpretation_____

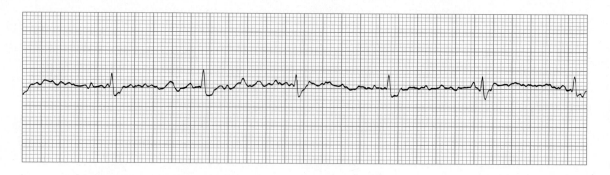

136. QRS complexes_____ Regularity_____ Heart rate_____

P waves_____

PR interval_____ QRS interval_____

Interpretation_____

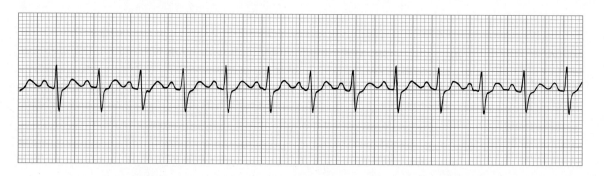

137. QRS complexes_____ Regularity_____ Heart rate_____

P waves_____

PR interval_____ QRS interval_____

Interpretation_____

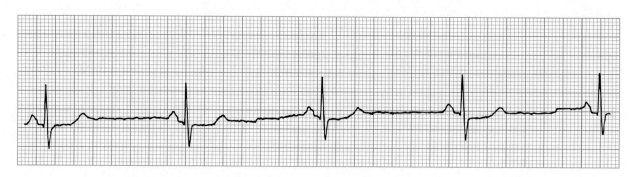

138. QRS complexes_____ Regularity_____ Heart rate_____

P waves_____

PR interval_____ QRS interval_____

Interpretation_____

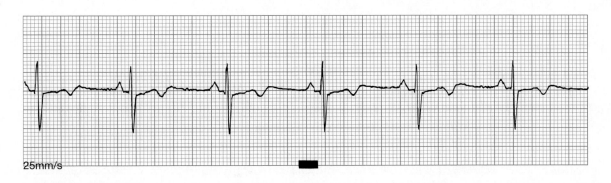

25mm/s

139. QRS complexes_____ Regularity_____ Heart rate_____

P waves_____

PR interval_____ QRS interval_____

Interpretation_____

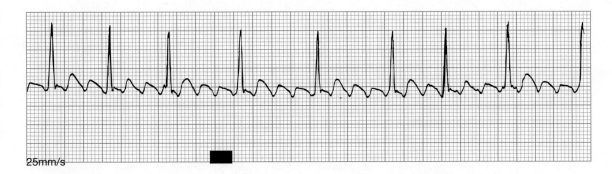

25mm/s

140. QRS complexes_____ Regularity_____ Heart rate_____

P waves_____

PR interval_____ QRS interval_____

Interpretation_____

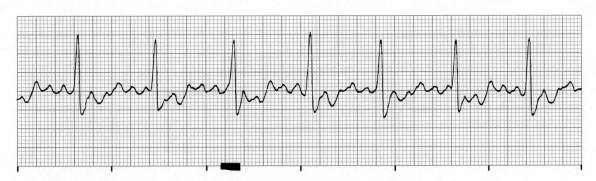

141. QRS complexes_____ Regularity_____ Heart rate_____

P waves_____

PR interval_____ QRS interval_____

Interpretation_____

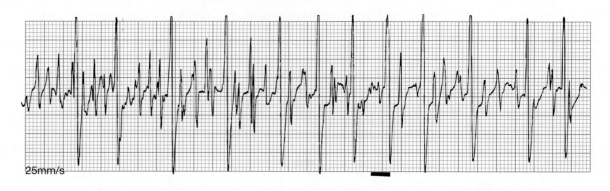

25mm/s

142. QRS complexes_____ Regularity_____ Heart rate_____

P waves_____

PR interval_____ QRS interval_____

Interpretation_____

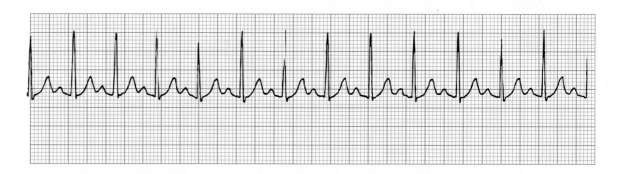

143. QRS complexes_____ Regularity_____ Heart rate_____

P waves_____

PR interval_____ QRS interval_____

Interpretation_____

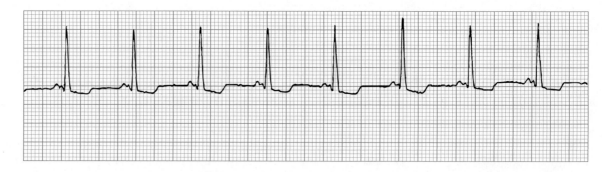

144. QRS complexes_____ Regularity_____ Heart rate_____

P waves_____

PR interval_____ QRS interval_____

Interpretation_____

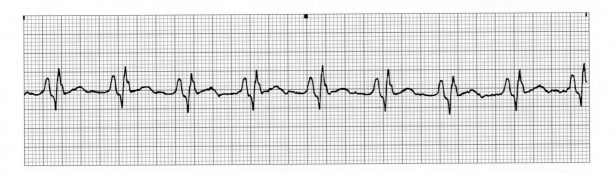

145. QRS complexes_____ Regularity_____ Heart rate_____

P waves_____

PR interval_____ QRS interval_____

Interpretation_____

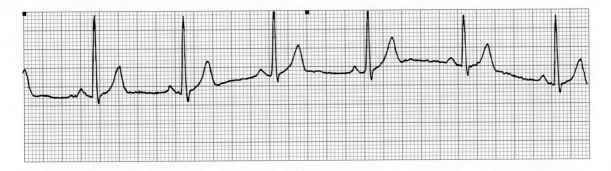

146. QRS complexes_____ Regularity_____ Heart rate_____

P waves_____

PR interval_____ QRS interval_____

Interpretation_____

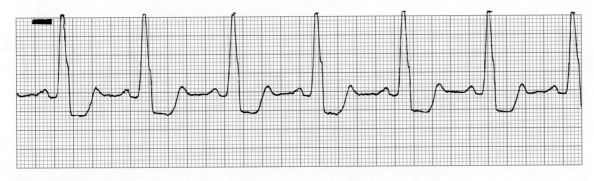

147. QRS complexes_____ Regularity_____ Heart rate_____

P waves_____

PR interval_____ QRS interval_____

Interpretation_____

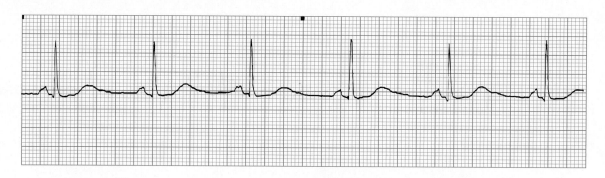

148. QRS complexes_____ Regularity_____ Heart rate_____

P waves_____

PR interval_____ QRS interval_____

Interpretation_____

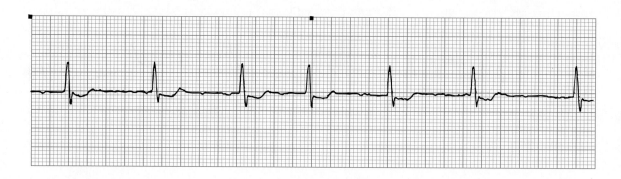

149. QRS complexes_____ Regularity_____ Heart rate_____

P waves_____

PR interval_____ QRS interval_____

Interpretation_____

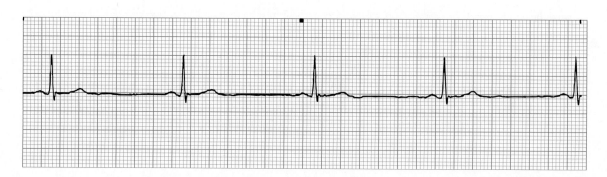

150. QRS complexes_____ Regularity_____ Heart rate_____

P waves_____

PR interval_____ QRS interval_____

Interpretation_____

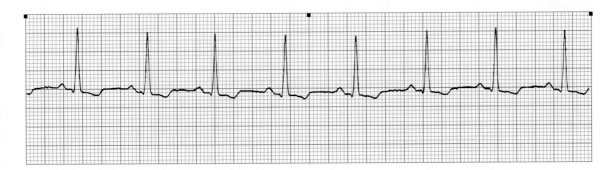

151. QRS complexes_____ Regularity_____ Heart rate_____

    P waves_____

    PR interval_____ QRS interval_____

    Interpretation_____

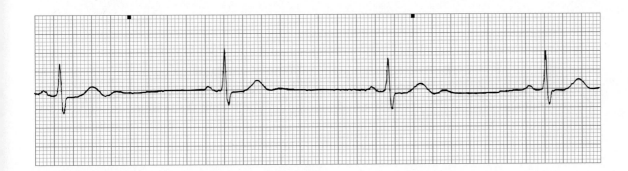

152. QRS complexes_____ Regularity_____ Heart rate_____

    P waves_____

    PR interval_____ QRS interval_____

    Interpretation_____

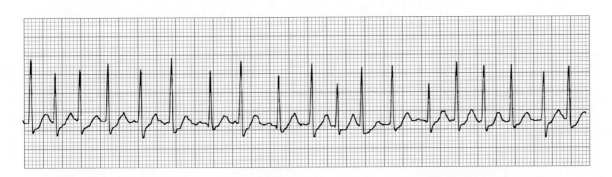

153. QRS complexes_____ Regularity_____ Heart rate_____

    P waves_____

    PR interval_____ QRS interval_____

    Interpretation_____

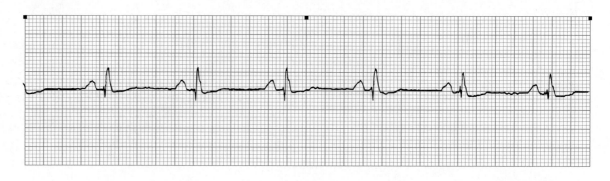

154. QRS complexes_____ Regularity_____ Heart rate_____

P waves_____

PR interval_____ QRS interval_____

Interpretation_____

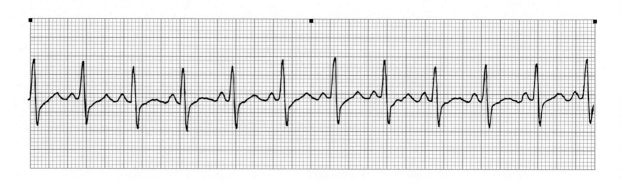

155. QRS complexes_____ Regularity_____ Heart rate_____

P waves_____

PR interval_____ QRS interval_____

Interpretation_____

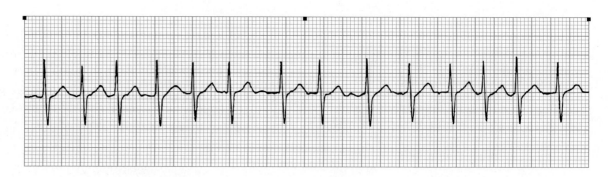

156. QRS complexes_____ Regularity_____ Heart rate_____

P waves_____

PR interval_____ QRS interval_____

Interpretation_____

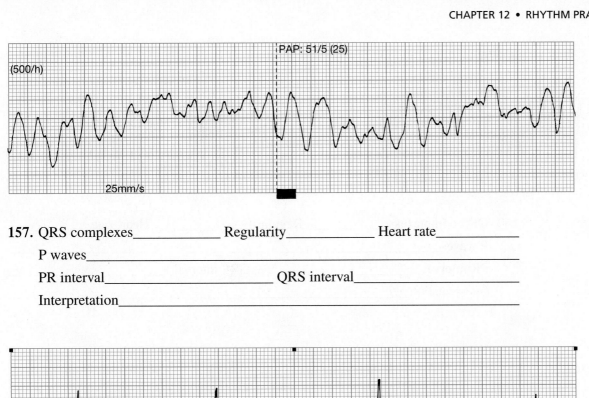

PAP: 51/5 (25)

(500/h)

25mm/s

157. QRS complexes_____ Regularity_____ Heart rate_____

P waves_____

PR interval_____ QRS interval_____

Interpretation_____

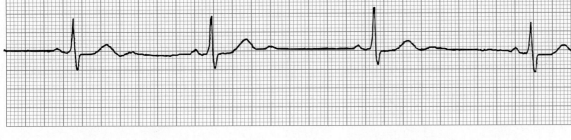

158. QRS complexes_____ Regularity_____ Heart rate_____

P waves_____

PR interval_____ QRS interval_____

Interpretation_____

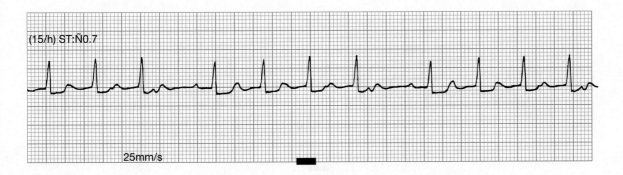

(15/h) ST:Ñ0.7

25mm/s

159. QRS complexes_____ Regularity_____ Heart rate_____

P waves_____

PR interval_____ QRS interval_____

Interpretation_____

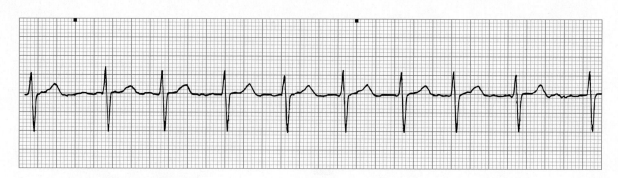

160. QRS complexes_____ Regularity_____ Heart rate_____

P waves_____

PR interval_____ QRS interval_____

Interpretation_____

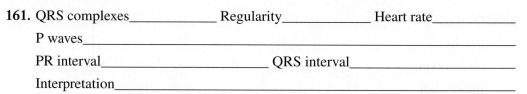

161. QRS complexes_____ Regularity_____ Heart rate_____

P waves_____

PR interval_____ QRS interval_____

Interpretation_____

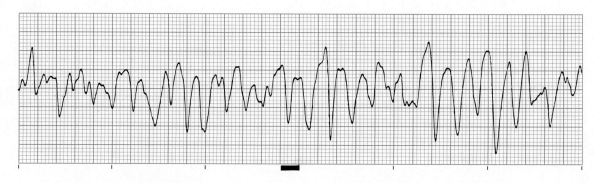

162. QRS complexes_____ Regularity_____ Heart rate_____

P waves_____

PR interval_____ QRS interval_____

Interpretation_____

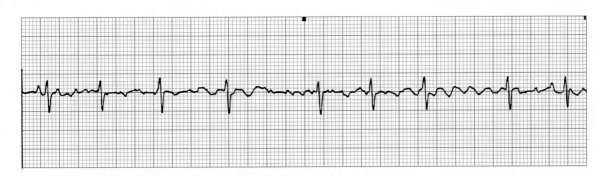

163. QRS complexes_____ Regularity_____ Heart rate_____

P waves_____

PR interval_____ QRS interval_____

Interpretation_____

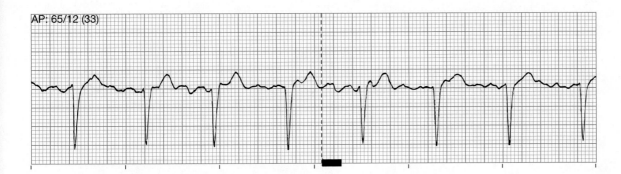

164. QRS complexes_____ Regularity_____ Heart rate_____

P waves_____

PR interval_____ QRS interval_____

Interpretation_____

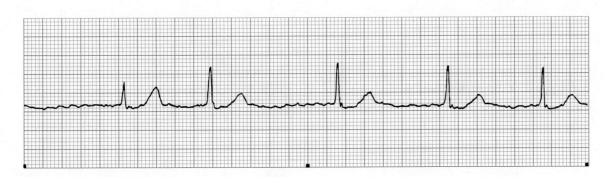

165. QRS complexes_____ Regularity_____ Heart rate_____

P waves_____

PR interval_____ QRS interval_____

Interpretation_____

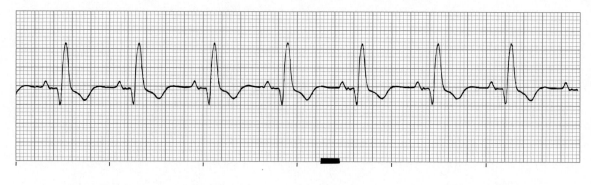

166. QRS complexes_____ Regularity_____ Heart rate_____

P waves_____

PR interval_____ QRS interval_____

Interpretation_____

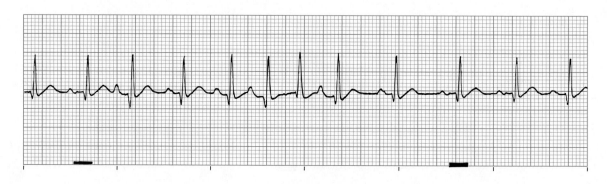

167. QRS complexes_____ Regularity_____ Heart rate_____

P waves_____

PR interval_____ QRS interval_____

Interpretation_____

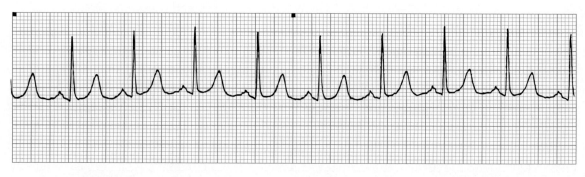

168. QRS complexes_____ Regularity_____ Heart rate_____

P waves_____

PR interval_____ QRS interval_____

Interpretation_____

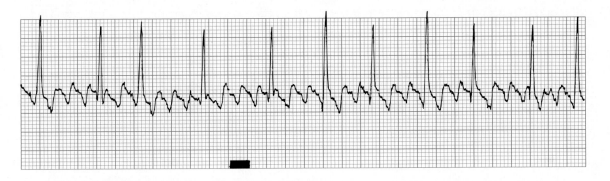

169. QRS complexes_____ Regularity_____ Heart rate_____

P waves_____

PR interval_____ QRS interval_____

Interpretation_____

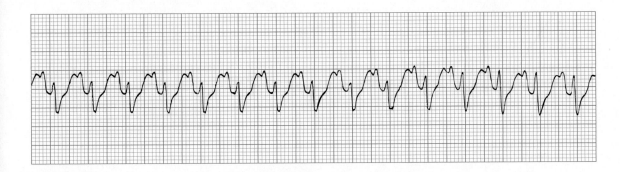

170. QRS complexes_____ Regularity_____ Heart rate_____

P waves_____

PR interval_____ QRS interval_____

Interpretation_____

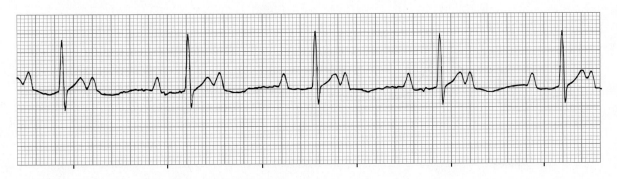

171. QRS complexes_____ Regularity_____ Heart rate_____

P waves_____

PR interval_____ QRS interval_____

Interpretation_____

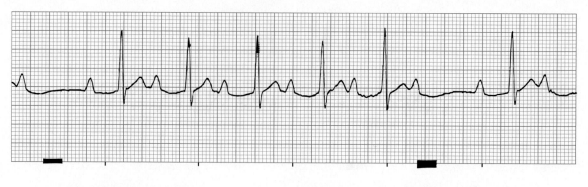

172. QRS complexes_____ Regularity_____ Heart rate_____

P waves_____

PR interval_____ QRS interval_____

Interpretation_____

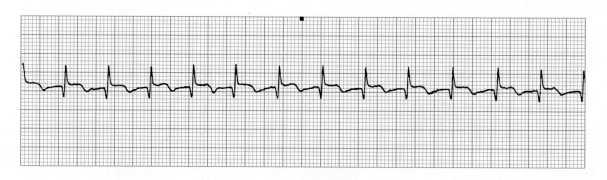

173. QRS complexes_____ Regularity_____ Heart rate_____

P waves_____

PR interval_____ QRS interval_____

Interpretation_____

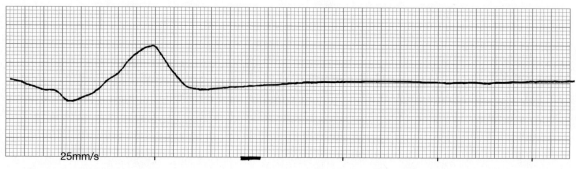

25mm/s

174. QRS complexes_____ Regularity_____ Heart rate_____

P waves_____

PR interval_____ QRS interval_____

Interpretation_____

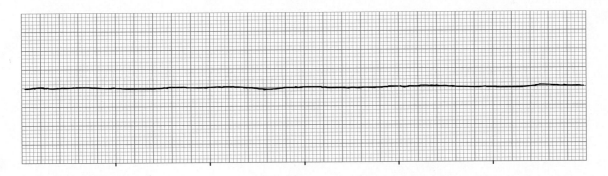

175. QRS complexes_____ Regularity_____ Heart rate_____

     P waves_____

     PR interval_____ QRS interval_____

     Interpretation_____

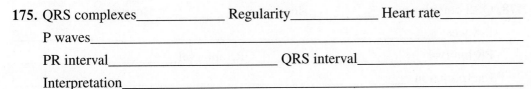

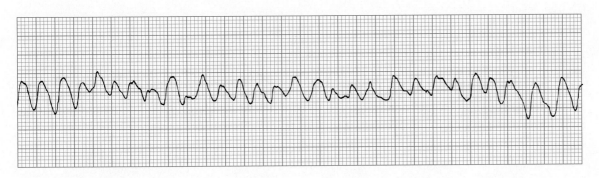

176. QRS complexes_____ Regularity_____ Heart rate_____

     P waves_____

     PR interval_____ QRS interval_____

     Interpretation_____

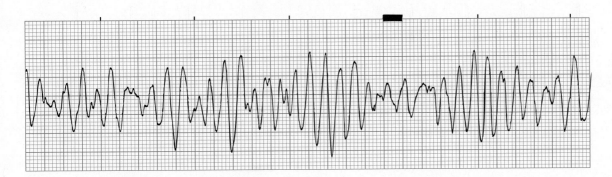

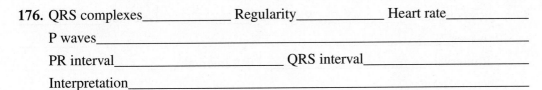

177. QRS complexes_____ Regularity_____ Heart rate_____

     P waves_____

     PR interval_____ QRS interval_____

     Interpretation_____

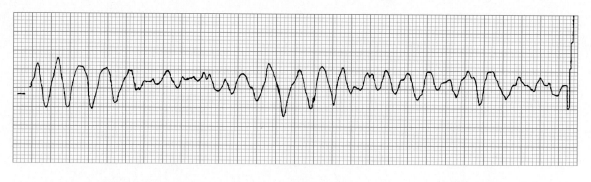

178. QRS complexes_____ Regularity_____ Heart rate_____

P waves_____

PR interval_____ QRS interval_____

Interpretation_____

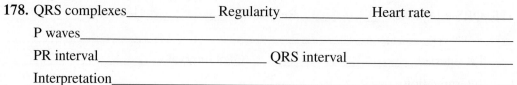

179. QRS complexes_____ Regularity_____ Heart rate_____

P waves_____

PR interval_____ QRS interval_____

Interpretation_____

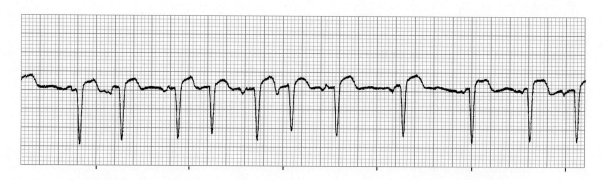

180. QRS complexes_____ Regularity_____ Heart rate_____

P waves_____

PR interval_____ QRS interval_____

Interpretation_____

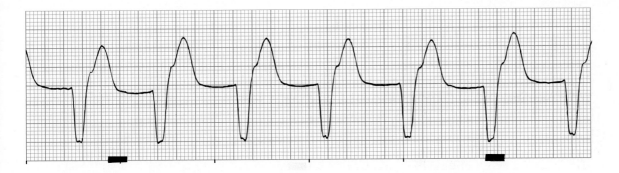

181. QRS complexes_____ Regularity_____ Heart rate_____

P waves_____

PR interval_____ QRS interval_____

Interpretation_____

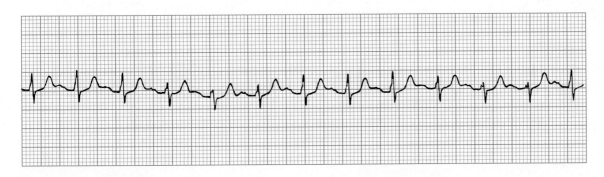

182. QRS complexes_____ Regularity_____ Heart rate_____

P waves_____

PR interval_____ QRS interval_____

Interpretation_____

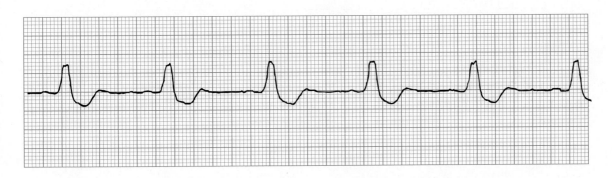

183. QRS complexes_____ Regularity_____ Heart rate_____

P waves_____

PR interval_____ QRS interval_____

Interpretation_____

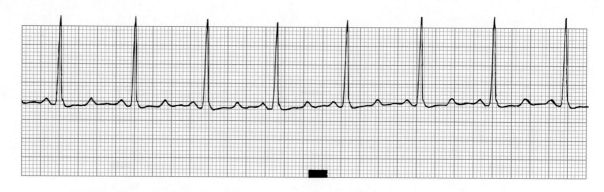

184. QRS complexes_____ Regularity_____ Heart rate_____

P waves_____

PR interval_____ QRS interval_____

Interpretation_____

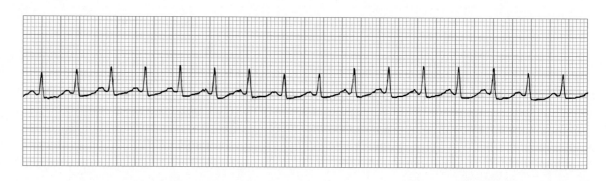

185. QRS complexes_____ Regularity_____ Heart rate_____

P waves_____

PR interval_____ QRS interval_____

Interpretation_____

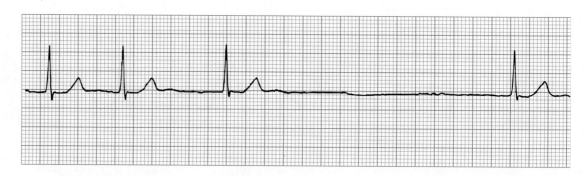

186. QRS complexes_____ Regularity_____ Heart rate_____

P waves_____

PR interval_____ QRS interval_____

Interpretation_____

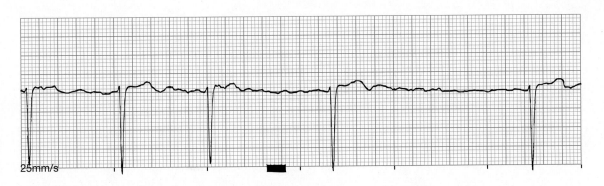

25mm/s

187. QRS complexes_____ Regularity_____ Heart rate_____

P waves_____

PR interval_____ QRS interval_____

Interpretation_____

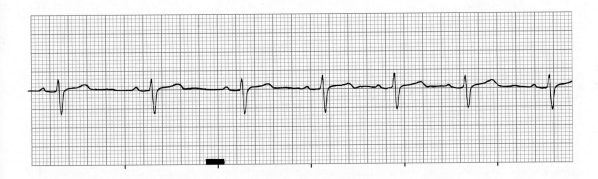

188. QRS complexes_____ Regularity_____ Heart rate_____

P waves_____

PR interval_____ QRS interval_____

Interpretation_____

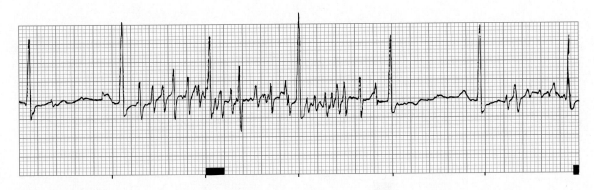

189. QRS complexes_____ Regularity_____ Heart rate_____

P waves_____

PR interval_____ QRS interval_____

Interpretation_____

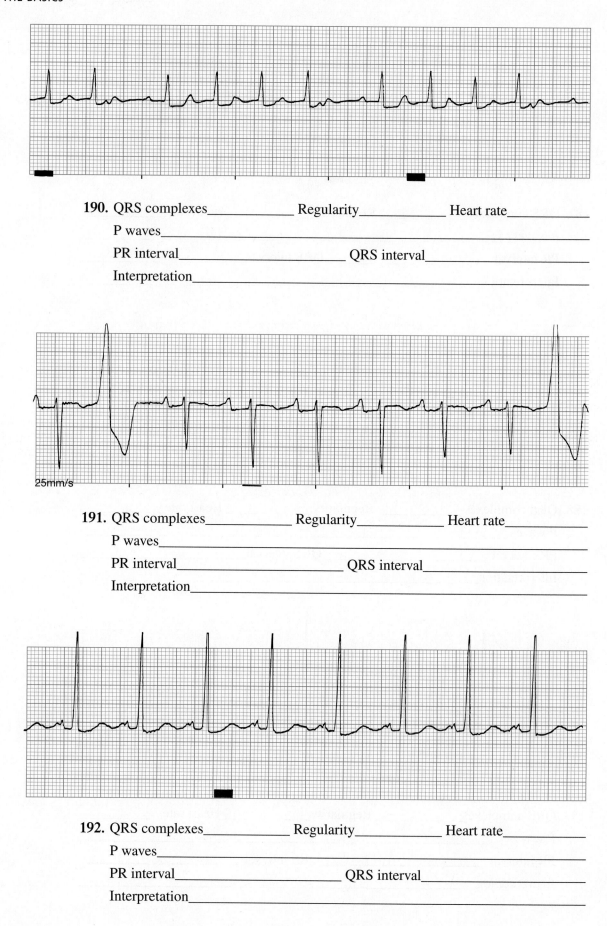

190. QRS complexes_____ Regularity_____ Heart rate_____

P waves_____

PR interval_____ QRS interval_____

Interpretation_____

191. QRS complexes_____ Regularity_____ Heart rate_____

P waves_____

PR interval_____ QRS interval_____

Interpretation_____

192. QRS complexes_____ Regularity_____ Heart rate_____

P waves_____

PR interval_____ QRS interval_____

Interpretation_____

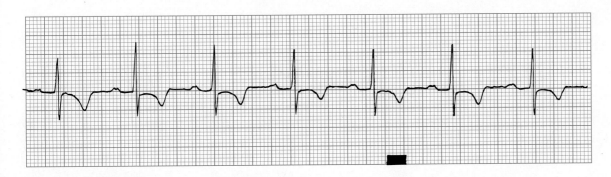

193. QRS complexes_____ Regularity_____ Heart rate_____

P waves_____

PR interval_____ QRS interval_____

Interpretation_____

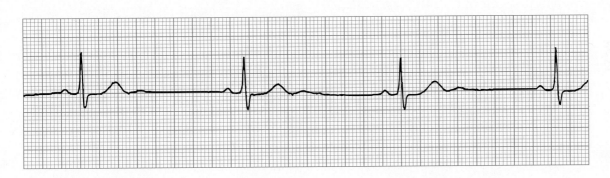

194. QRS complexes_____ Regularity_____ Heart rate_____

P waves_____

PR interval_____ QRS interval_____

Interpretation_____

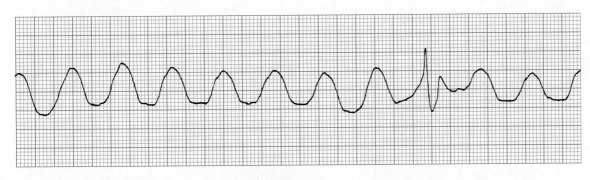

195. QRS complexes_____ Regularity_____ Heart rate_____

P waves_____

PR interval_____ QRS interval_____

Interpretation_____

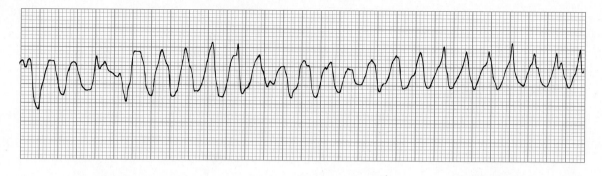

196. QRS complexes_____ Regularity_____ Heart rate_____

P waves_____

PR interval_____ QRS interval_____

Interpretation_____

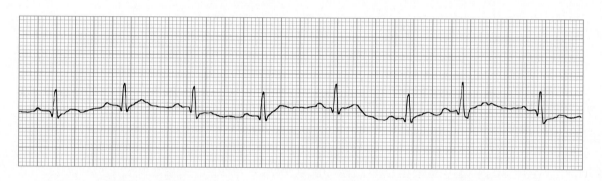

197. QRS complexes_____ Regularity_____ Heart rate_____

P waves_____

PR interval_____ QRS interval_____

Interpretation_____

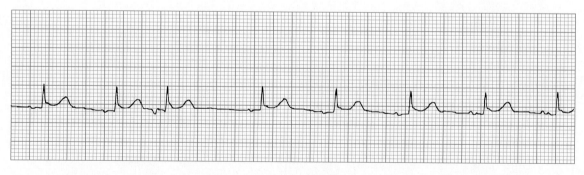

198. QRS complexes_____ Regularity_____ Heart rate_____

P waves_____

PR interval_____ QRS interval_____

Interpretation_____

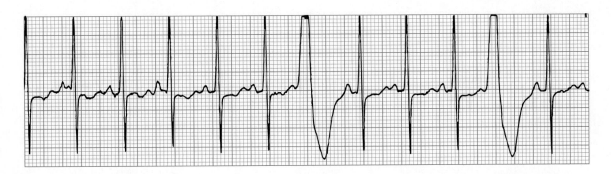

199. QRS complexes_____ Regularity_____ Heart rate_____

P waves_____

PR interval_____ QRS interval_____

Interpretation_____

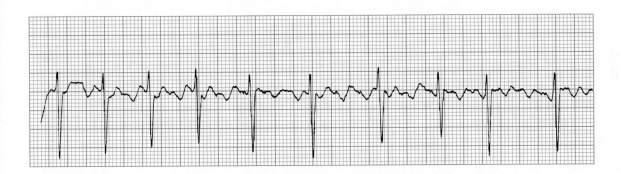

200. QRS complexes_____ Regularity_____ Heart rate_____

P waves_____

PR interval_____ QRS interval_____

Interpretation_____

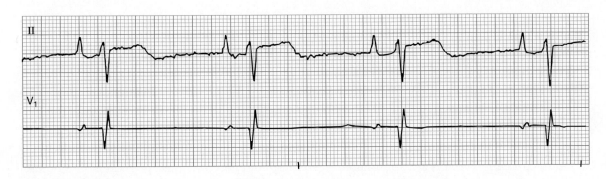

201. QRS complexes_____ Regularity_____ Heart rate_____

P waves_____

PR interval_____ QRS interval_____

Interpretation_____

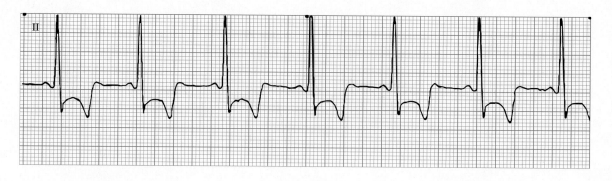

202. QRS complexes_____ Regularity_____ Heart rate_____

P waves_____

PR interval_____ QRS interval_____

Interpretation_____

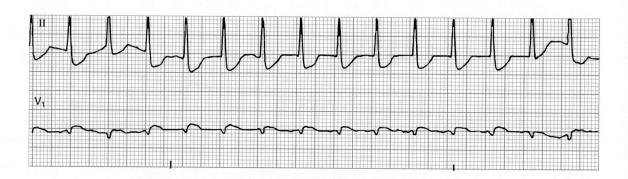

203. QRS complexes_____ Regularity_____ Heart rate_____

P waves_____

PR interval_____ QRS interval_____

Interpretation_____

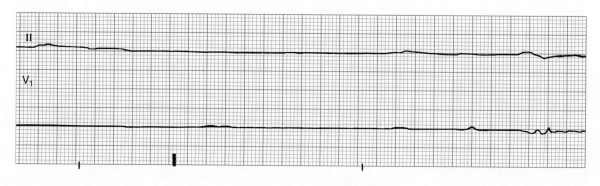

204. QRS complexes_____ Regularity_____ Heart rate_____

P waves_____

PR interval_____ QRS interval_____

Interpretation_____

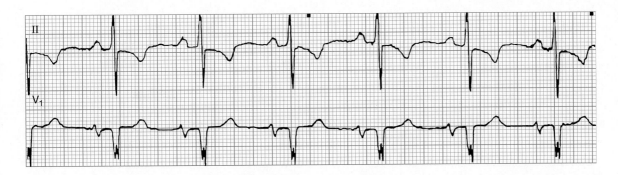

205. QRS complexes_____ Regularity_____ Heart rate_____

P waves_____

PR interval_____ QRS interval_____

Interpretation_____

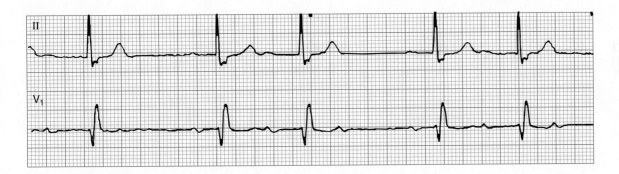

206. QRS complexes_____ Regularity_____ Heart rate_____

P waves_____

PR interval_____ QRS interval_____

Interpretation_____

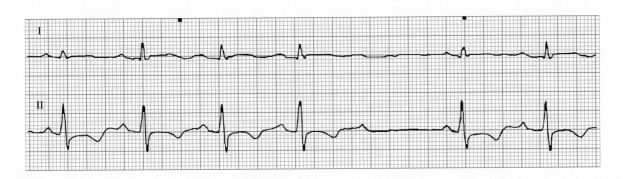

207. QRS complexes_____ Regularity_____ Heart rate_____

P waves_____

PR interval_____ QRS interval_____

Interpretation_____

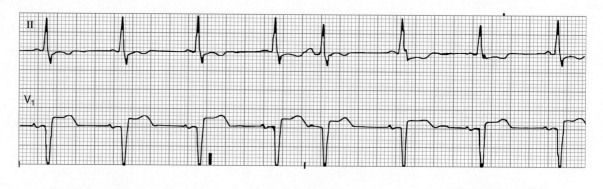

208. QRS complexes_____ Regularity_____ Heart rate_____

P waves_____

PR interval_____ QRS interval_____

Interpretation_____

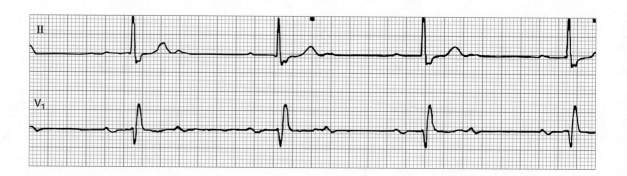

209. QRS complexes_____ Regularity_____ Heart rate_____

P waves_____

PR interval_____ QRS interval_____

Interpretation_____

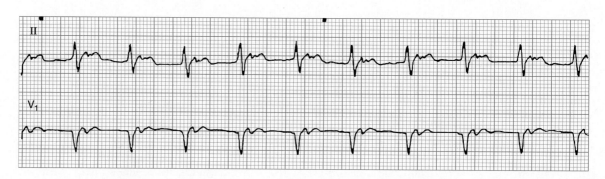

210. QRS complexes_____ Regularity_____ Heart rate_____

P waves_____

PR interval_____ QRS interval_____

Interpretation_____

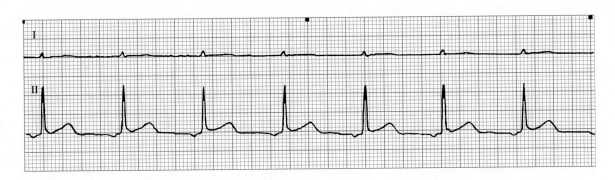

211. QRS complexes_____ Regularity_____ Heart rate_____

P waves_____

PR interval_____ QRS interval_____

Interpretation_____

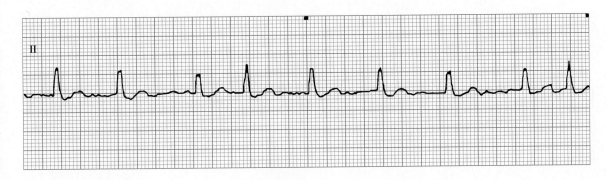

212. QRS complexes_____ Regularity_____ Heart rate_____

P waves_____

PR interval_____ QRS interval_____

Interpretation_____

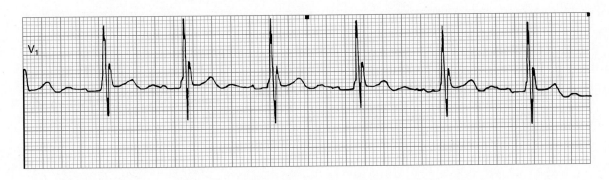

213. QRS complexes_____ Regularity_____ Heart rate_____

P waves_____

PR interval_____ QRS interval_____

Interpretation_____

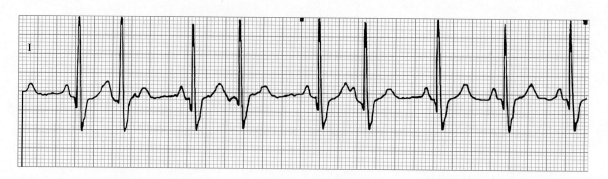

214. QRS complexes_____ Regularity_____ Heart rate_____

P waves_____

PR interval_____ QRS interval_____

Interpretation_____

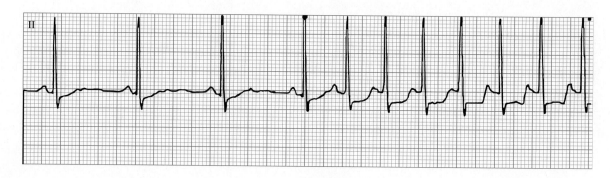

215. QRS complexes_____ Regularity_____ Heart rate_____

P waves_____

PR interval_____ QRS interval_____

Interpretation_____

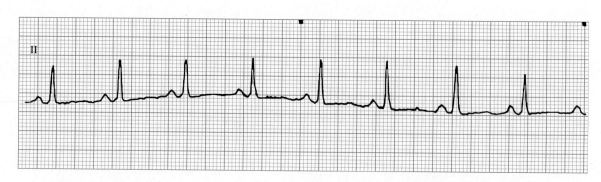

216. QRS complexes_____ Regularity_____ Heart rate_____

P waves_____

PR interval_____ QRS interval_____

Interpretation_____

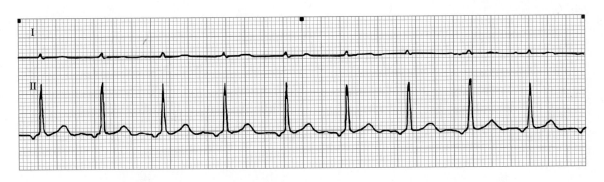

217. QRS complexes_____ Regularity_____ Heart rate_____

P waves_____

PR interval_____ QRS interval_____

Interpretation_____

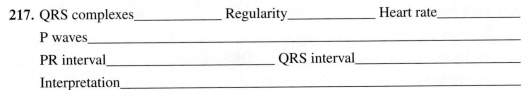

218. QRS complexes_____ Regularity_____ Heart rate_____

P waves_____

PR interval_____ QRS interval_____

Interpretation_____

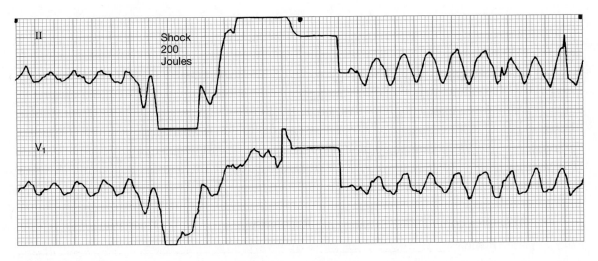

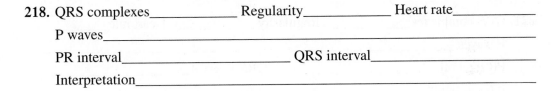

219. QRS complexes_____ Regularity_____ Heart rate_____

P waves_____

PR interval_____ QRS interval_____

Interpretation_____

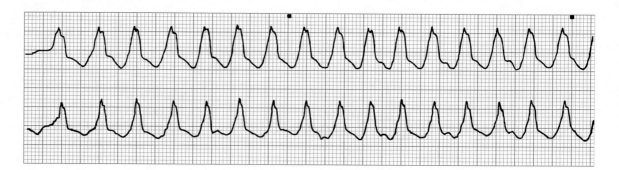

220. QRS complexes_____ Regularity_____ Heart rate_____

P waves_____

PR interval_____ QRS interval_____

Interpretation_____

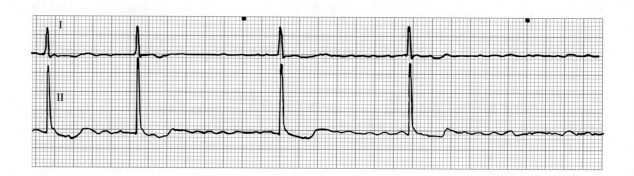

221. QRS complexes_____ Regularity_____ Heart rate_____

P waves_____

PR interval_____ QRS interval_____

Interpretation_____

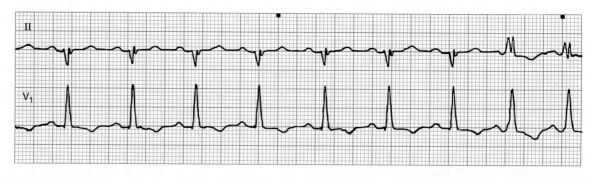

222. QRS complexes_____ Regularity_____ Heart rate_____

P waves_____

PR interval_____ QRS interval_____

Interpretation_____

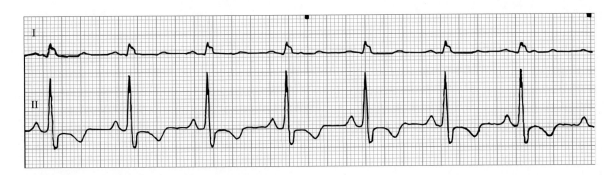

223. QRS complexes_____ Regularity_____ Heart rate_____

P waves_____

PR interval_____ QRS interval_____

Interpretation_____

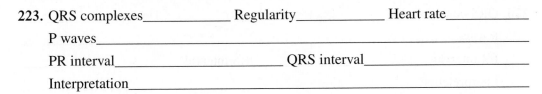

224. QRS complexes_____ Regularity_____ Heart rate_____

P waves_____

PR interval_____ QRS interval_____

Interpretation_____

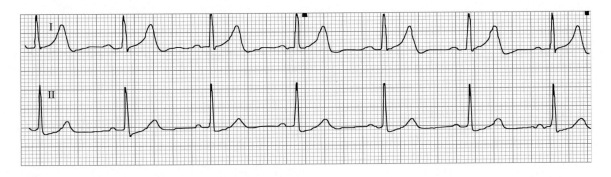

225. QRS complexes_____ Regularity_____ Heart rate_____

P waves_____

PR interval_____ QRS interval_____

Interpretation_____

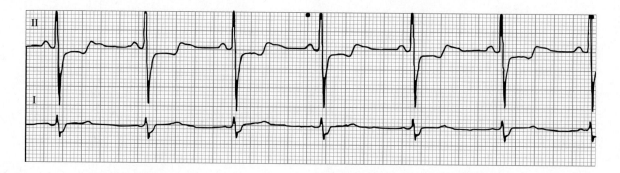

226. QRS complexes_____ Regularity_____ Heart rate_____

P waves_____

PR interval_____ QRS interval_____

Interpretation_____

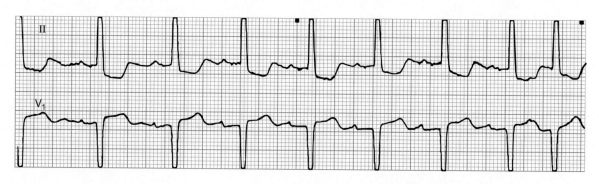

227. QRS complexes_____ Regularity_____ Heart rate_____

P waves_____

PR interval_____ QRS interval_____

Interpretation_____

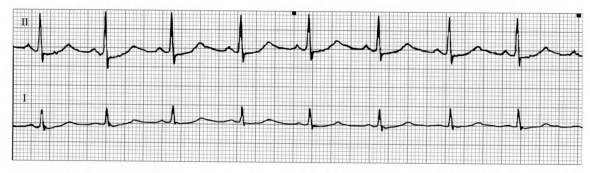

228. QRS complexes_____ Regularity_____ Heart rate_____

P waves_____

PR interval_____ QRS interval_____

Interpretation_____

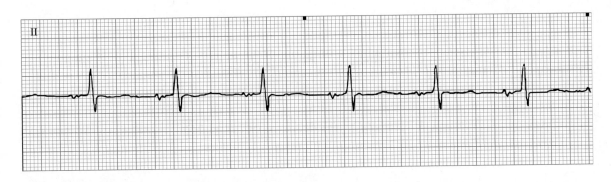

229. QRS complexes_____ Regularity_____ Heart rate_____

P waves_____

PR interval_____ QRS interval_____

Interpretation_____

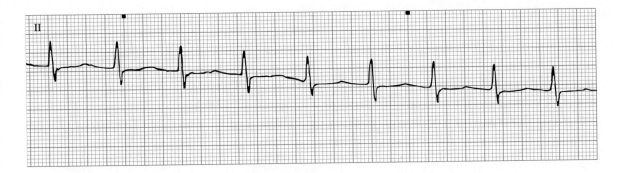

230. QRS complexes_____ Regularity_____ Heart rate_____

P waves_____

PR interval_____ QRS interval_____

Interpretation_____

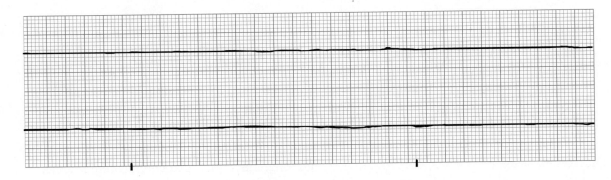

231. QRS complexes_____ Regularity_____ Heart rate_____

P waves_____

PR interval_____ QRS interval_____

Interpretation_____

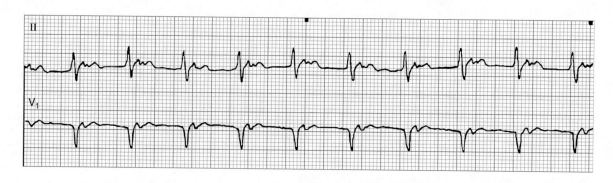

232. QRS complexes_____ Regularity_____ Heart rate_____

P waves_____

PR interval_____ QRS interval_____

Interpretation_____

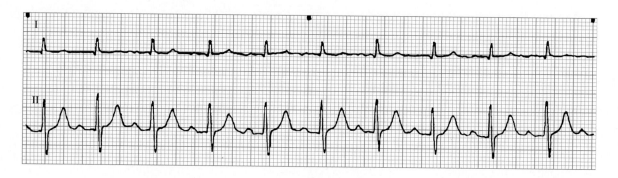

233. QRS complexes_____ Regularity_____ Heart rate_____

P waves_____

PR interval_____ QRS interval_____

Interpretation_____

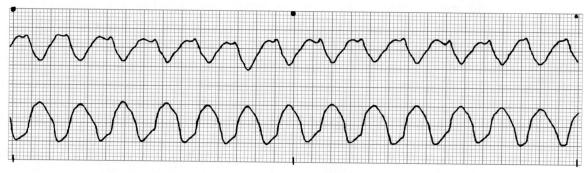

234. QRS complexes_____ Regularity_____ Heart rate_____

P waves_____

PR interval_____ QRS interval_____

Interpretation_____

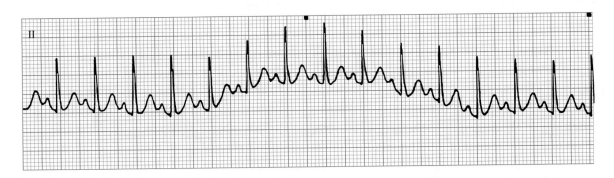

235. QRS complexes_____ Regularity_____ Heart rate_____

P waves_____

PR interval_____ QRS interval_____

Interpretation_____

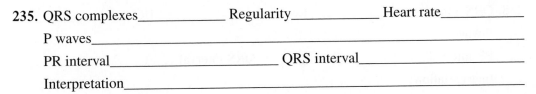

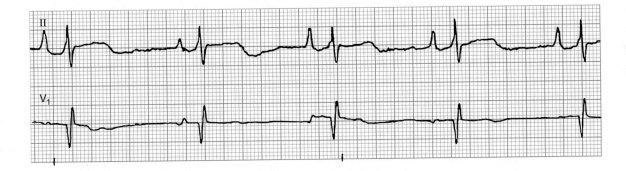

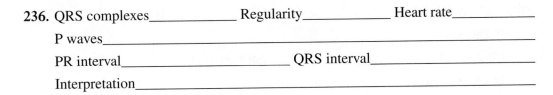

236. QRS complexes_____ Regularity_____ Heart rate_____

P waves_____

PR interval_____ QRS interval_____

Interpretation_____

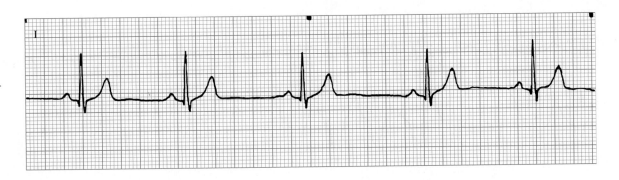

237. QRS complexes_____ Regularity_____ Heart rate_____

P waves_____

PR interval_____ QRS interval_____

Interpretation_____

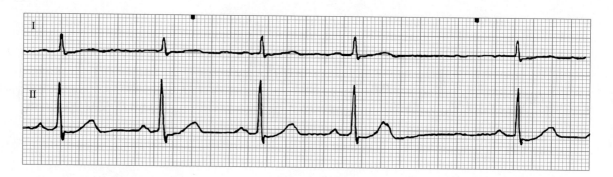

238. QRS complexes_____ Regularity_____ Heart rate_____

P waves_____

PR interval_____ QRS interval_____

Interpretation_____

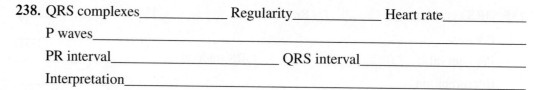

239. QRS complexes_____ Regularity_____ Heart rate_____

P waves_____

PR interval_____ QRS interval_____

Interpretation_____

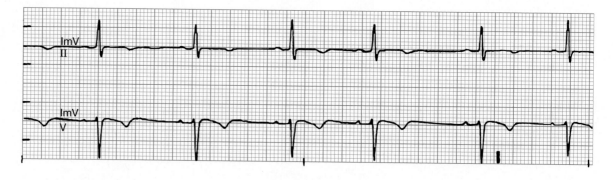

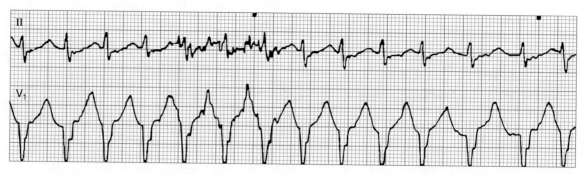

240. QRS complexes_____ Regularity_____ Heart rate_____

P waves_____

PR interval_____ QRS interval_____

Interpretation_____

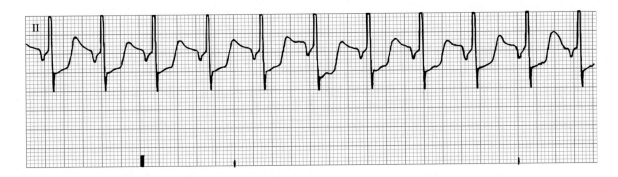

241. QRS complexes_____ Regularity_____ Heart rate_____

P waves_____

PR interval_____ QRS interval_____

Interpretation_____

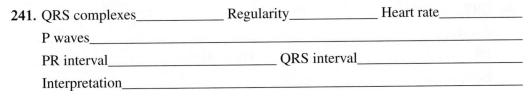

242. QRS complexes_____ Regularity_____ Heart rate_____

P waves_____

PR interval_____ QRS interval_____

Interpretation_____

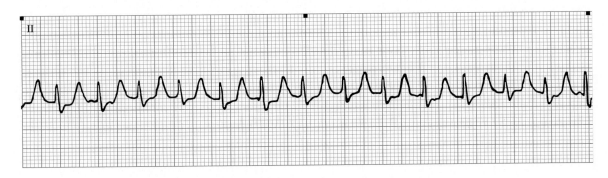

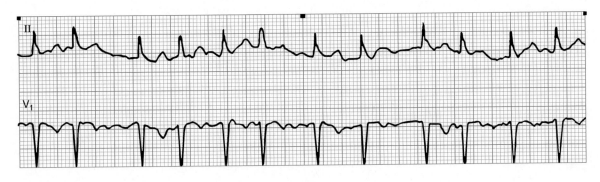

243. QRS complexes_____ Regularity_____ Heart rate_____

P waves_____

PR interval_____ QRS interval_____

Interpretation_____

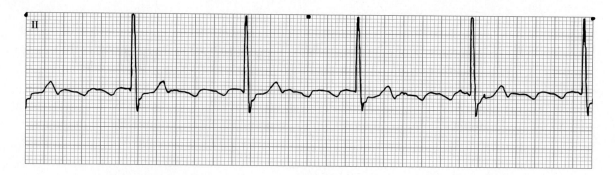

244. QRS complexes_____ Regularity_____ Heart rate_____

P waves_____

PR interval_____ QRS interval_____

Interpretation_____

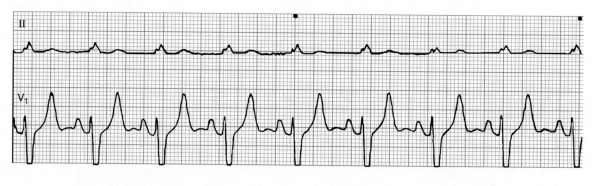

245. QRS complexes_____ Regularity_____ Heart rate_____

P waves_____

PR interval_____ QRS interval_____

Interpretation_____

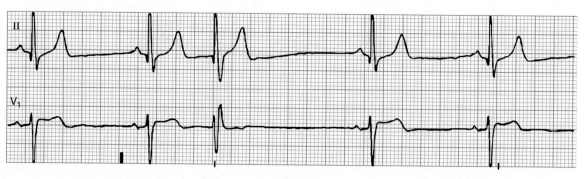

246. QRS complexes_____ Regularity_____ Heart rate_____

P waves_____

PR interval_____ QRS interval_____

Interpretation_____

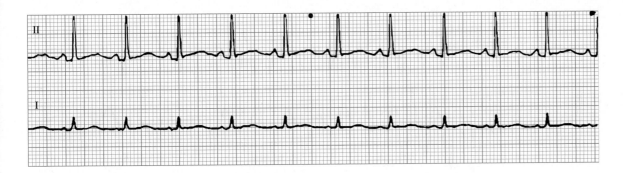

247. QRS complexes_____ Regularity_____ Heart rate_____

P waves_____

PR interval_____ QRS interval_____

Interpretation_____

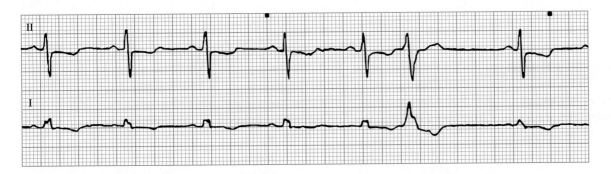

248. QRS complexes_____ Regularity_____ Heart rate_____

P waves_____

PR interval_____ QRS interval_____

Interpretation_____

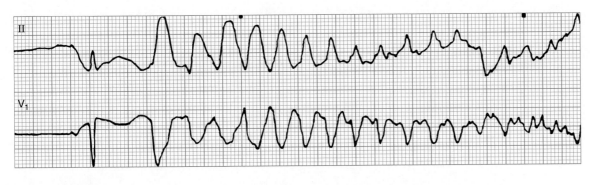

249. QRS complexes_____ Regularity_____ Heart rate_____

P waves_____

PR interval_____ QRS interval_____

Interpretation_____

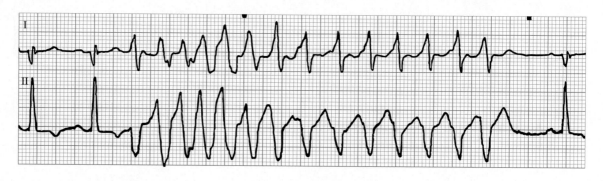

250. QRS complexes_____ Regularity_____ Heart rate_____

    P waves_____

    PR interval_____ QRS interval_____

    Interpretation_____

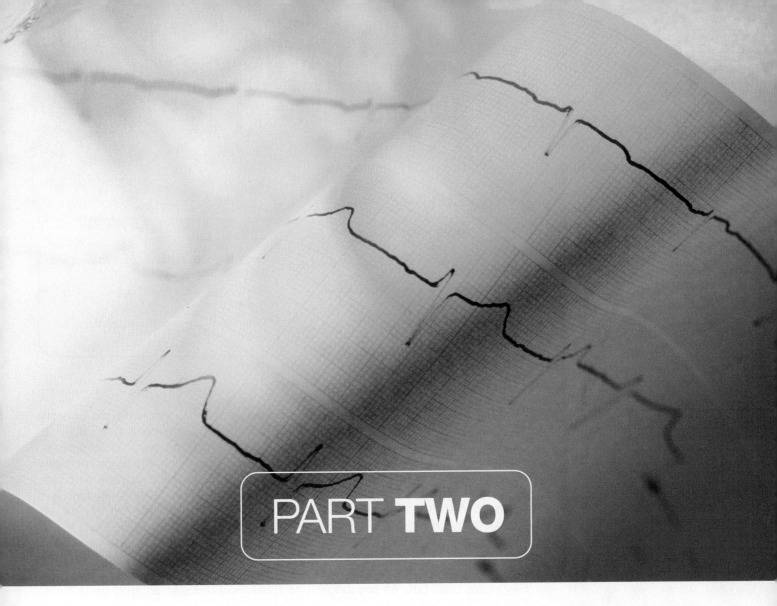

PART **TWO**

Advanced Concepts

How to Interpret a 12-Lead EKG

Upon completion of this chapter, the student will be able to:

- List the 6 steps to 12-lead EKG interpretation.
- Determine the axis quadrant on a variety of practice EKGs.
- Determine if right or left bundle branch blocks exist.

- Determine the presence of left anterior and left posterior hemiblocks.
- Identify right and left ventricular hypertrophy.
- Determine if any miscellaneous effects are present.

What It's All About

Mr. Seybourne is in the ICU complaining that he feels extremely weak. He has a history of kidney failure, and his doctors have been telling him he will soon need dialysis. "I'm trying to hold off on it as long as I can," Mr. Seybourne tells his nurse Erin. Erin draws some blood for lab work and does an EKG, on which she notes markedly tall pointy T waves consistent with hyperkalemia. She alerts the physician, who tells Mr. Seybourne that based on the EKG it looks like his potassium level is very high and he may need to start dialysis tonight. "You can tell how my labs are going to look just by looking at my EKG?" Mr. Seybourne asks the physician. "Yes, the EKG can tell us a lot of information about other things besides the heart," the physician answers. Soon the lab results are back and the potassium level is indeed alarmingly high. Other labs are also markedly elevated, so the physician alerts the dialysis nurse to come out. Mr. Seybourne can't hold off any longer—he starts his dialysis emergently tonight.

Introduction

The 12-lead EKG is a diagnostic test done primarily to identify the presence of myocardial infarction or ischemia, but it is also useful in identifying arrhythmias, electrolyte imbalances, drug toxicities, and other conditions. It is done with the patient at rest, usually in the **supine** (back-lying) position. As with rhythm interpretation, it is important to use a systematic method of assessment.

The Six Steps to 12-Lead EKG Interpretation

Use these steps in order:

1. **Interpret the basics—rhythm, heart rate, and intervals (PR, QRS, QT).** These were covered in Part I of the text. If the EKG has a rhythm strip at the bottom, assess the basics here. Otherwise, pick any lead (Leads II and V_1 are the best ones to evaluate for rhythm). Do the intervals fall within normal limits or are they abnormally shortened or prolonged?
2. **Determine the axis quadrant.** Is it normal or is there axis deviation? **Axis** is simply a method of determining the mean direction of current flow in the heart.
3. **Check for bundle branch blocks and hemiblocks (a block of a branch of the left bundle branch).**
4. **Check for ventricular hypertrophy (overgrowth of myocardial tissue).** Use V_1 and V_{5-6} to check the QRS complexes for signs of ventricular hypertrophy.

5. **Determine the presence of miscellaneous effects.**   Examine all leads for disturbances in calcium or potassium levels in the bloodstream and for digitalis effects.
6. **Check for myocardial infarction/ischemia.**   For this you'll look at all leads except aVR. You'll look for ST elevation or depression, inverted T waves, and significant Q waves. You'll also note R wave progression in the precordial leads. This will be covered in depth in Chapter 14.

Let's get started.

Axis Determination

The electrical axis is a method of determining the direction of the heart's electrical current flow. Recall that the heart's current starts normally in the sinus node and travels downward toward the left ventricle. If we drew an arrow depicting this current flow, it would point downward to the left. In abnormal hearts or abnormal rhythms, this current may travel in an unusual direction, resulting in an axis deviation (the arrow would point in a different direction).

Causes of Axis Deviations

- *Normal variant.*   It may be normal for some individuals to have an abnormal axis. In these patients, tests have ruled out any pathology as a cause.
- *Myocardial infarction.*   Infarcted (dead) tissue does not conduct electrical current, so the current travels away from this dead tissue, shifting the axis away.
- *Ventricular hypertrophy.*   Hypertrophied tissue needs more current to depolarize it, so the current shifts toward the hypertrophied area.
- *Arrhythmias.*   Arrhythmias can cause axis deviation. Ventricular rhythms, for example, start in the ventricle and send their current upward toward the atria. The axis would then point upward rather than downward.
- *Advanced pregnancy or obesity.*   Either or both conditions physically push the diaphragm and the heart upward, causing the axis to shift upward to the left.
- *Chronic lung disease and pulmonary embolism.*   These conditions cause a rightward axis shift because they enlarge the right ventricle.
- *Hemiblocks.*   These blocks of one of the branches of the left bundle branch cause impulses to travel in an alternate direction, resulting in either a right axis deviation or a left axis deviation.

Determining the Axis Quadrant

Since the axis is concerned with direction, axis calculation requires a compass. A compass has lines delineating north, south, east, and west. In axis calculation, our compass is the hexiaxial diagram superimposed on the heart, as seen in Figure 13–1. Review Chapter 2 if you need a refresher on the leads. The hexiaxial diagram has lines depicting the frontal leads—I, II, III, aVR, aVL, and aVF. Lead I runs right to left, and aVF runs up and down. The other leads are points in between. The leads are separated from one another by 30° increments. The **axis circle** is made by joining the ends of these lead lines. Note the degree markings in Figure 13–1. Current of the heart flowing from the sinus node to the left ventricle would yield an axis of about 60°. That's a normal axis.

If we use Leads I and aVF to divide the axis circle into four quadrants, normal axis would be between 0 to +90°. Left axis deviation is between 0 to −90°. Right axis deviation is between +90 to ±180°. Indeterminate axis (so-called because it cannot be determined whether it is an extreme left axis deviation or an extreme right axis deviation) is between −90 and ±180°. Note the axis quadrants in Figure 13–1.

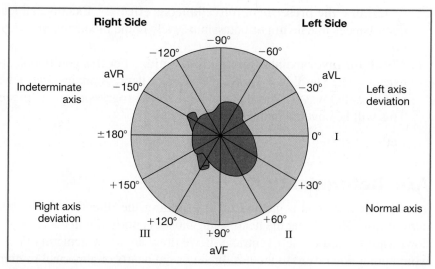

FIGURE 13-1

Axis circle and quadrants.

Look at the QRS in Leads I and aVF to determine the axis quadrant. Since Lead I connects right and left arms, it tells us whether the heart's current is traveling to the right or left; aVF is located on the leg, so it tells us whether the heart's current is traveling upward or downward. If the QRS in both Leads I and aVF is positive, the axis is normal. If Lead I is positive and aVF is negative, it's left axis deviation (LAD). If Lead I and aVF are both negative, it's indeterminate axis. If Lead I is negative but aVF is positive, it's right axis deviation (RAD). See Figure 13–2.

Quick Tip

If Leads I and aVF are both upright, you could say they're "on the up and up" and that's always good (normal).

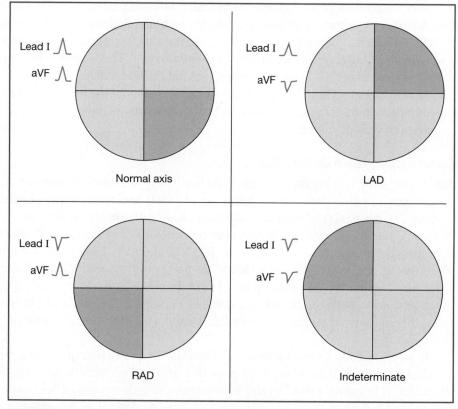

FIGURE 13-2

Determining the axis quadrant.

Axis Practice EKGs

Determine the axis quadrant on the following EKGs.

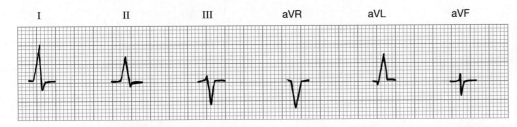

1. Axis quadrant = ___LAD___

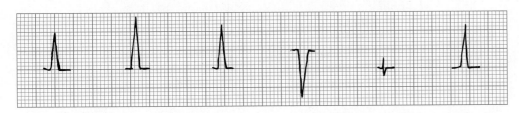

2. Axis quadrant = ___normal___

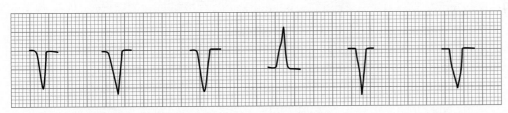

3. Axis quadrant = ~~RAD~~ indeterminant

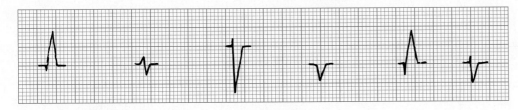

4. Axis quadrant = LAD

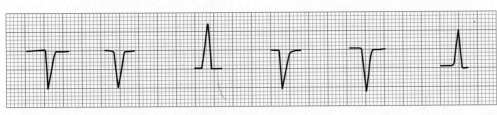

5. Axis quadrant = ~~indeterminant~~ RAD

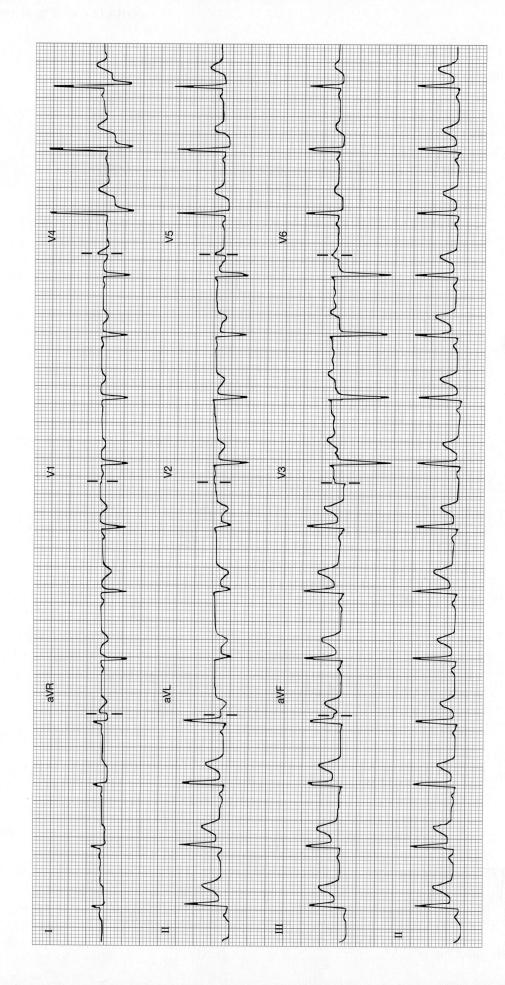

6. Axis quadrant = _____

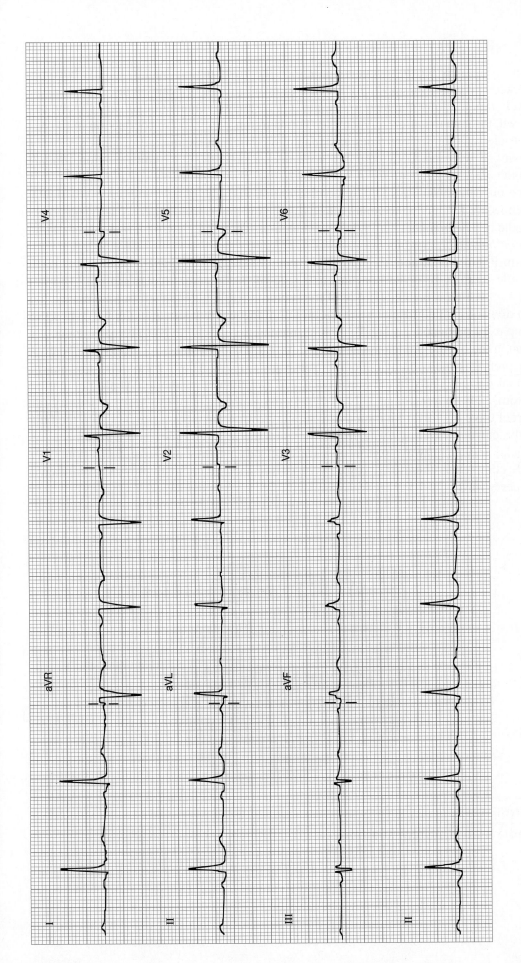

7. Axis quadrant = *normal*

Bundle Branch Blocks

Bundle branch blocks occur when either the right or left bundle branch becomes blocked and unable to conduct impulses, often as a result of heart disease. The impulse travels rapidly down the healthy bundle branch and then must trudge very slowly, cell by cell, through the affected ventricle. This difference in impulse conduction in the two ventricles causes the ventricles to depolarize consecutively instead of simultaneously, causing a widened QRS complex with a characteristic QRS configuration. *Bundle branch blocks are seen only in supraventricular (sinus, atrial, or junctional) rhythms,* since only these rhythms require conduction through the bundle branches. Ventricular rhythms are formed in the ventricular tissue below the bundle branch system and do not use the bundle branches for impulse conduction. Therefore, *ventricular rhythms cannot exhibit bundle branch blocks.*

In Figure 13–3, note the normal anatomy of the bundle branch system. The right bundle branch is located on the right side of the interventricular septum. The left bundle branch is on the left side of the septum. You'll note the left bundle branch has two divisions called fascicles. Fascicles are branches. In order to understand the QRS complexes produced by bundle branch blocks, let's first review normal conduction through the bundle branch system. We'll look at Lead V_1 since this lead is the best for interpreting bundle branch blocks. See Figure 13–4. You'll recall that the heart's normal current starts in the sinus node and travels toward the left ventricle—top to bottom, right to left. Since V_1's electrode sits to the right of the heart, it sees a little current traveling toward it (across the septum toward the right ventricle), then the bulk of the current traveling away from it toward the left ventricle. You'll recall that an impulse traveling away from a positive electrode writes a negative deflection. V_1's QRS complex is therefore primarily negative, showing a small R wave and then a deeper S wave.

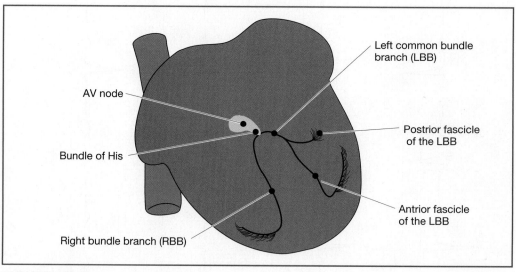

FIGURE 13–3

Bundle branch system anatomy.

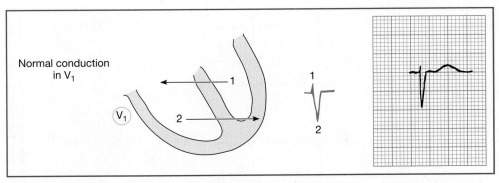

FIGURE 13–4

Normal conduction in V₁: (1) septal and beginning right ventricular activation, (2) left ventricular activation.

Right Bundle Branch Block (RBBB)

See Figure 13–5. In *right bundle branch block* (RBBB), the QRS complex typically starts out looking normal—primarily negative—indicating initial normal travel through the heart via the healthy left bundle branch. But then the QRS has an extra R wave at the end, signifying the current that's slogging slowly, cell by cell, through the right ventricle toward V₁'s electrode. Thus, V₁ has an R wave, an S wave, then another R wave. This second R wave is called **R prime** and is written R′. Occasionally a RBBB will lose its initial R wave and will instead have a small Q wave and then a prominent R wave.

All bundle branch blocks will have a QRS interval of ≥0.12 seconds and a T wave that slopes off opposite the terminal wave of the QRS complex. If the terminal wave of the QRS is upward, for example, the T wave will be inverted. If the terminal wave of the QRS is downward, the T wave will be upright. See Figure 13–5. In V₁, the QRS interval is 0.14 secs and the terminal wave of the QRS is upright, so the T wave is inverted. It is important to recognize these bundle-related T waves so as not to misinterpret them as signs of ischemia. See Figure 13–6 for a RBBB on a 12-lead EKG.

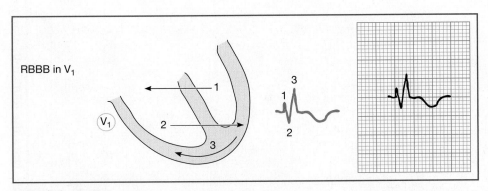

FIGURE 13–5

RBBB in V₁: (1) septal and beginning right ventricular activation, (2) left ventricular activation, (3) final right ventricular activation.

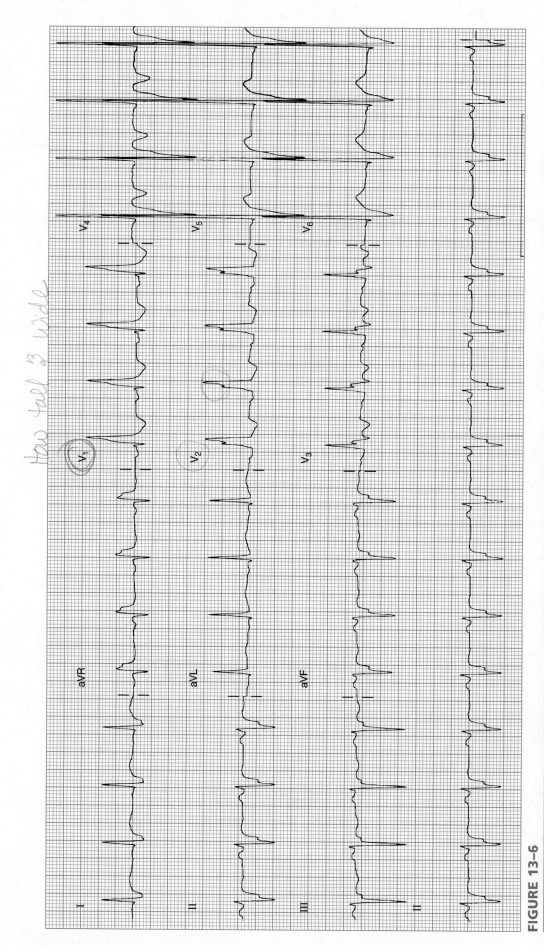

How tall 3 wide

FIGURE 13–6

Right bundle branch block. Note the RSR′ in V$_1$ along with the QRS interval ≥0.12 seconds and the T waves opposite the terminal QRS wave.

Left Bundle Branch Block (LBBB)

Left bundle branch block (LBBB) can occur in two ways: There can be a block of the left common bundle branch (the part of the left bundle branch before it divides into its fascicles) or a block of both fascicles. In either case, depolarization of the septum cannot occur normally in LBBB. See Figure 13–7. Septal depolarization must go backward, right to left, sending its current away from V_1's positive electrode. When the current reaches the left ventricle, it finds the bundle branch blocked and must traverse the left ventricular tissue slowly, one cell at a time. Meanwhile, right ventricular activation is occurring normally through the healthy right bundle branch. In Figure 13–7, numbers 1 and 2 are swallowed up inside number 3, as the huge amount of current required to activate the left ventricle dwarfs the current traveling to the septum and right ventricle. The slowed travel through the left ventricle results in a wider-than-normal S wave. LBBB in V_1 thus presents as a large, deep QS complex in V_1. On occasion, there may be a small R wave preceding the deep S wave. As with a RBBB, the QRS interval of a LBBB will be ≥0.12 secs, and the T wave will be opposite the terminal wave of the QRS complex. See Figure 13–8 for a LBBB on a 12-lead EKG.

Rate-Related BBB

Bundle branch blocks seen only at certain heart rates are known as rate-related bundle branch blocks, and the rate at which the BBB appears is called the critical rate. In this disorder, conduction through the bundle branches is normal at heart rates below the critical rate. Once the critical rate is reached, however, one of the bundle branches becomes incapable of depolarizing rapidly enough to allow normal conduction, and a BBB results. When the heart rate falls below the critical rate, bundle branch depolarization returns to normal and the BBB disappears.

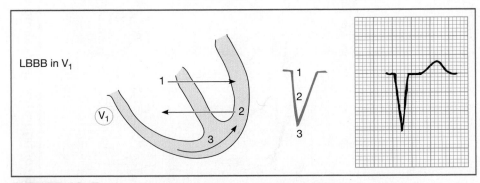

FIGURE 13–7

LBBB in V_1: (1) septal and beginning left ventricular activation, (2) right ventricular activation, (3) final left ventricular activation.

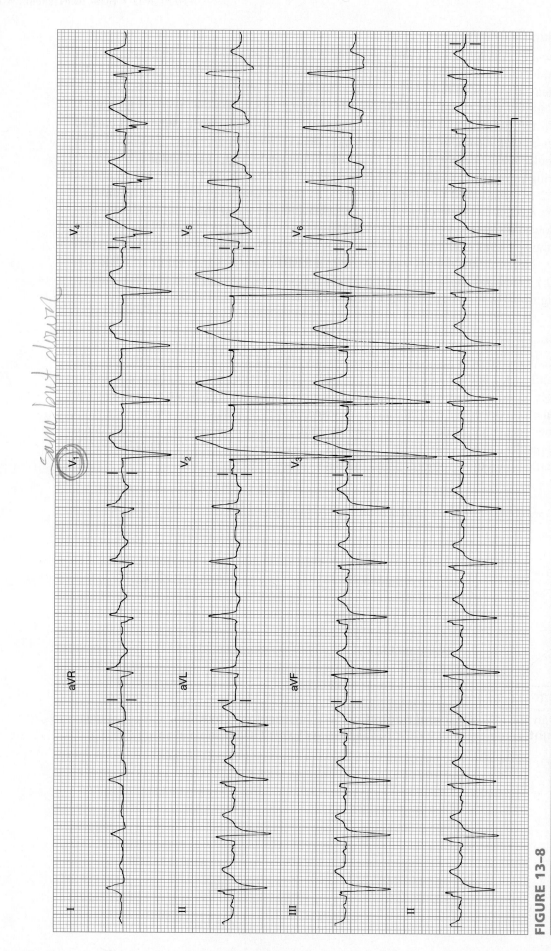

FIGURE 13-8

Left bundle branch block. Note the RS configuration in V_1 along with the widened QRS interval ($\geq$0.12 seconds) and the T wave opposite the terminal wave of the QRS.

Clinical Implications of BBB

Bundle branch blocks do not cause symptoms. In fact, they *are* a symptom of an impaired conduction system. The question is what's causing the BBB? Although RBBB can be seen in normal healthy hearts, LBBB almost always implies extensive cardiac disease. Patients with bundle branch block are at risk for developing severe AV blocks (e.g., if both bundle branches become blocked simultaneously), so it is important to observe their rhythm closely for further signs of conduction disturbance, such as a new first-degree AV block. *A new bundle branch block should prompt an immediate assessment of the patient.* A 12-lead EKG should be done in an effort to determine the cause of the BBB. Remember—*the BBB is a symptom of another problem.* For example, the BBB might be a result of an MI in progress. Also remember that BBBs cause T wave changes that can be misinterpreted as ischemia. Certain kinds of MIs usually cannot be diagnosed in the presence of an LBBB, as the bundle-related changes mask the MI. See Figure 13–9 for a summary of the criteria and causes of bundle branch blocks.

Type of BBB	QRS configuration in V_1	QRS interval	T wave	Causes
RBBB	RSR' 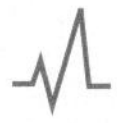	≥0.12 secs	Opposite the terminal QRS	• Coronary artery disease • Condition system lesion • Normal variant • Right ventricular hypertrophy • Congenital heart disease • Right ventricular dilatation
LBBB	QS or RS 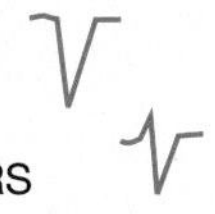	≥0.12 secs	Opposite the terminal QRS	• Coronary artery disease • Condition system lesion • Hypertension • Other organic heart disease

FIGURE 13–9

Summary of criteria and causes of bundle branch blocks.

chapter CHECKUP

We're about halfway through this chapter. To evaluate your understanding of the material thus far, answer the following questions. If you have trouble with them, review the material again before continuing.

1. Name the steps to EKG interpretation.
2. State the causes of axis deviation.
3. Determine the axis quadrant if the QRS is positive in Leads I and aVF, and if both are negative.
4. State the criteria for RBBB and LBBB.

Hemiblock

Before we leave bundle branch blocks, let's briefly discuss hemiblocks. A *hemiblock* is a block of one of the fascicles of the left bundle branch. There are two kinds of hemiblocks: **left anterior hemiblock** (LAHB), a block in the left anterior fascicle of the left bundle branch, and **left posterior hemiblock** (LPHB), a block in the posterior fascicle.

Unlike bundle branch blocks, hemiblocks do not cause QRS widening, but they do cause axis deviation. Left anterior hemiblock results in left axis deviation, and left posterior hemiblock results in right axis deviation. LAHB is much more common than LPHB because LPHB has a dual blood supply—the circumflex and right coronary arteries—and LAHB has only a single blood supply—the left anterior descending coronary artery. Hemiblocks that occur alone are not usually clinically significant. If they occur simultaneously with RBBB, however, they can predispose the patient to AV blocks because that means that two of the conduction pathways to the ventricle are blocked. Hemiblocks are caused by the same factors that cause bundle branch blocks. Treatment is not required for hemiblocks per se, but treat AV blocks if they occur. See Figure 13–10 for hemiblock configurations.

Now let's look at an algorithm for bundle branch blocks and hemiblocks. You can use Figure 13–11 to help decide if there's a BBB and/or hemiblock, and what kind it is. Look back at Figure 13–6. We know there's a RBBB there but there's also a hemiblock. Can you tell what kind?

It's LAHB. See the left axis deviation along with the RBBB?

Now let's practice. Look for BBBs and hemiblocks.

> **Quick Tip**
>
> Hemiblocks can accompany right bundle branch blocks but not left bundle branch blocks. LBBB already implies that both fascicles are blocked.

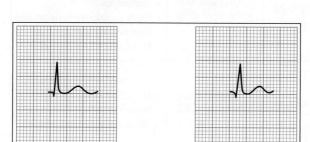

Lead I   Lead III

Normal QRS configuration in leads I and III.

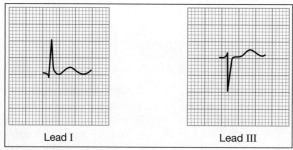

Lead I   Lead III

QRS configuration in LAHB.

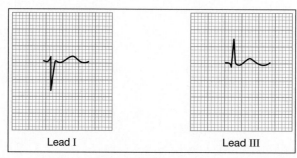

Lead I   Lead III

QRS configuration in LPHB.

FIGURE 13–10

QRS configuration in hemiblocks.

Bundle Branch Block/Hemiblock Algorithm

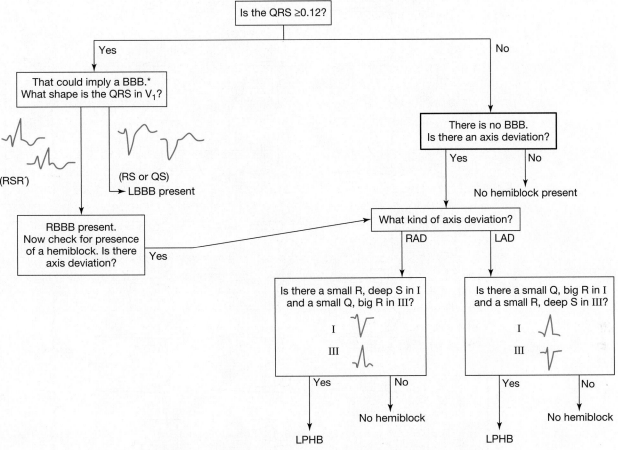

*Wide QRS complexes could be ventricular in origin, rather than a BBB.

FIGURE 13–11

Bundle branch block/hemiblock algorithm.

BBB Practice

1. Type of BBB/HB (if any): _____

1. wide QRS
  w/ R waves (normal)
2. T waves opposite QRS

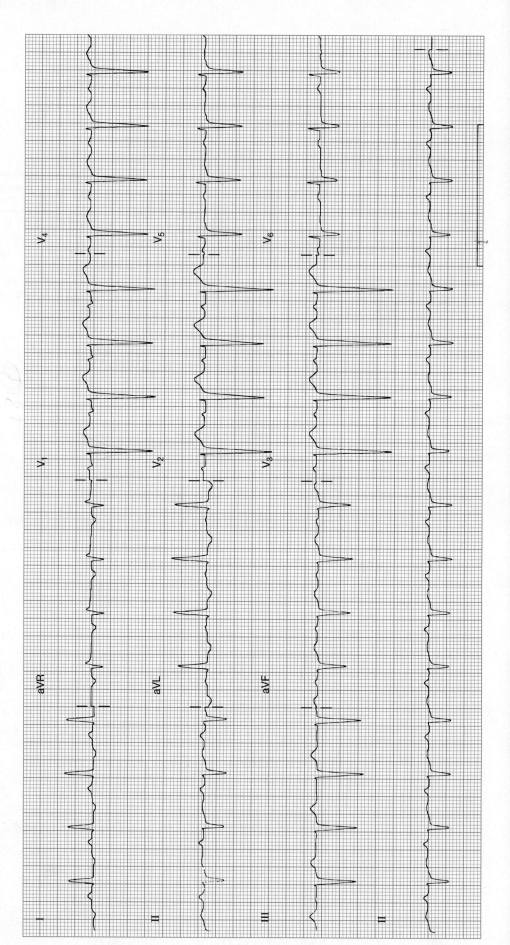

I

II

III

II

aVR

aVL

aVF

V1

V2

V3

V4

V5

V6

2. Type of BBB/HB (if any): _____

I   aVR   V₁   V₄
II   aVL   V₂   V₅
III aVF   V₃   V₆
II

279

3. Type of BBB/HB (if any): _____

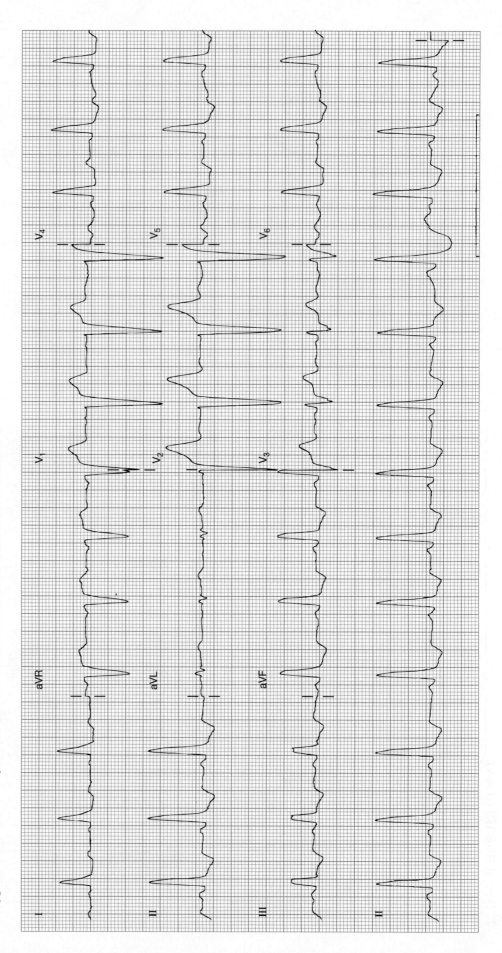

4. Type of BBB/HB (if any): _____

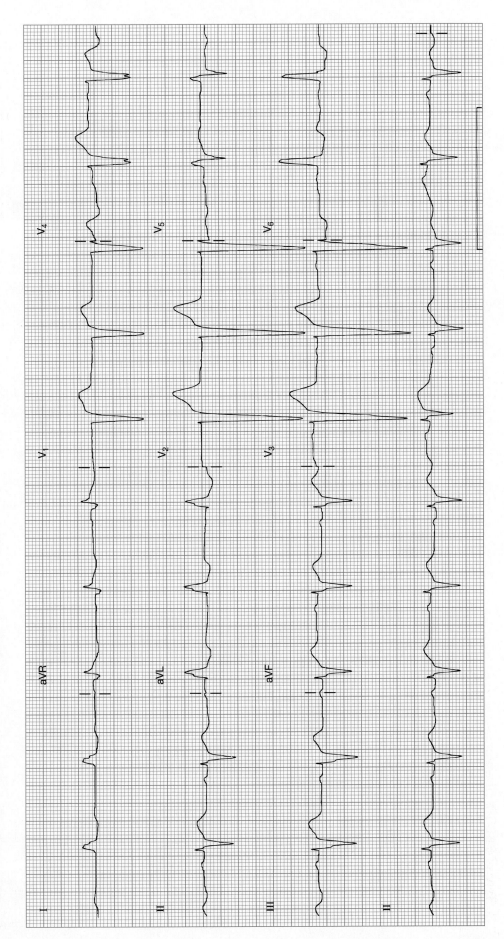

5. Type of BBB/HB (if any): _____

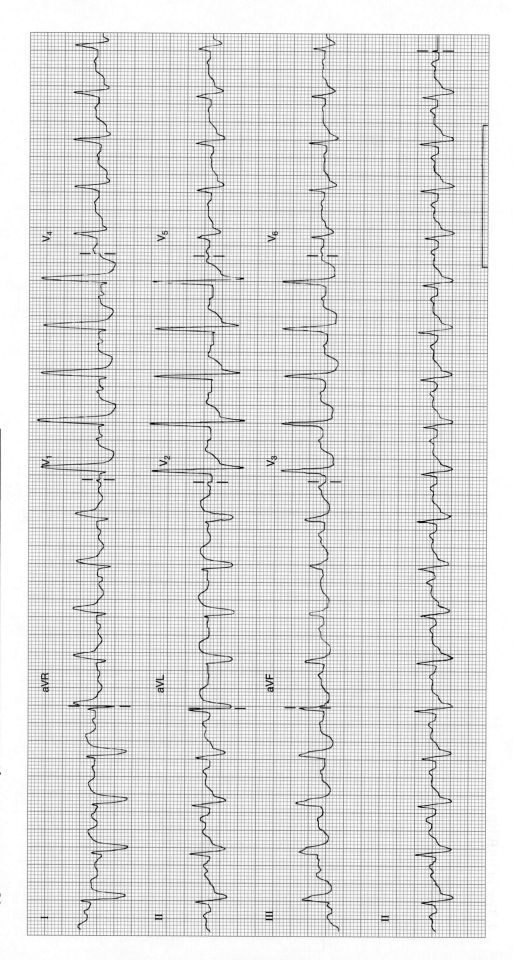

6. Type of BBB/HB (if any): _____

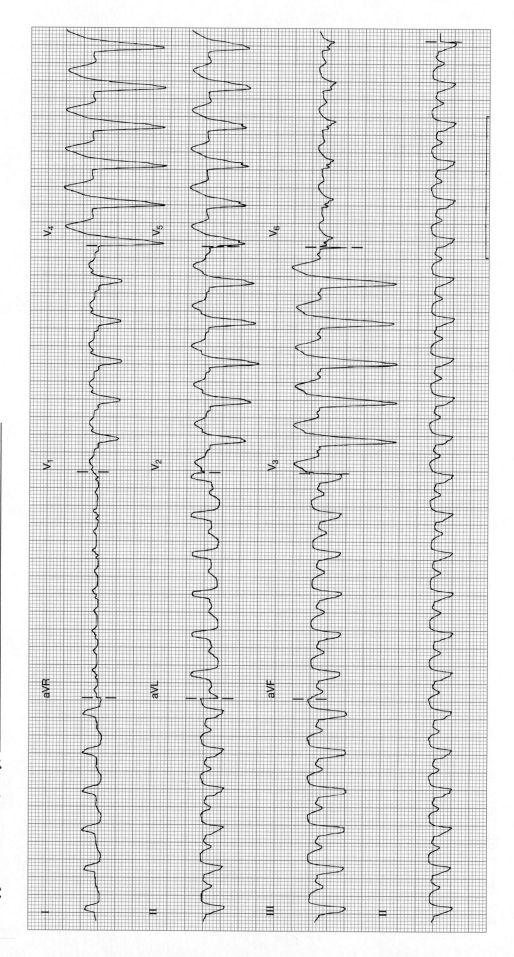

7. Type of BBB/HB (if any): _____

284

8. Type of BBB/HB (if any): _____

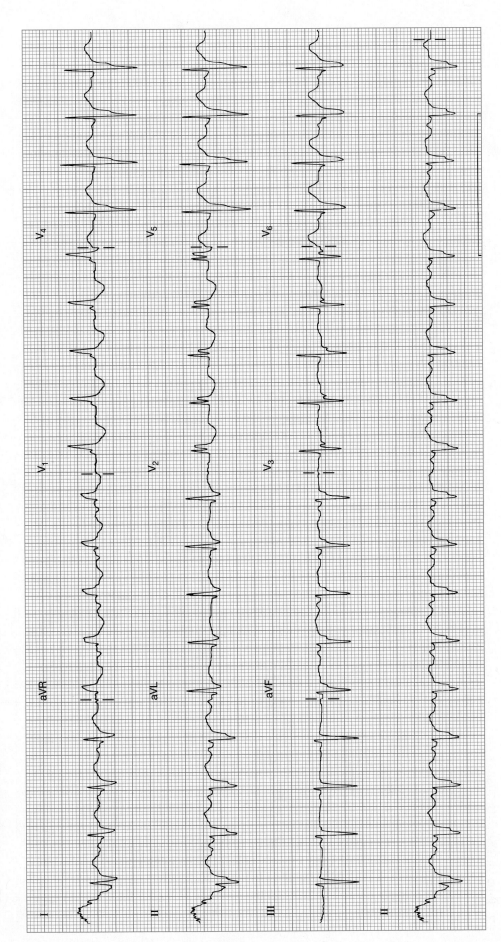

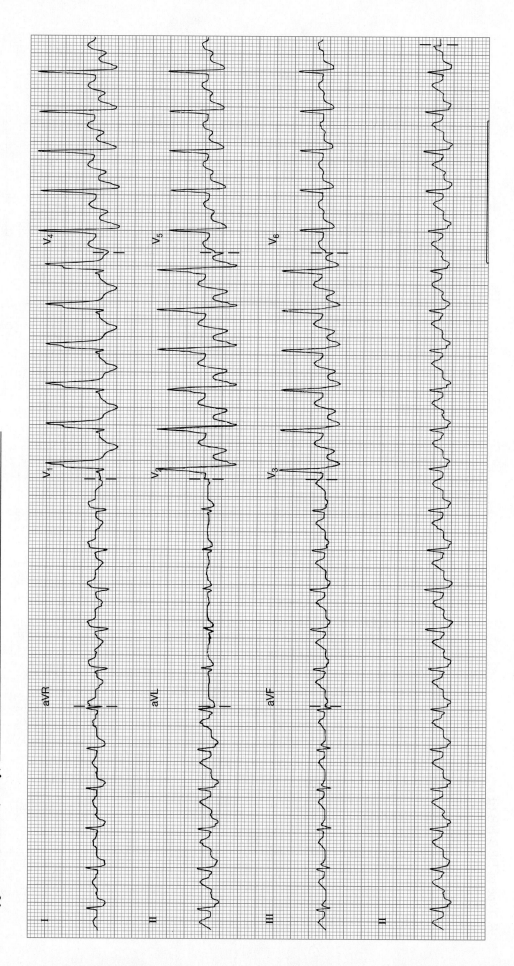

9. Type of BBB/HB (if any): _____

10. Type of BBB/HB (if any): _____

287

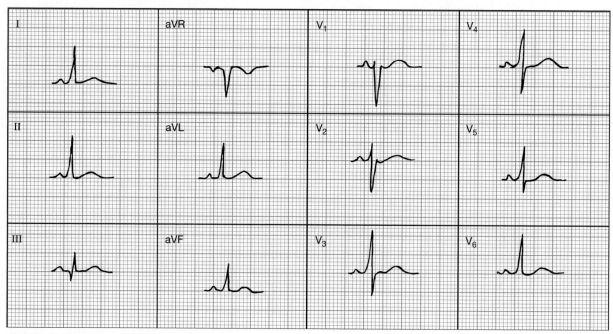

FIGURE 13–12

Normal QRS amplitude (voltage).

Ventricular Hypertrophy

Hypertrophy refers to excessive growth of tissue. In ventricular hypertrophy, the muscle mass of the right or left ventricle (or both) is thickened, usually as a result of disease. This thickened tissue requires more current to depolarize it and thus causes greater-than-normal amplitude (voltage) of the QRS complexes in the leads over the hypertrophied ventricle. Let's look at an example of normal QRS amplitude. See Figure 13–12. *The normal QRS complex should be no taller or deeper than 13 mm high (13 small blocks) in any lead.*

Right Ventricular Hypertrophy (RVH)

Right ventricular hypertrophy (RVH) is evidenced on the EKG by a tall R wave in V_1 (greater than or equal to the size of the S wave), accompanied by a right axis deviation and, often noted but not required, T wave inversion. Since the R wave in V_1 represents depolarization of the right ventricle, it will be taller than normal if the right ventricle is enlarged. The most common cause of RVH is chronic lung disease, which forces the right ventricle to bulk up in order to force its blood out into the now high-pressure lung system. See Figure 13–13 for an example of the typical QRST configuration in RVH in V_1.

Now let's see what RVH looks like on a 12-lead EKG. See Figure 13–14.

Left Ventricular Hypertrophy (LVH)

Left ventricular hypertrophy (LVH) is most commonly caused by hypertension (high blood pressure), which causes the left ventricle to bulk up in order to expel its blood against the great resistance of the abnormally high blood pressure.

LVH has several possible criteria but the one most commonly used is the following:

R wave in V_5 or V_6 (whichever is taller) + the S wave in $V_1 \geq 35$ mm

FIGURE 13–13

QRST configuration typical of RVH in V_1.

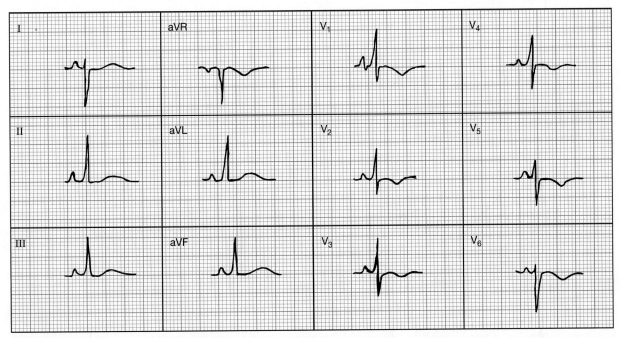

FIGURE 13–14

Right ventricular hypertrophy. Note that the R wave in V₁ is taller than the S wave is deep; there are right axis deviation and T wave inversion.

In LVH, Leads I, aVL, V$_5$, and V$_6$ will have taller-than-normal R waves as the current travels toward their positive electrodes; Leads V$_1$ and V$_2$ will have deeper-than-normal S waves as the current travels away from their positive electrode. See Figure 13–15. Add the height of the R wave in V$_5$ to the depth of the S wave in V$_1$. The result is ≥35 mm. This is LVH by voltage criteria. See Figure 13–16 for a 12-lead EKG example of LVH.

Ventricular hypertrophy does not usually prolong the QRS interval beyond normal limits.

Low-Voltage EKGs

It should be immediately obvious, when checking for hypertrophy, whether there is abnormally *low voltage* of the QRS complexes. Some people have abnormally low-voltage EKGs, in which the waves and complexes are shorter than usual. See Figure 13–17. Note the difference in voltage between this EKG and the normal one in Figure 13–12. Low-voltage EKGs, contrary to what may seem logical, do not imply that the heart is smaller than normal, or that it is generating less current than normal. It is usually caused by an outside influence that affects the heart's current on its way to the electrodes on the skin.

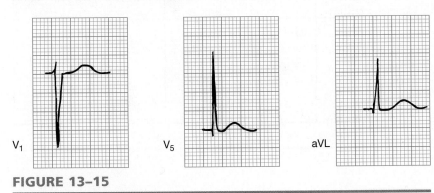

FIGURE 13–15

LVH by voltage criteria.

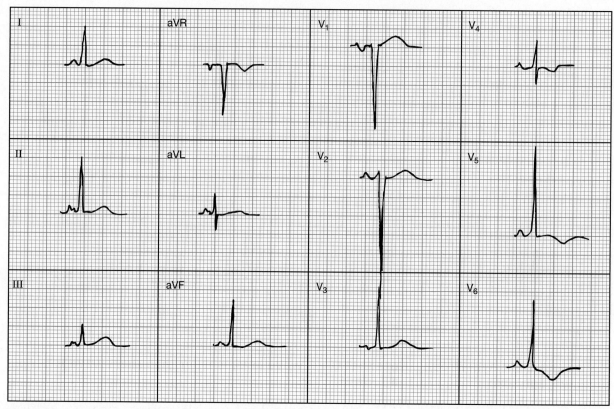

FIGURE 13–16

Left ventricular hypertrophy. Note the S wave in V_1 is 22 mm deep, and the R in V_5 is 24 mm tall, for a total voltage of 46 mm. This meets and exceeds the criteria for LVH.

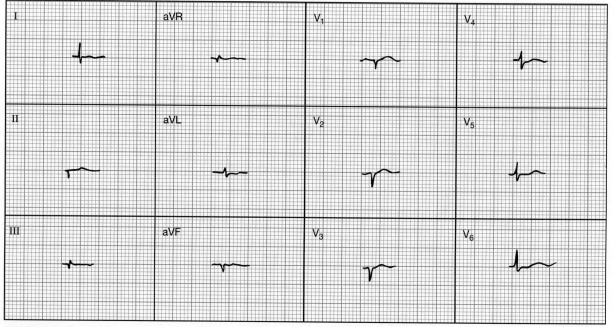

FIGURE 13–17

Low-voltage EKG.

Some causes of a low-voltage EKG are the following:

- *Obesity.*   Fatty tissue muffles the cardiac impulse on its way to the electrodes on the skin.
- *Emphysema.*   Air trapping in the lungs muffles the impulse.
- *Myxedema.*   The thyroid gland function is abnormally low, causing decreased voltage.
- *Pericardial effusion.*   Excessive fluid inside the pericardial sac surrounding the heart muffles the impulse on its way to the skin.

Clinical Implications of Hypertrophy

Hypertrophy is the heart's way of attempting to meet a contractile demand that cannot be met by normal-size heart muscle. Unfortunately, hypertrophy also places increased demands on the coronary circulation to feed that extra muscle bulk. When that increased blood and oxygen demand cannot be adequately met, ischemia results. Hypertrophy increases the likelihood of ischemia and infarction simply by increasing the amount of muscle to be nourished by the coronary arteries.

Ventricular dilatation, a stretching of the myocardial fibers that results from overfilling of the ventricles or inadequate pumping of blood out of the ventricles, can also result in a hypertrophy pattern on the EKG.

Hypertrophy Practice

Look for hypertrophy and low voltage on the following EKGs. Your answer will be one of these: RVH, LVH, low voltage, or normal.

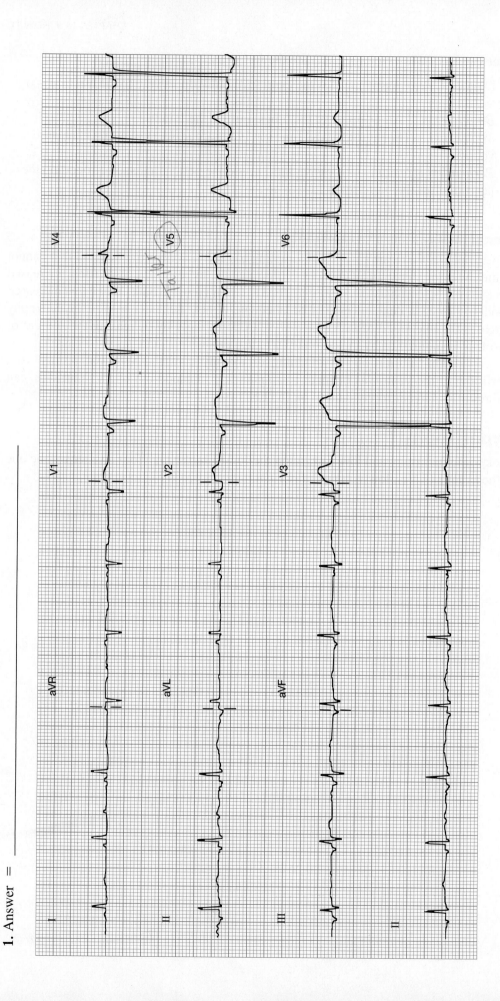

1. Answer = _____

2. Answer = _____

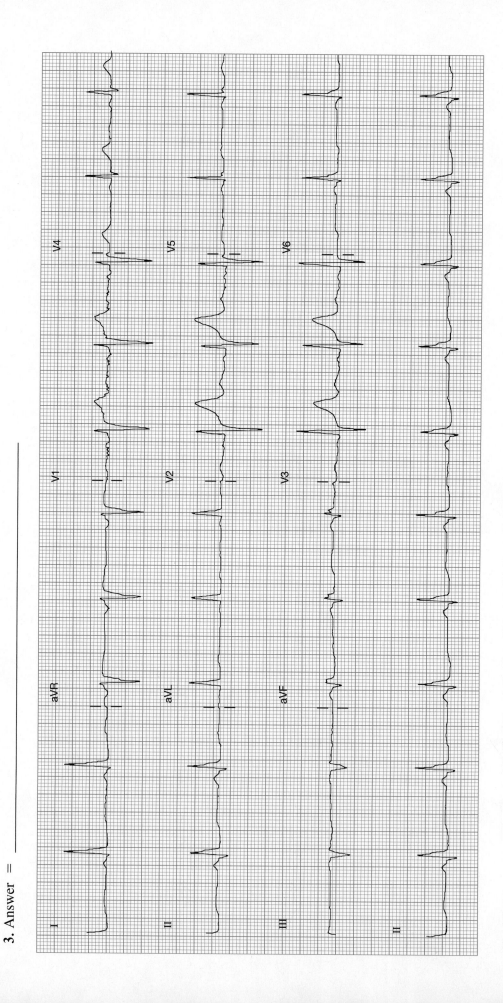

3. Answer = _____

4. Answer = _____

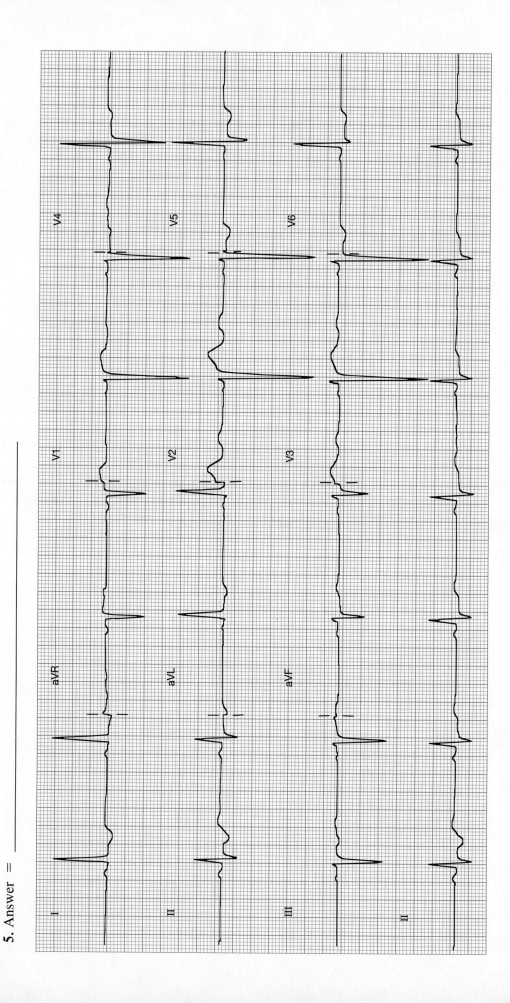

5. Answer = _____

Miscellaneous Effects

Electrolyte (blood chemicals) abnormalities and certain medications can affect the EKG. Let's look at some of these effects.

Digitalis Effect

Digitalis is a medication given to increase the force of myocardial contraction in patients with heart failure, or to slow the heart rate in patients with tachycardias. Digitalis medications are notorious for causing sagging ST segment depression (also called a scooping ST segment) that is easily misinterpreted as ischemia. The cause of this ST segment change is still not understood. Digitalis also prolongs the PR interval because it slows conduction through the AV node. These effects are not necessarily indicative of digitalis toxicity (excessive digitalis in the bloodstream), as they also occur at normal therapeutic levels. See Figure 13–18. See the sagging, very rounded ST segments and prolonged PR interval? This is typical of the digitalis effect.

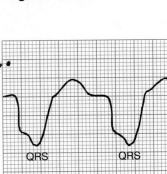

FIGURE 13–18

Digitalis effect.

Electrolyte Abnormalities

Hyperkalemia

Hyperkalemia, a high potassium level in the blood-stream, has two main EKG effects. First, potassium levels of about 6 cause tall, pointy, narrow T waves. (Normal blood potassium level is around 3.5 to 5.) As the potassium level rises to around 8, the tall T wave is replaced by a widened QRS complex. This widened QRS is a sign that cardiac arrest may be imminent if the potassium level is not lowered quickly. These EKG effects are due to potassium's effect on depolarization and repolarization and will return to normal once the potassium level is normalized. One way to remember potassium's effect on the T wave is to think of the T wave as a tent containing potassium: the more potassium, the taller the tent. See Figure 13–19. In Figure 13–19A, note the tall, pointy T waves. In Figure 13–19B, note the widened QRS complex.

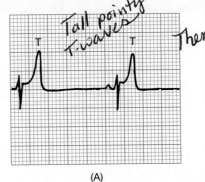

(A)

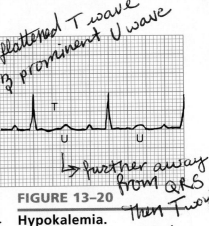

(B)

FIGURE 13–19

Hyperkalemia.

Hypokalemia

A low potassium level in the bloodstream results in a prominent U wave and flattened T waves. The potassium tent is almost empty, so it flattens out. These effects occur because repolarization, especially phase 3 of the action potential, is disturbed by the potassium deficit. See Figure 13–20.

Note the flattened T wave and the prominent U wave in Figure 13–20. Recall the U wave is not usually seen on the EKG, but if it is present it follows the T wave. T waves always follow QRS complexes. *If there are no obvious T waves on the strip, be sure the QRS complexes are really QRS complexes and not artifact.* Then, if you still can't see T waves following those QRS complexes, you can be reasonably sure the potassium level is quite low, usually around a blood level of 2.0. T waves will improve after supplemental potassium is given.

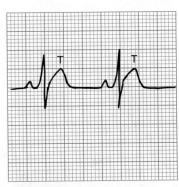

FIGURE 13–20

Hypokalemia.

Hypercalcemia

Hypercalcemia, an elevated blood calcium level, causes the ST segment to shorten to such an extent that the T wave seems to be almost on top of the QRS. This effect occurs because the elevated calcium level shortens the repolarization phase of the action potential. See Figure 13–21.

In Figure 13–21, note the extremely short ST segment that results in a short QT interval. The ST segment and QT interval will return to normal once the calcium level is normalized.

FIGURE 13–21

Hypercalcemia.

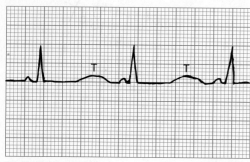

FIGURE 13–22

Hypocalcemia.

Hypocalcemia

Hypocalcemia, low calcium levels in the bloodstream, prolong repolarization and cause a prolonged ST segment, thus prolonging the QT interval.

In Figure 13–22, note how far the T wave is from the QRS complex. This demonstrates a very prolonged ST segment and QT interval.

See Figure 13–23 for a summary of miscellaneous effects.

We now can evaluate *almost all* of a 12-lead EKG with one very important exception—we need to know if our patient is having an MI. Let's check that out in the next chapter.

EFFECT	EKG CHANGE
Digitalis effect	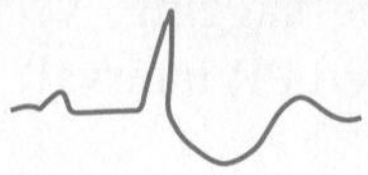 Prolonged PR interval, sagging ST segment depression
Hyperkalemia	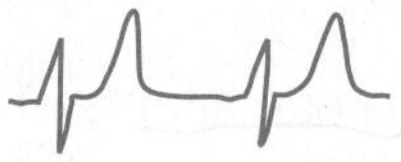 Tall, narrow, pointy T waves
Severe hyperkalemia	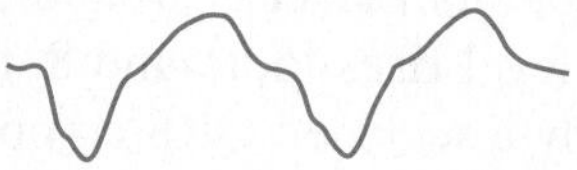 Widened QRS complex
Hypokalemia	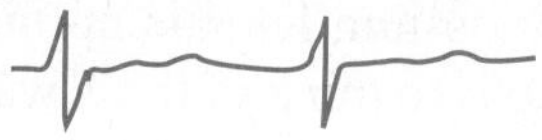 Flattened T wave, prominent U wave
Hypercalcemia	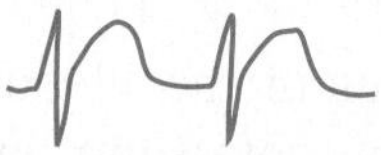 Shortened, almost nonexistent, ST segment causing shortened QT interval
Hypocalcemia	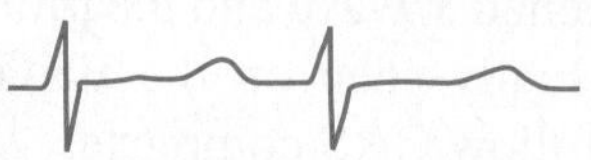 Prolonged ST segment, causing prolonged QT interval

FIGURE 13–23

Miscellaneous effects summary.

chapter thirteen notes TO SUM IT ALL UP . . .

- **Six steps to 12-lead EKG interpretation:**
  - *The basics*—Rhythm, heart rate, intervals
  - Axis quadrant
  - Bundle branch blocks/hemiblocks
  - Ventricular hypertrophy
  - Miscellaneous effects
  - MI/ischemia
- **Causes of axis deviation:**
  - Normal variant
  - MI
  - Ventricular hypertrophy
  - Arrhythmias
  - Advanced pregnancy or obesity
  - Chronic lung disease, pulmonary embolus
  - Hemiblocks
- **Axis quadrants:**
  - *Normal*—Leads I and aVF both positive, axis 0 to +90 degrees
  - *LAD*—Lead I positive, aVF negative, axis 0 to −90 degrees
  - *RAD*—Lead I negative, aVF positive, axis +90 to ±180 degrees
  - *Indeterminate*—Leads I and aVF both negative, axis −90 to ± 180 degrees
- **Right bundle branch block**—RSR′ in V_1; QRS ≥ 0.12 secs. Caused by coronary artery disease, conduction system lesions, right ventricular hypertrophy, congenital heart disease, right ventricular dilatation. Can be normal.

- **Left bundle branch block**—RS or QS in V_1; QRS ≥ 0.12 secs. Caused by coronary artery disease, hypertension, conduction system lesion, other heart disease. Is *never* normal.
- **Rate-related BBB**—Occurs at a critical rate—when bundle branches can't depolarize fast enough to keep up.
- **Hemiblock**—Block of one of the fascicles of the left bundle branch.
  - *LAHB*—Small Q in Lead I, small R in Lead III, left axis deviation, QRS <0.12 secs
  - *LPHB*—Small R in Lead I, small Q in Lead III, right axis deviation, QRS <0.12 secs
- **Right ventricular hypertrophy**—Tall R in V_1 (≥S wave), right axis deviation; may or may not have inverted T wave
- **Left ventricular hypertrophy**—R wave in V_5 or V_6 + S in V_1 ≥ 35
- **Low voltage EKGs caused by:**
  - Obesity
  - Emphysema
  - Myxedema
  - Pericardial effusion
- **Hypertrophy strains the heart and causes ventricular enlargement or dilatation.**
- **Digitalis effect**—Sagging or scooping ST segments
- **Hyperkalemia**—Tall, pointy T waves, then eventually widened QRS complexes
- **Hypokalemia**—Prominent U waves, flattened T waves
- **Hypercalcemia**—Shortened ST segment
- **Hypocalcemia**—Prolonged ST segment

Practice Quiz

1. If the QRS complexes in Leads I and aVF are both negative, in what quadrant is the axis?

_____

2. True or False. Right bundle branch block almost always implies cardiovascular disease.

3. Sagging ST segments are associated with which miscellaneous effect?

_____

4. True or False. Tall, pointy T waves are typical of RBBB.

5. Name three causes of axis deviations.

_____

6. Write the voltage criteria for LVH.

_____

7. True or False. RVH is always associated with an inverted T wave.

8. Define *hypertrophy.* _____

_____

9. Hypokalemia has what effect on the T wave?

_____

10. In a BBB, the QRS interval must be at least_____ seconds.

Putting It All Together—Critical Thinking Exercises

These exercises may consist of diagrams to label, scenarios to analyze, brain-stumping questions to ponder, or other challenging exercises to boost your understanding of the chapter material.

1. If both the right and left bundle branches became blocked simultaneously and no lower pacemaker took over to control the ventricles, which rhythm would result?

   _____

2. Draw the characteristic QRS configuration of a RBBB and a LBBB in V_1.

3. Your patient is a 29-year-old female who has a 6-month-old baby and 8-year-old twins. She had an EKG about 7 months ago and again today. In the first EKG, Lead I was positive and aVF was negative. Today Leads I and aVF are both positive. Explain what happened. _____

   _____

   _____

Myocardial Infarction

14

CHAPTER 14 OBJECTIVES

Upon completion of this chapter, the student will be able to:

- Describe the difference between ST elevation MI (STEMI) and non-ST elevation MI (NSTEMI).
- State the symptoms of MI.
- Describe the three Is of infarction.
- Describe what EKG changes are associated with ischemia, injury, and infarction.
- Draw the different kinds of ST segment abnormalities and explain what each implies.
- Draw the different T wave abnormalities and explain what each implies.
- Describe how a significant Q wave differs from a normal Q wave.
- Describe normal R wave progression.
- Identify the transition zone in a variety of EKGs.
- Describe where the transition zone is for clockwise and counterclockwise rotation.

- Describe the EKG changes associated with MI evolution and give the timeline associated with each change.
- Explain how to determine the age of an MI.
- Name the four walls of the left ventricle.
- Name the leads that look at each of the four walls of the left ventricle.
- Describe an easy way to find posterior MIs.
- Name the coronary artery that feeds each of the four walls of the left ventricle.
- Describe how to determine if a right ventricular infarction is present.
- Describe precordial lead placement for a right-sided EKG.
- Describe how pericarditis and early repolarization mimic an MI.
- Describe the EKG complications of MI.
- State the routine treatment for STEMI and NSTEMI.

What It's All About

Mr. Bacon has a nasty case of indigestion. It didn't go away with antacids, and it kept him up all last night even though he propped the head of his bed up with three pillows. Now he's starting to feel nauseated and short-winded. His daughter tells him he looks terrible. "You're pale as a ghost; why don't you go see your doctor," she suggests. Mr. Bacon calls the doctor's office but can't get an appointment until next month. That's a lot of help, he thinks—I could be dead by then. Oh well, I can't do anything about it. So he settles down in front of the TV with his bottle of antacid and watches his favorite shows. His daughter returns later after some errands and finds her dad still in his chair but he doesn't look right. "Oh my gosh, he's not breathing!" She calls 911 and the paramedics arrive and find Mr. Bacon in ventricular fibrillation. They defibrillate him and run an EKG. He's having an MI right now. The paramedics rush Mr. Bacon to the closest hospital that can do percutaneous coronary intervention and he's rushed into the cardiac catheterization lab where his occluded coronary artery is ballooned open. He goes to the ICU afterward. Jill is the nurse caring for him. Mr. Bacon is awake and talking about his close call. Jill explains that his indigestion was not really indigestion. It was chest discomfort often seen—and misinterpreted—with an MI. She teaches him the warning signs of an MI and makes him promise to call her if he has any more chest discomfort, shortness of breath, or other distress. At 3 A.M., Mr. Bacon puts on his call light and tells Jill he's having that indigestion feeling again. Jill runs an EKG and sees changes from the previous one. Concluding that Mr. Bacon's MI is extending from the anterior wall into the lateral wall, she alerts the cardiologist to the EKG changes, and he comes in to examine the patient and the EKG. He agrees with Jill. The MI is definitely extending. So off to the cath lab goes Mr. Bacon for the second time. Again an occluded coronary artery is successfully ballooned open and Mr. Bacon spends the rest of his hospital stay learning about all things cardiac while Jill basks in the glow of having impressed a cardiologist with her ability to read an EKG.

Introduction

Myocardial infarctions (MIs) involve death of myocardial tissue in an area deprived of blood flow by an occlusion (blockage) of a coronary artery. Actual death of tissue is the end of a process that begins with ischemia and injury.

There are two types of myocardial infarctions: ST elevation MIs (**STEMI**) and non-ST elevation MIs (NSTEMI).

- STEMIs tend to be transmural (i.e., they usually, though not always, damage the entire thickness of the myocardium in a certain area of the heart). STEMIs result in ST segment elevation, T wave inversion, and significant Q waves, along with the usual symptoms of an MI. STEMIs were formerly called Q wave or transmural MIs.
- The NSTEMI tends to be subendocardial or incomplete, damaging only the innermost layer of the myocardium just beneath the endocardium. This kind of MI typically does less damage than a STEMI and does not result in the typical EKG changes associated with STEMIs. NSTEMIs can be difficult to diagnose. They sometimes present with widespread ST segment depression and T wave inversion. At other times, the MI is diagnosed only by patient history, ST segment changes, and elevated lab values that indicate myocardial damage. With NSTEMIs, the patient will have the usual symptoms of an MI and will typically go on to have a STEMI within a few months if treatment for the coronary artery blockage is not rendered. NSTEMIs were formerly called non-Q wave or subendocardial MIs. See Figure 14–1.

This chapter will focus on recognition of STEMIs, since they are the most common type of MI and require urgent recognition and treatment.

Symptoms of MI

The classic symptom of an MI, whether STEMI or NSTEMI, is chest pain. It's often described as left-sided chest tightness, heaviness, pressure, "an elephant sitting on the chest," or some variation of those. This sensation can even extend into the jaw, the right chest, the neck, the back, or down the arm (usually the left arm). It can even present as a stubborn toothache. See Figure 14–2. Keep in mind that patients with long-time diabetes may not have chest or other discomfort with their MI. They can have a condition called neuropathy, which results in diminished pain sensation. Diabetics are notorious for having "silent MIs," those that show up, perhaps on a routine EKG at the physician's office, without the typical signs and symptoms. Also important to note is *that females in general are more likely to have atypical symptoms when they infarct.* Be suspicious when a female, especially one who is postmenopausal, complains of fatigue,

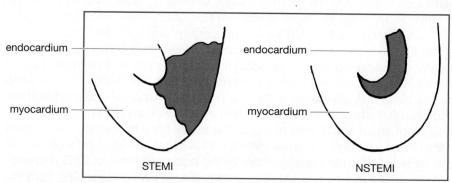

FIGURE 14–1

STEMIs and NSTEMIs.

EARLY SIGNS OF ACUTE CORONARY SYNDROME (HEART ATTACK)

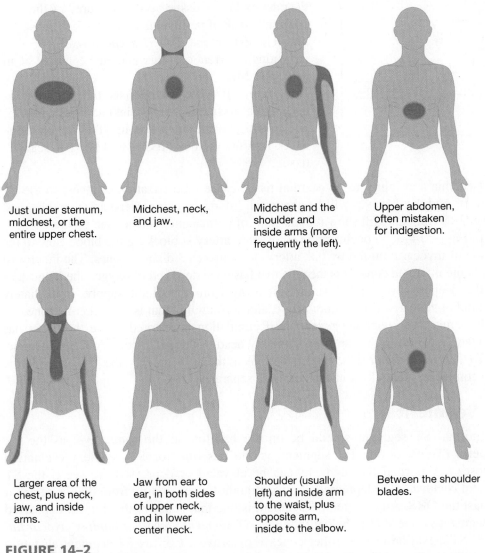

Just under sternum, midchest, or the entire upper chest.

Midchest, neck, and jaw.

Midchest and the shoulder and inside arms (more frequently the left).

Upper abdomen, often mistaken for indigestion.

Larger area of the chest, plus neck, jaw, and inside arms.

Jaw from ear to ear, in both sides of upper neck, and in lower center neck.

Shoulder (usually left) and inside arm to the waist, plus opposite arm, inside to the elbow.

Between the shoulder blades.

FIGURE 14–2

Chest pain locations.

shortness of breath, or other vague symptoms. It could be her version of chest pain—what cardiologists call women's **anginal equivalent**. (**Angina** means chest pain.)

Other signs and symptoms (S&S) of MI are shortness of breath, nausea/vomiting, pallor, diaphoresis, and arrhythmias. Not all patients with MI will have all these S&S.

An unfortunate symptom seen too often with MI is sudden cardiac death from an arrhythmia, usually V-fib. Many individuals with MI never make it to the hospital.

For those who do, it is crucial that we offer the best care possible. Let's learn more about MIs.

The Three Is of Infarction

The sequence of events that occurs when a coronary artery becomes occluded is known as the *three Is of infarction:*

- **Ischemia**   Experiments on dogs have shown that almost immediately after a coronary artery becomes occluded, the *T wave inverts* in the EKG leads overlooking the occluded area. This indicates that myocardial tissue is ischemic, starving for blood and oxygen due to the lack of blood flow. Myocardial tissue becomes pale and whitish in appearance.

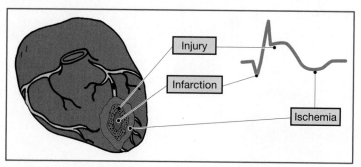

FIGURE 14–3

The three Is of infarction.

- **Injury** Soon, as the coronary occlusion continues, the once-ischemic tissue becomes injured by the continued lack of perfusion. The tissue becomes bluish in appearance. The *ST segment rises,* indicating a current of injury and the beginning of an acute STEMI.
- **Infarction** If occlusion persists, the jeopardized myocardial tissue **necroses** (dies) and turns black. *Significant Q waves develop* (in STEMIs) on the EKG. In time, the dead tissue will become scar tissue.

Ischemia and injury to myocardial tissue cause repolarization changes, so the ST segments and the T waves will be abnormal. Infarction causes depolarization changes, so the QRS complex will show telltale signs of permanent damage. See Figure 14–3.

In Figure 14–3, an occlusion in a coronary artery is blocking the blood flow to the portion of myocardium fed by that artery. This creates 3 distinct zones. The innermost zone is the infarcted zone. It is the area that has been deprived of oxygen the longest, as it's the deepest layer and thus farthest away from the blood supply. Immediately surrounding that area is the injured zone, and surrounding that is the ischemic zone.

Ischemia and injury are reversible if circulation is restored. Once the tissue has infarcted, however, the tissue is permanently dead. Myocardial cells do not regenerate.

To determine if an MI is present, we look at the ST segments, the T waves, and the QRS complexes. Let's look at each of those separately.

ST Segment

The normal ST segment should be on the baseline at the same level as the PR segment. (Think of the PR segment as the baseline for ST segment evaluation purposes.) Abnormal ST segments can be elevated or depressed. To see if the ST segment is elevated or depressed, draw a straight line extending from the PR segment out past the QRS. An elevated ST segment is one that is above this line. A depressed ST segment is one that is below this line. *ST segment elevation implies myocardial injury.* ST elevation can be either concave or convex. Convex ST segment elevation (also called a **coved ST segment**) is most often associated with a STEMI in progress. Concave ST elevation is often associated with **pericarditis**, an inflammation of the pericardium and the myocardium immediately beneath it, but it can also be seen in STEMIs. *ST depression implies ischemia or reciprocal changes opposite the area of infarct.* See Figure 14–4.

In Figure 14–4, note how the ST segment is right on line with the PR segment in the normal ST example.

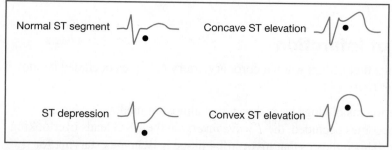

FIGURE 14–4

ST segment abnormalities.

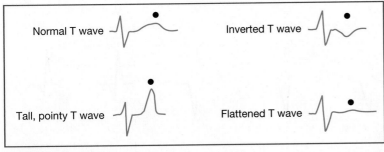

FIGURE 14–5

T wave abnormalities.

T Wave

The normal T wave should be rounded with an amplitude less than or equal to 5 mm in the frontal leads and should be upright in all leads except aVR and V_1; aVR's T wave should be negative. V_1's T wave can be flat, inverted, or upright. See Figure 14–5.

All the abnormal T waves in Figure 14–5 can imply myocardial ischemia. The tall, pointy T can also signal hyperkalemia or hyperacute changes of an MI in progress. Hyperacute changes are those that accompany an MI in its earliest stages.

QRS Complexes

We look for significant Q waves and poor R wave progression as clues to an MI. Normal Q waves imply septal and right ventricular depolarization. A significant (i.e., pathological) Q wave implies myocardial necrosis. For a Q wave to be significant, it must be *either* 0.04 seconds (one little block) wide *or* at least one-third the size of the R wave. In Figure 14–6, see the difference between a normal Q and a significant Q.

R Wave Progression and Transition

In the precordial *chest* leads, you'll recall that the QRS starts out primarily negative in V_1 and goes through a transition around V_3 or V_4, where the QRS is isoelectric. The QRS then ends up primarily positive by V_6. Thus the R waves progress from very small in V_1 to very large in V_6. If the R waves do not get progressively larger in the precordial leads, as they should, this can imply myocardial infarction. Sometimes poor R wave progression is the only electrocardiographic evidence of an MI.

The transition zone is the lead in which the QRS becomes isoelectric. This transition should occur between V_3 and V_4. A transition in V_1 or V_2 is called counterclockwise; a transition in V_5 or V_6 is clockwise. See Figure 14–7.

In Figure 14–7, look at the R wave progression in the normal transition example. The R waves grow progressively taller across the precordium, and the transition zone is in V_4. See how V_4's QRS complex is mostly isoelectric? Here, V_1 through V_3 are mostly negative, V_5 and V_6 are positive, and V_4 is where the transition from negative to positive occurs.

In the counterclockwise example, the transition zone is between V_1 and V_2. There is no real isoelectric complex. V_1 is negative and V_2 is already positive, so the transition

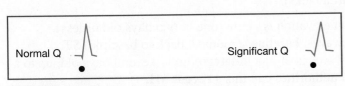

FIGURE 14–6

Normal versus significant Q waves.

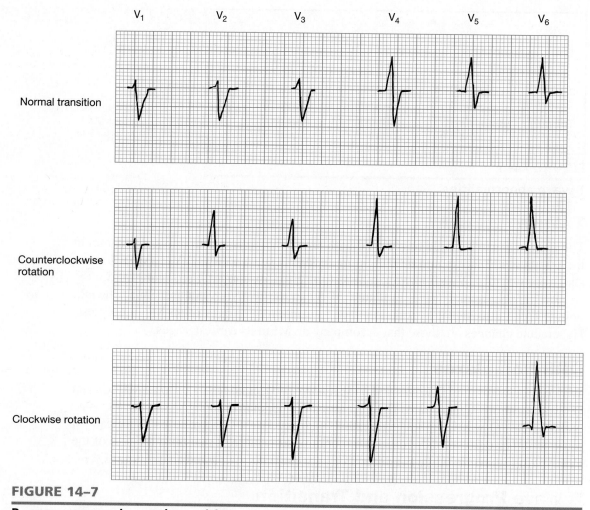

FIGURE 14–7

R wave progression and transition zones in the precordial leads.

zone would have to be between the two. The R wave progression is abnormal. The R waves progress from very small in V_1 to unusually large in V_2.

In the clockwise example, the transition zone is between V_5 and V_6. R wave progression is abnormal—the R wave is small in V_5 and very tall in V_6.

Evolution of a STEMI

STEMIs occur over a period of time. The EKG changes over the course of a STEMI are its evolution. See Figure 14–8.

Determining the Age of an MI

When an EKG is interpreted, the interpreter does not necessarily know the patient's clinical status and therefore must base determination of the MI's age on the indicative changes present on the EKG. The age of an MI is determined as follows (see website for a video on the topic of heart attacks):

- An MI that has ST segment elevation is acute (one to two days old or less).
- An MI with significant Q waves, baseline (or almost back to baseline) ST segments, and inverted T waves is of age indeterminate (several days old, up to a year in some cases). Some authorities call this a **recent MI.**
- The MI with significant Q waves, baseline ST segments, and upright T waves is *old* (weeks to years old).

TIMELINE	AGE OF MI	EKG CHANGE	IMPLICATION
Immediately before the actual MI starts		T wave inversion ✓	Cardiac tissue is ischemic, as evidenced by the newly inverted T waves.
Within hours after the MI's start	Acute	Marked ST elevation + upright T wave ✓	Acute MI has begun, starting with myocardial injury.
Hours later	Acute	Significant Q + ST elevation + upright T ✓	Some of the injured myocardial tissue has died, while other tissue remains injured.
Hours to a day or two later	Acute	Significant Q + less ST elevation + marked T inversion ✓	Infarction is almost complete. Some injury and ischemia persist at the infarct edges.
Days to weeks later (in some cases this stage may last up to a year)	Age indeterminate	Significant Q + T wave inversion	Infarction is complete. Though there is no more ischemic tissue (it has either recovered or died), the T wave inversion persists.
Weeks, months, years later	Old	Significant Q only	The significant Q wave persists, signifying permanent tissue death.

FIGURE 14–8

Evolution of a STEMI.

Walls of the Left Ventricle

Although it is possible to have an infarction of the right ventricle, infarctions occur mostly in the left ventricle, since it has the greatest oxygen demand and thus is impacted more adversely by poor coronary artery flow. MIs can affect any of the four walls of the left ventricle (see Figure 14–9):

- **Anterior wall** The front wall—fed by the left anterior descending coronary artery.
- **Inferior wall** The bottom wall—fed by the right coronary artery.
- **Lateral wall** The left side wall of the heart—fed by the circumflex coronary artery.
- **Posterior wall** The back wall—fed by the right coronary artery.

Each of these left ventricular walls can be "seen" by our EKG electrodes. You'll recall that the positive pole of Leads II, III, and aVF sit on the left leg. They look at the heart from the bottom. Which wall of the heart would they see? Good for you if you said the inferior wall.

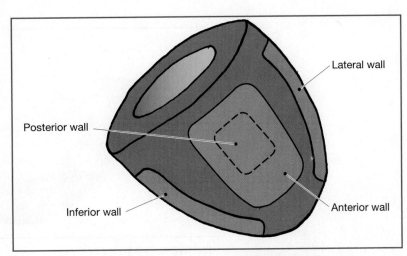

FIGURE 14–9

Walls of the left ventricle.

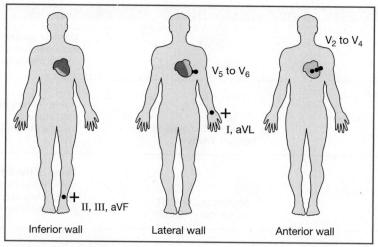

FIGURE 14–10

Leads looking at the anterior, inferior, and lateral walls of the left ventricle.

What about Leads I, aVL, and V$_5$ and V$_6$? They sit on the heart's left side, so they look at the lateral wall.

Leads V$_2$ through V$_4$ sit right in the front of the heart, looking at the anterior wall. See Figure 14–10.

What about the posterior wall? Unlike the other infarct locations, there are no leads looking directly at the posterior wall because we do not put EKG electrodes on the patient's back for a routine 12-lead EKG. Therefore, the only way to look at the posterior wall is to look *through* the anterior wall. See Figure 14–11.

The ventricles depolarize from endocardium to epicardium (from inside to outside). You'll note on Figure 14–11 that the vectors (arrows) representing depolarization of the anterior and posterior walls are opposite each other. Therefore, *the only way to diagnose a posterior MI is to look for changes opposite those that would be seen with an anterior MI*. We use leads V$_1$ and V$_2$ since they sit almost directly opposite the posterior wall. What's the opposite of a Q wave? An R wave. What's opposite ST elevation? ST depression. What's opposite T wave inversion? Upright T wave. Those are what we look for with a posterior infarct.

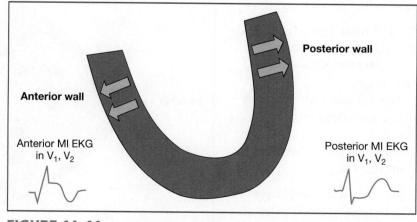

FIGURE 14–11

Posterior wall MI changes.

An easy way to find posterior MIs is to turn the EKG upside down (make the top the bottom) and look at V₁ and V₂ from the back of the EKG. This mimics what the EKG would look like if we had leads directly over the posterior wall. If there is a significant Q wave and T wave inversion in V_1 and V_2 in this upside-down reverse approach, there is a posterior MI. The ST segment may be elevated or at baseline, depending on the age of the MI. Also keep in mind that posterior MIs almost always accompany an inferior MI, so always look for a posterior MI when an inferior MI is present.

Myocardial Infarction Locations

A STEMI is diagnosed on the EKG by indicative changes (i.e., ST elevation, T wave inversion, and significant Q waves) in the leads for that area. Depending on the age of the infarct, not all of those indicative changes will be present.

In the area electrically opposite the infarct area are **reciprocal changes** (i.e., ST depression). Reciprocal ST depression is seen only when there is ST elevation in the indicative leads.

Let's look at the EKG changes associated with the different infarction locations. It is not necessary to have every single change listed in order to determine the kind of infarction, but most of the criteria should be met. Note the coronary artery involved. See Table 14–1.

The MIs in Table 14–1 involve only one wall of the left ventricle. MIs can extend across into other walls as well. For example, a patient might have an inferior-lateral MI, which would involve the inferior leads as well as the lateral leads. Combination MIs such as this do not always involve every one of the usual leads. For example, an inferior-lateral MI might involve the inferior leads and only a few lateral leads. An anterior-lateral MI might include the anterior leads and only a few lateral leads.

On the next several pages, you'll find helpful ways of determining the kind of MI you're seeing. First there are infarction squares, then MI pictorials, and then an MI algorithm. Let's check them out.

TABLE 14–1   Infarction Locations

Location of STEMI	EKG Changes	Coronary Artery
Anterior	Indicative changes in V_2 to V_4 Reciprocal changes in II, III, aVF	Left anterior descending (LAD)
Inferior	Indicative changes in II, III, aVF Reciprocal changes in I, aVL, and V leads	Right coronary artery (RCA)
Lateral	Indicative changes in I, aVL, V_5 to V_6 May see reciprocal changes in II, III, aVF	Circumflex
Posterior	No indicative changes, since no leads look directly at posterior wall Diagnosed by reciprocal changes in V_1 and V_2 (large R wave, upright T wave, and possibly ST depression). Seen as a mirror image of an anterior MI.	RCA or circumflex
Extensive anterior (sometimes called *extensive anterior-lateral*)	Indicative changes in I, aVL, V_1 to V_6 Reciprocal changes in II, III, aVF	LAD or left main
Anteroseptal	Indicative changes in V_1 plus any anterior lead(s) Usually no reciprocal changes	LAD

We're about halfway through this chapter. To evaluate your understanding of the material thus far, answer the following questions. If you have trouble with them, review the material again before continuing.

Mrs. Uhura has chest pain radiating to her left arm. She is nauseated and short of breath. An EKG shows ST segment elevation in Leads II, III, and aVF.

Lab results are positive for an MI.

1. Is it a STEMI or a NSTEMI?
2. Which wall of the heart is damaged?
3. In which leads would you expect to see reciprocal changes?

Infarction Squares

In Table 14–2, each lead square is labeled with the wall of the heart at which it looks. When you analyze an EKG, note which leads have ST elevation and/or significant Q waves. Then use the infarction squares to determine the type of infarction. For example, if there were ST elevation in Leads II, III, aVF, and V_5 and V_6, you would note that the MI involves inferior and lateral leads. The MI would be inferior-lateral.

Next let's look at some MI pictorials. Ignore the QRS width in these pictorials—the drawings are just to illustrate what these types of MIs look like.

TABLE 14–2 Infarction Squares

I Lateral	aVR Ignore this lead when looking for MIs	V_1 Septal (posterior if mirror image)	V_4 Anterior
II Inferior	aVL Lateral	V_2 Anterior (posterior if mirror image)	V_5 Lateral
III Inferior	aVF Inferior	V_3 Anterior	V_6 Lateral

MI Pictorials

Anterior STEMI

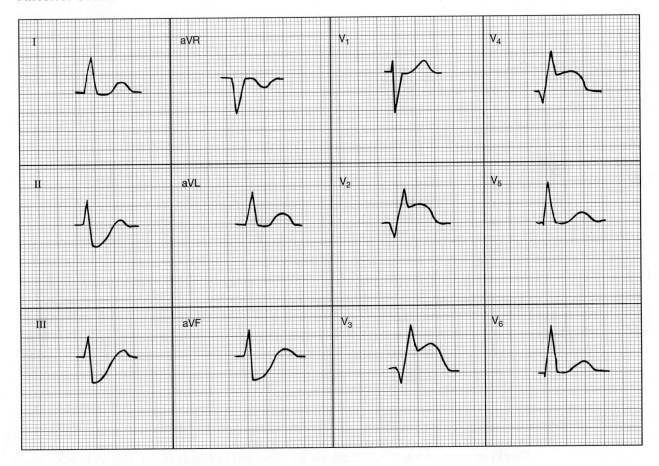

This is an *acute anterior MI,* as evidenced by the ST elevation in V_2 to V_4. Also note the reciprocal ST depression in Leads II, III, and aVF.

If this MI were *age indeterminate,* it would have more normal ST segments, significant Q waves, and T wave inversions in V_2 to V_4.

If this MI were *old,* it would have only the significant Q wave remaining. The ST segment would be back at baseline and the T wave would be upright.

Inferior STEMI

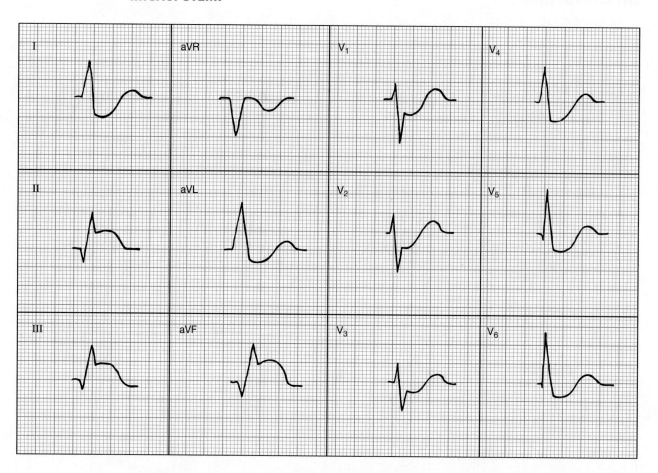

This is an *acute inferior MI*. Note the ST elevation in Leads II, III, and aVF. Note also the reciprocal ST segment depression in Leads I, aVL, and V_1 to V_6.

The *age indeterminate inferior MI* would have more normal ST segments along with significant Q waves and inverted T waves in Leads II, III, and aVF.

The *old inferior MI* would have only significant Q waves in II, III, and aVF. The ST segments would be at baseline and T waves would be upright.

Lateral Wall STEMI

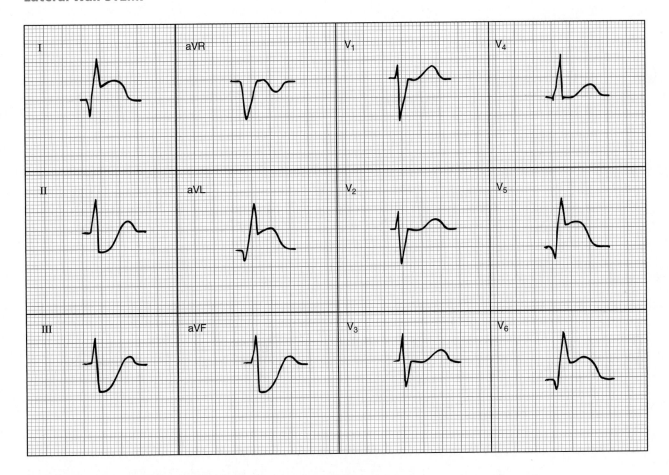

This is an *acute lateral wall MI,* as evidenced by the ST elevation in Leads I, aVL, and V_5 to V_6. Note also the reciprocal ST depression in Leads II, III, and aVF.

If this were an *age indeterminate lateral MI,* there would be more normal ST segments along with significant Q waves and inverted T waves in I, aVL, and V_5 to V_6.

An *old lateral wall MI* would have baseline ST segments, significant Q waves, and upright T waves in I, aVL, and V_5 to V_6.

Posterior MI

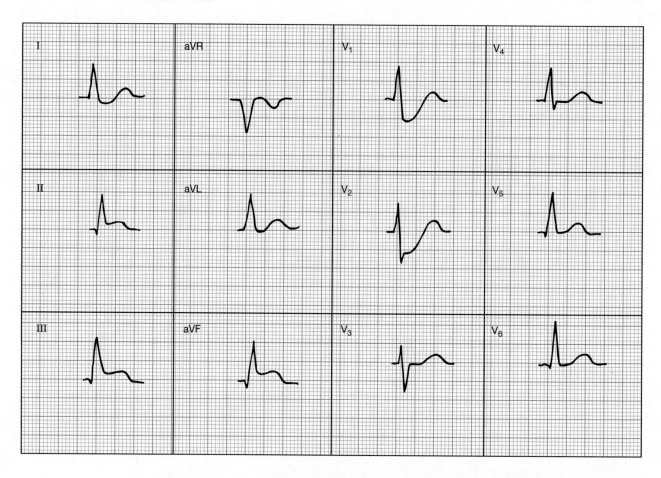

This is an *acute posterior wall MI.* Note the tall R wave in V_1 to V_2 along with ST segment depression and an upright T wave. Remember, a posterior MI is diagnosed by a mirror image of the normal indicative changes of an MI in V_1 to V_2. Note that there is an acute inferior MI as well.

An *age indeterminate posterior MI* would have more normal ST segments, a tall R wave, and an upright T wave.

The *old posterior MI* would have only the tall R wave remaining. The ST segments would be at baseline and the T wave would be inverted.

Extensive Anterior STEMI

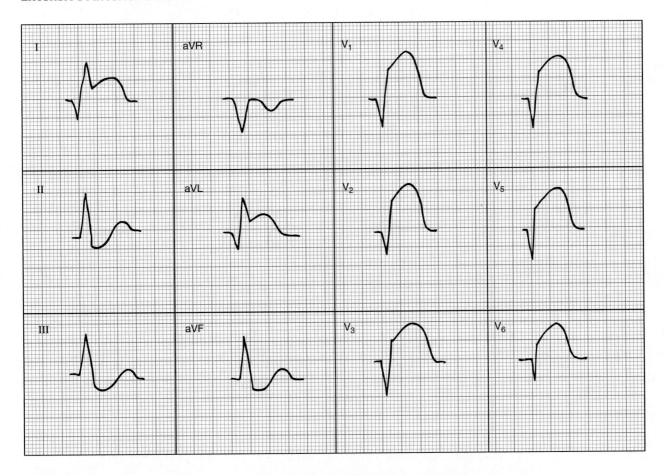

Here we have a huge MI, the *acute extensive anterior MI*. Note the significant Q waves and ST elevation in I, aVL, and V_1 to V_6 along with the reciprocal ST depression in II, III, and aVF.

The *age indeterminate extensive anterior MI* would have more normal ST segments along with significant Q waves and T wave inversion.

The *old extensive anterior MI* would have baseline ST segments, significant Q waves, and upright T waves in I, aVL, and V_1 to V_6.

Anteroseptal STEMI

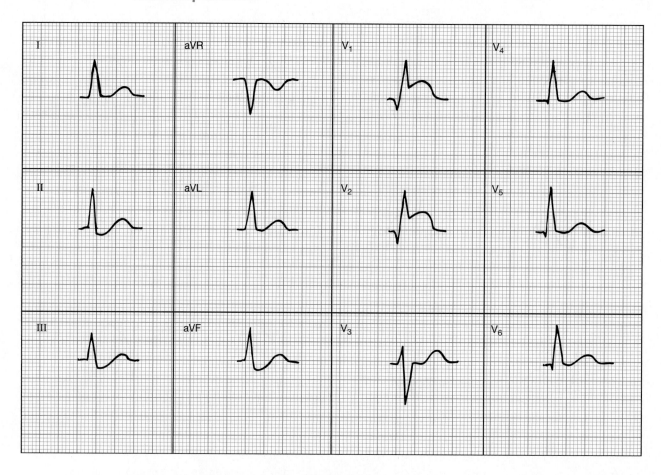

This is an *acute anteroseptal MI.* Note the ST elevation in Leads V_1 to V_2. Recall V_1 is a septal lead and V_2 is an anterior lead. *The combination of V_1 plus any anterior lead results in an anteroseptal MI.*

If this were an *age indeterminate anteroseptal MI,* it would have more normal ST segments, significant Q waves, and inverted T waves in V_1 to V_2.

If this were an *old anteroseptal MI,* it would have only significant Q waves remaining in V_1 to V_2. The ST segments would be at baseline and the T waves would be upright.

NSTEMI

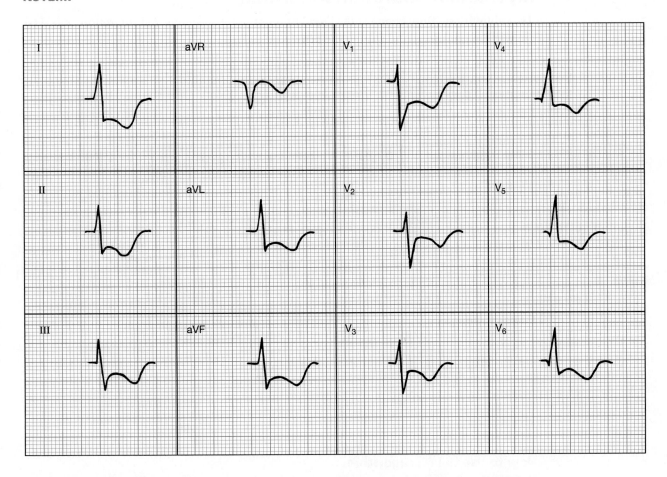

This is an *acute NSTEMI*. It is characterized by widespread ST depression and T wave inversions. NSTEMIs are diagnosed only in the acute phase, as they do not cause significant Q waves, and their T waves are already inverted.

Myocardial Infarction Algorithm

This algorithm (flow chart) is designed to point out the myocardial infarction area. Just answer the questions and follow the arrows.

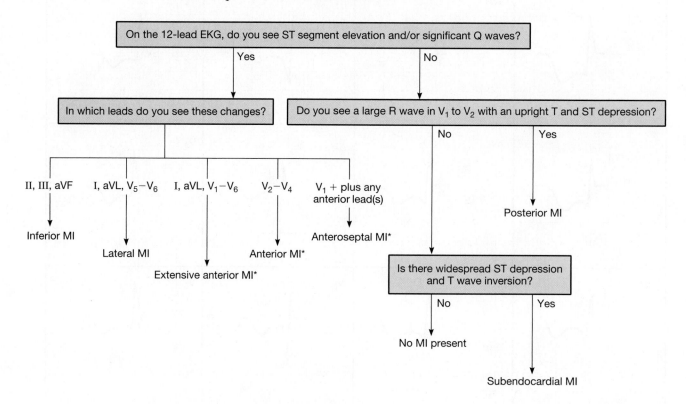

How to Use the MI Algorithm

Refer to the EKG in Figure 14–12. Do you see any ST segment elevation or significant Q waves? Yes, there are significant Q waves, and also there is ST elevation.

In which leads do you see these changes? These are noted in V_1 to V_4. The arrow points to anteroseptal MI.

Right Ventricular Infarction

On occasion, an inferior MI will be accompanied by a right ventricular (RV) infarction. RV infarctions occur when the blockage to the right coronary artery system is so extensive that damage extends into the right ventricle. RV infarctions are not detectable by the routine 12-lead EKG, which looks at the left ventricle. To diagnose an RV infarction, two conditions must be met: First, there must be electrocardiographic evidence of an inferior wall MI on a standard 12-lead EKG. Second, a right-sided EKG must reveal ST elevation in V_3R and/or V_4R. This right-sided EKG is done only if an RV infarction is suspected (i.e., the patient exhibits symptoms, particularly hypotension, beyond what is expected with just an inferior MI).

A right-sided EKG is done with the limb leads in their normal places, but with the precordial leads placed on the right side of the chest instead of the left. See lead placement for a right-sided EKG in Figure 14–13.

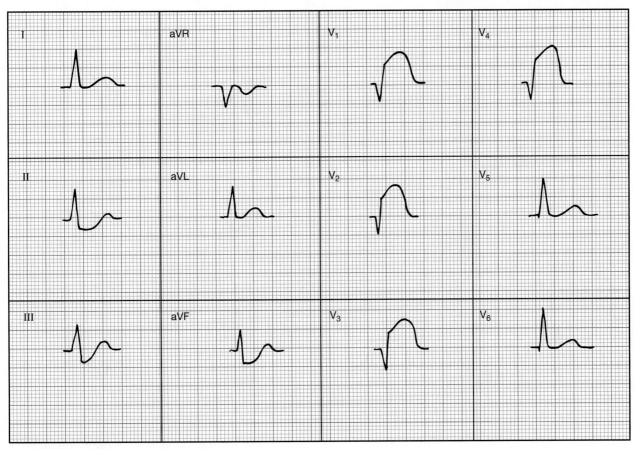

FIGURE 14–12

MI for algorithm.

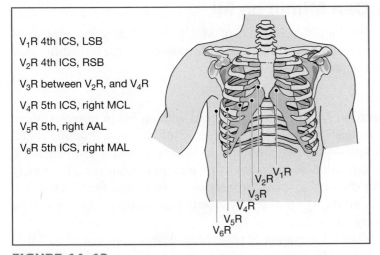

V_1R 4th ICS, LSB

V_2R 4th ICS, RSB

V_3R between V_2R, and V_4R

V_4R 5th ICS, right MCL

V_5R 5th, right AAL

V_6R 5th ICS, right MAL

FIGURE 14–13

Lead placement for a right-sided EKG.

Right Ventricular Infarction (Right-Sided EKG)

See Figure 14–14. On this right-sided EKG, note the ST elevation in Leads V_3R to V_4R. This proves there is an RV infarction. You'll note also that there is ST elevation in Leads II, III, and aVF that indicates an inferior MI. Remember, the right-sided EKG leaves the limb leads in their normal place but moves the precordial leads to the right side of the chest. So the inferior MI will still be obvious on the right-sided EKG.

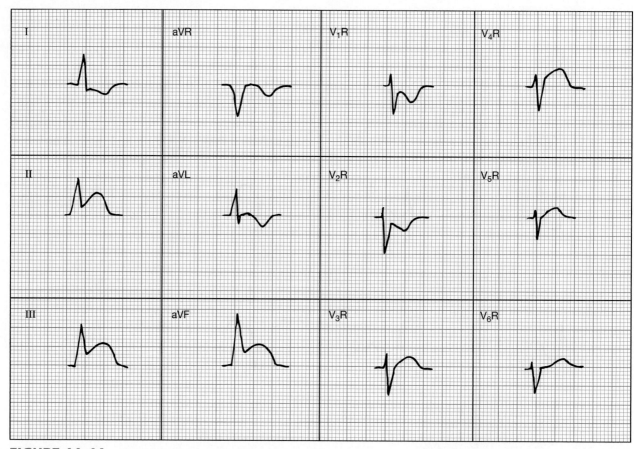

FIGURE 14–14

Right ventricular infarction (right-sided EKG).

Conditions That Can Mimic an MI

Now that you have a feel for the different kinds of MIs, let's look at some conditions that can cause EKG changes that look just like an MI. In most cases, the only difference is in the patient's medical symptoms and history.

Acute Pericarditis

Although ST segment elevation is most often associated with an MI in progress, there are times when it may instead imply an inflammation of the pericardium, called pericarditis. In acute pericarditis, the pericardium and the myocardium just beneath it are inflamed, causing repolarization abnormalities that present as concave ST segment elevation. Since pericarditis does not involve coronary artery blockage, the ST elevation will not be limited to leads overlying areas fed by a certain coronary artery—it will be widespread throughout many leads.

The ST elevation of pericarditis differs from that of an MI in that an MI usually produces *convex* ST elevation, whereas pericarditis produces *concave* elevation. These are often referred to as the *smiley-face* and *frowny-face* ST segments. The smiley face is concave ST elevation. The frowny face is convex. See Figure 14–15.

Like an MI, pericarditis also causes chest pain, and it is crucial to differentiate between the two, as treatment differs greatly. See Figure 14–16.

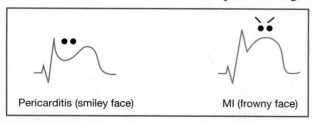

Pericarditis (smiley face)   MI (frowny face)

FIGURE 14–15

Smiley-face (concave) and frowny-face (convex) ST elevations.

In Figure 14–16, note the widespread concave ST elevation in Leads I, II, III, aVL, aVF, and V_1 to V_6. This is *not* typical of an MI because it is so widespread. Is it possible this is a huge MI instead of pericarditis? Sure. But based on the concave ST elevation

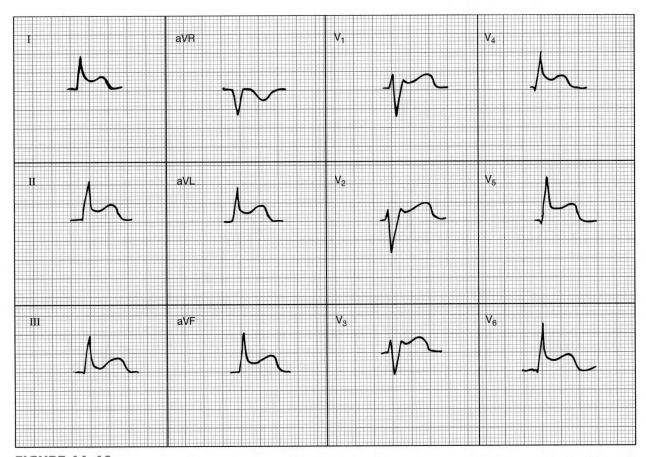

FIGURE 14–16

Pericarditis.

scattered across many leads, it's more likely that it's pericarditis. Only by examining the patient would we know for sure.

Early Repolarization

A normal variant sometimes seen in young people, especially young black males, early repolarization results in ST elevation that may be <u>convex</u> or <u>concave</u>. Repolarization begins so early in this condition that the ST segment appears to start even before the QRS complex has finished, making it appear that the ST segment is mildly elevated. Often there is a "fishhook" at the end of some of the QRS complexes that makes recognition of early repolarization easier. Note the ST elevation and the fishhook (see arrow) in Figure 14–17.

It is not always possible to distinguish early repolarization from an MI based on only a single EKG. A series of EKGs would reveal the typical evolutionary changes if an MI is present, and they would remain unchanged if early repolarization is present. The ST segment elevations of early repolarization are most often evident in Leads V_2 to V_4, although they may be more widespread. Of great help in differentiating early repolarization from an MI are the age and presentation of the patient. A 20-year-old black male with no cardiac complaints who has mild ST elevations probably has early repolarization. A 65-year-old male with chest pain and ST elevation is more likely to have an MI in progress. Only by examining the patient can the definitive diagnosis of early repolarization versus MI be made. See Figure 14–18.

In Figure 14–18, note the mild ST segment elevation in almost all leads and the fishhook in V_3 to V_6 (see arrows). This is typical of early repolarization.

Now it's time for some practice. The EKGs that follow all represent standard left-sided EKGs. The first 5 EKGs are like the MI pictorials, consisting of only one beat in each lead box. The last 5 are genuine 12-lead EKGs. Use the infarction squares and/or the MI algorithm if you need help.

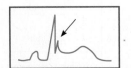

FIGURE 14–17

Fishhook of early repolarization.

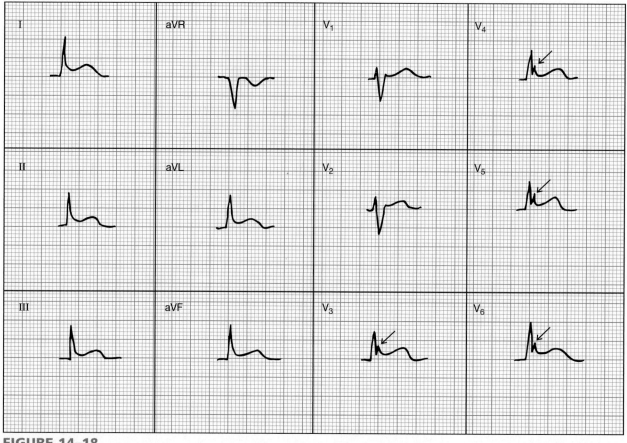

FIGURE 14–18

Early repolarization.

MI Practice

Tell which wall of the heart is affected and how old the MI is (if there is indeed an MI).

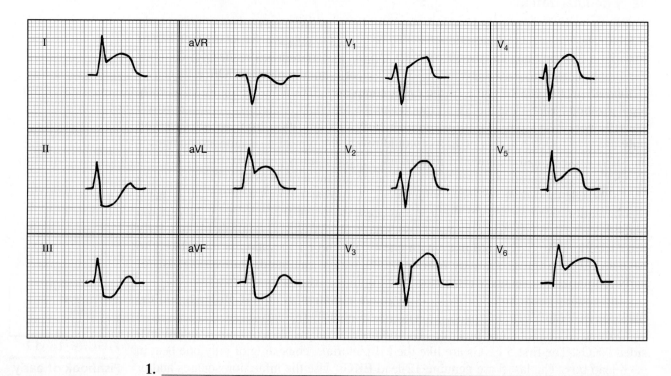

1. _____

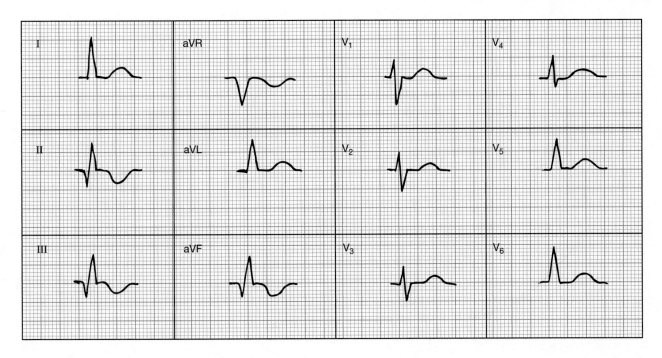

2. _____

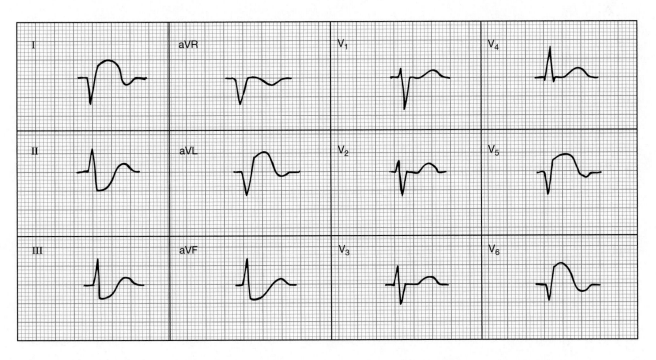

3. _____

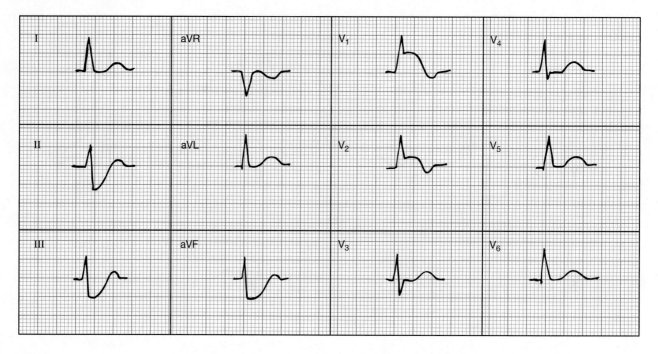

4. _____

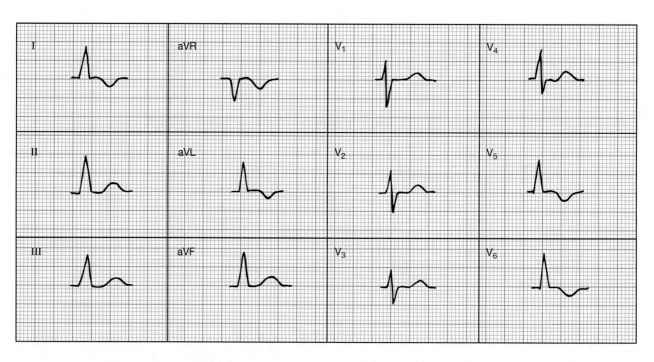

5. _____

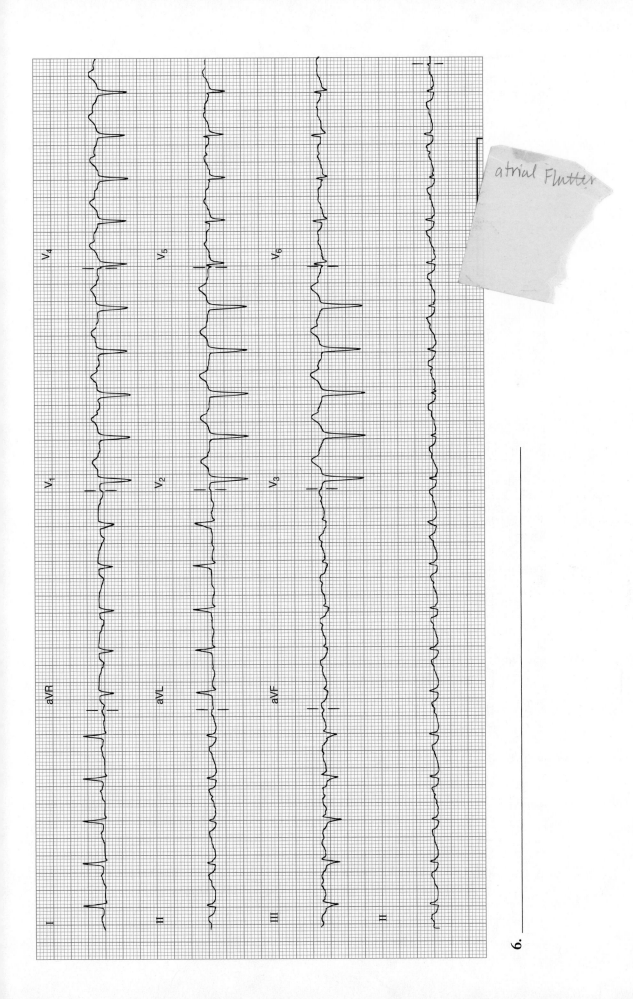

atrial Flutter

6.

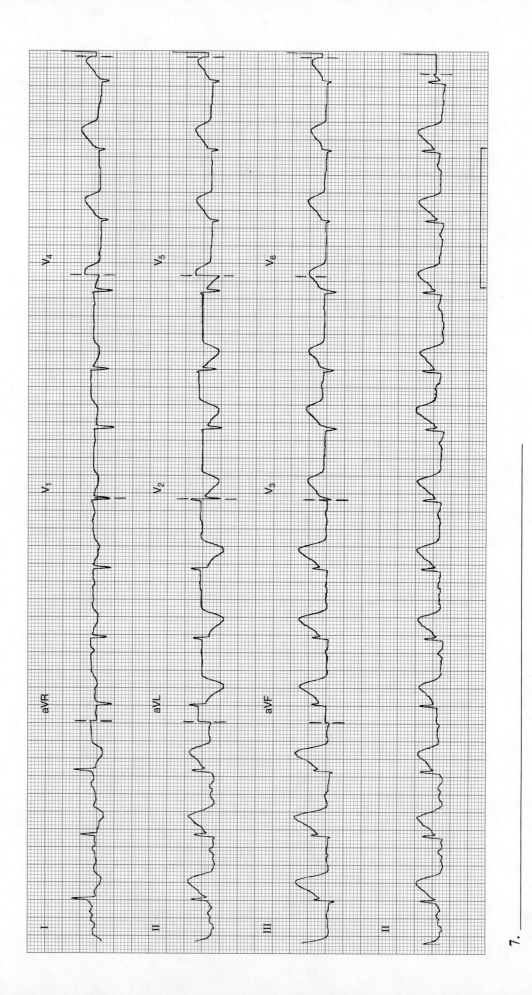

7.

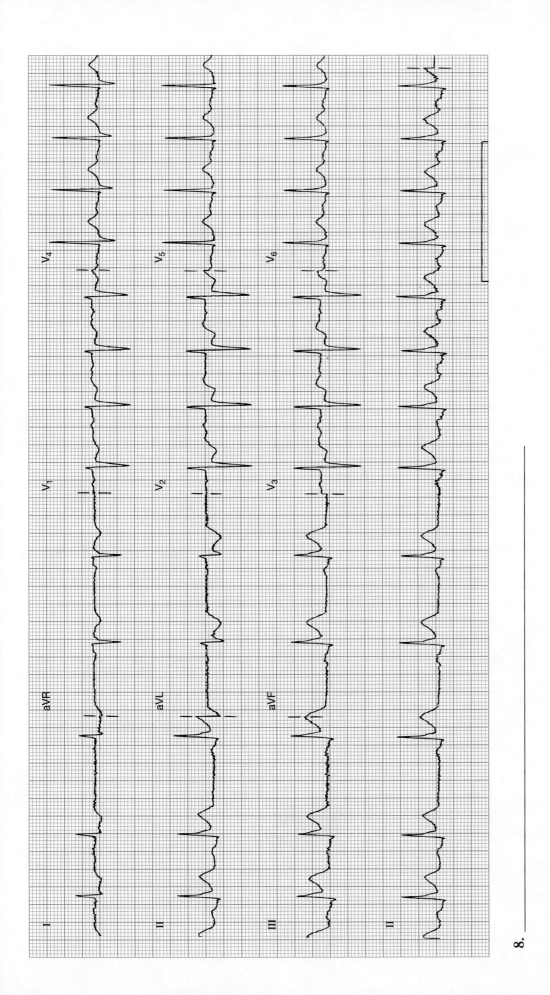

8.

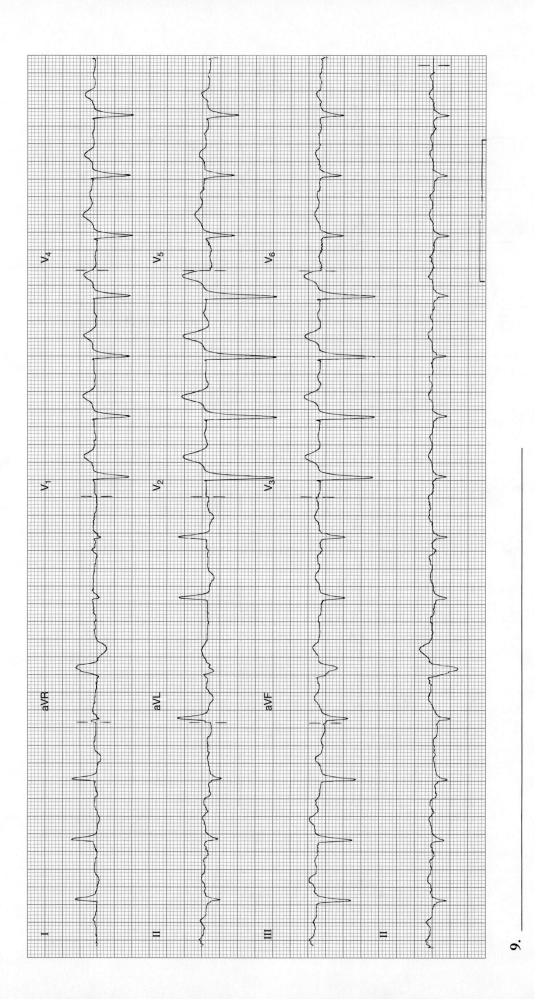

9.

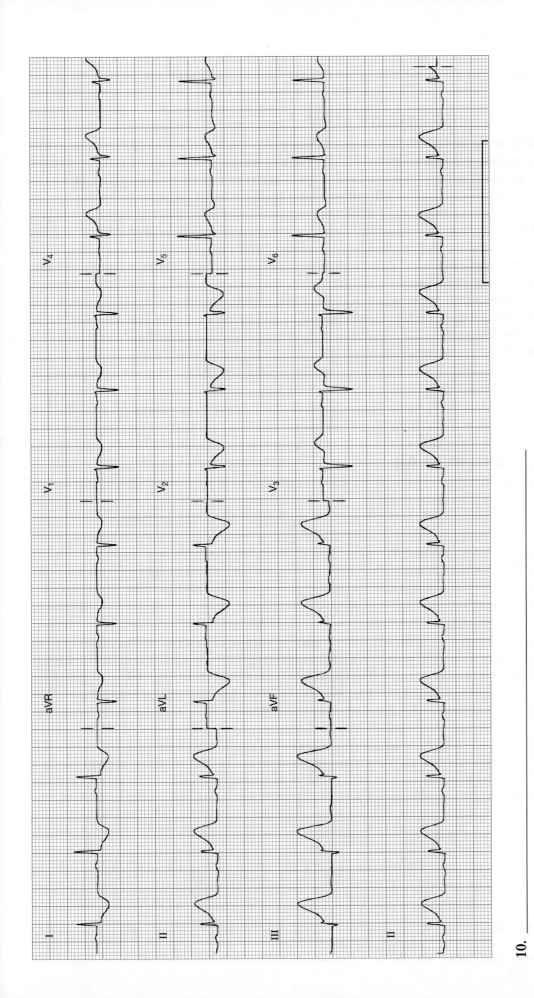

10.

Now that we know how to identify MIs, let's briefly discuss the EKG complications that can occur with the most common MI types—anterior wall MI and inferior wall MI.

EKG Complications of MI

Because the myocardium is damaged during an MI, it is not unusual for some degree of heart failure (decreased pumping efficiency) to occur. Since the heart can't pump out as much blood as before, it compensates by pumping more often—this in an attempt to maintain cardiac output. Therefore, sinus tachycardia is common following an MI. Unfortunately this effort by the heart to maintain cardiac output may actually backfire. If the heart rate rises too high, there is not enough time in between beats for the heart to fill up with blood—referred to as decreased diastolic filling time—so the cardiac output drops even more. This can lead to cardiogenic shock, a type of shock caused by catastrophic heart failure.

Arrhythmias are common following MI. Ventricular fibrillation is often seen (and too often fatal) in the first hours after MI and in fact is sometimes the first clue that the person had an MI. The myocardium is very irritable during/after MI and ventricular arrhythmias often result.

Other EKG disturbances occur as well. See Table 14–3 for EKG complications of the most common types of MIs—the anterior and inferior wall MIs.

So now that we can identify MIs and their EKG complications, how do we treat the MI?

Treatment of MI

Patients suspected of having an MI should have a 12-lead EKG and blood drawn to determine if an MI is in progress. Certain enzymes (Troponin and CPK in particular) are released into the bloodstream by damaged myocardial cells during an MI and can be noted on lab values. Patients will be started on oxygen by nasal cannula to decrease the heart's workload. They'll be given *nitroglycerine* and perhaps *morphine* for chest pain. The nitroglycerine dilates (opens up) the narrowed coronary artery, allowing more blood flow to the stricken myocardium. This can relieve the pain. If that is ineffective, morphine, a narcotic that has cardiac benefits (it modestly decreases return of venous blood to the heart, helping treat/prevent heart failure) can be used to relieve MI pain. Pain is dangerous for the MI patient, since it increases heart rate and stresses the heart even more. Relieving pain is extremely important. MI patients will be given an *aspirin* to chew (yes, chew) to help decrease platelet aggregation (clumping of platelets). Platelet aggregation forms clots. Preventing this aggregation helps prevent any blood clot that's already in the coronary artery from growing larger. *These meds are given only*

TABLE 14–3   EKG Complications of MI

MI Wall	EKG Complications
Anterior	Mobitz II second degree AV block, third-degree AV block with wide QRS, bundle branch blocks, sinus tachycardia, ventricular arrhythmias, V-fib in the first hours after infarct, AIVR, right bundle branch block, left posterior hemiblock
Inferior	Bradycardias, first-degree AV block, Wenckebach, ventricular arrhythmias, V-fib in the first hours after infarct, accelerated junctional rhythm, junctional bradycardia, AIVR, third-degree AV block with narrow QRS
Anteroseptal	Same as anterior, with increased chance of V-fib occurring greater than 48 hours after MI

if there are no contraindications. For example, a patient with bleeding ulcers in his or her stomach may not be given the aspirin, since it would increase the chance of bleeding. The above combination of meds is referred to as *MONA: morphine-oxygen-nitro-aspirin.*

Treatment of STEMIs and NSTEMIs differs after initial treatment and diagnostic workup. NSTEMIs are treated less aggressively early on, since these MIs do still allow some coronary artery flow distal to (beyond) the narrowed area. NSTEMI patients may receive antiplatelet or anticoagulant medications to thin the blood and prevent recurrences of the MI. They may be started on beta blockers to decrease the heart's workload, and they will likely eventually have an angiogram done to determine where the coronary artery blockage is. Further treatment can then be determined based on the angiogram results.

Treatment of STEMIs is more emergent since the coronary artery blockage is complete, and myocardial necrosis is a certainty without treatment. The American Heart Association and American College of Cardiology recommend that STEMI patients arriving in the emergency department be taken immediately to the cardiac catheterization lab for reperfusion via PCI (percutaneous coronary intervention), a balloon procedure to open the blocked coronary artery. A wire mesh called a stent may then be placed at the site of the former blockage to serve as a sort of scaffold to keep the artery open. The goal of PCI is a door-to-balloon time of 90 minutes, meaning the STEMI patient should be having the PCI procedure within 90 minutes of arrival at the hospital. At some smaller hospitals without cardiac catheterization labs, PCI is not possible, so STEMI patients at these facilities can either be transported to a nearby facility that can do the PCI within the 90 minutes or they can be treated with thrombolytic medications (medications that dissolve blood clots) within 30 minutes of arrival at the smaller hospital. Thrombolytics dissolve the blood clot causing the MI, but they can be given only to a closely screened population of patients because of the increased risk of bleeding, which can cause strokes or other problems.

Patients with an uncomplicated course following their MI may be home from the hospital in less than a week.

chapter fourteen notes TO SUM IT ALL UP . . .

- **MI**—Death of myocardial tissue—caused by occlusion of a coronary artery.
- **Two types of MI:**
  - *STEMI*—ST elevation MI
  - *NSTEMI*—Non-ST elevation MI
- **Symptoms of MI** (patient may have any or all of these):
  - Chest pain, pressure, or discomfort that can radiate to the arms, jaw, neck, back
  - Pallor
  - Nausea
  - Feeling of impending doom
  - Shortness of breath
  - Lightheadedness or dizziness
- **Females and diabetics are notorious for having atypical symptoms (or no symptoms at all) of their MI.**
- **Three Is of infarction:**
  - *Ischemia*—Decreased blood flow to heart muscle—tissue pale whitish—inverted T wave on EKG.
  - *Injury*—Tissue injured by continued lack of blood flow—tissue bluish—ST segment elevation.
- *Infarction*—Tissue dies and turns black—significant Q waves.
- **ST segment**—Convex (coved) implies STEMI. Concave seen with pericarditis.
- **Hyperacute T waves**—Unusually tall T waves seen in earliest stages of MI.
- **Significant Q wave**—Must be at least 0.04 seconds wide or one-third the size of the R wave.
- **R wave progression**—R waves start out small in V_1 and get larger as they move toward V_6. Transition zone V_3 to V_4.
- **Age of STEMI:**
  - *Acute* = ST elevation
  - *Age indeterminate* = Significant Q wave, ST back (or almost back) to baseline, T wave inverted
  - *Old* = Significant Q wave, ST at baseline, T wave upright
- **Walls of left ventricle:**
  - *Anterior*—Fed by left anterior descending coronary artery
  - *Inferior*—Fed by right coronary artery
  - *Lateral*—Fed by circumflex
  - *Posterior*—Fed by right coronary artery

- ■ **STEMI criteria:**
  - Anterior MI—ST elevation V_2 to V_4
  - Inferior—ST elevation II, III, aVF
  - Lateral—ST elevation I, aVL, V_5 to V_6
  - Posterior—ST depression and large R wave in V_1 to V_2
  - Extensive anterior—ST elevation I, aVL, all V leads
  - Anteroseptal—ST elevation V_1 plus any other lead from V_2 to V_4
- ■ **Right ventricular infarction**—Accompanies inferior wall MI—diagnosed by seeing ST elevation in V_3 to V_4R on right-sided EKG.
- ■ **Pericarditis**—Inflammation of pericardial sac—also inflames myocardium—causes concave ST elevation (smiley face). ST elevation widespread.
- ■ **Early repolarization**—Common in young people, especially young black males—causes mild ST elevation—sometimes see "fishhook" at end of QRS complexes in the V leads.

- ■ **EKG Complications of MI:**
  - Anterior MI—Mobitz II second-degree AV block, third-degree AV block with wide QRS, V-fib in early hours, RBBB, LPHB, AIVR, sinus tachycardia, ventricular arrhythmias
  - Inferior MI—Bradycardias, first-degree AV block, Wenckebach, third-degree AV block with narrow QRS, accelerated junctional rhythm, junctional bradycardia, AIVR, ventricular arrhythmias, V-fib in early hours
  - Anteroseptal—Same as anterior but with increased chance of V-fib occurring late (greater than 48 hours after infarct)
- ■ **MI treatment:**
  - All suspected MIs—MONA (morphine-oxygen-nitroglycerine-aspirin)
  - STEMI—PCI or thrombolytics
  - NSTEMI—Medications such as beta blockers, anti-coagulants or anti-platelet agents, eventual angiogram

Practice Quiz

1. List the three Is of infarction. _____
   ischemia, injury, infarction

2. State the differences between a STEMI and a NSTEMI. *STEMI = ST↑, T wave ↓, sig Q on EKG*
   NSTEMI = does not cause sig. Q waves

3. Which coronary artery's occlusion results in an anterior wall MI? *LAD coronary artery*

4. Name the three normal indicative changes of an MI.
   ST elevation, sig. Q waves
   T wave inversions

5. Reciprocal changes are seen in which area of the heart? *area electrically opposite the*
   damaged area

6. If there is marked ST elevation in Leads II, III, and aVF, how old is the MI and in which wall of the heart?
   Acute inferior

7. If there is a significant Q wave in V_1 to V_3 with baseline ST segments and upright T waves, how old is the MI and in which wall of the heart? _____
   old ? antereo sep septal

8. If the transition zone of the precordial leads is in V_1 to V_2, which kind of rotation is the heart said to have? *counter clockwise rotation*
   of the heart

9. The kind of MI that can be diagnosed by inverting the EKG and looking at Leads V_1 and V_2 from behind is the *posterior MI*

10. Which coronary artery supplies the lateral wall of the left ventricle? *C-flex*

Putting It All Together—Critical Thinking Exercises

These exercises may consist of diagrams to label, scenarios to analyze, brain-stumping questions to ponder, or other challenging exercises to boost your understanding of the chapter material.

1. Draw and label the evolution of EKG changes seen from immediately before the actual STEMI starts to a STEMI that is weeks, months, or years old.

2. If Mr. Milner, a 69-year-old man with a history of chest pain, arrives in your ER with newly inverted T waves in Leads II, III, and aVF, what do you suspect is happening? _____

   _____

3. If an hour later Mr. Milner is doubled over with crushing chest pain and his EKG now shows marked ST elevation in II, III, aVF and V_5 to V_6, what is happening?_____

   _____

   _____

   The following is a scenario that will provide you with information about a fictional patient and ask you to analyze the situation, answer questions, and decide on appropriate actions.

   Mr. Jones is a 79-year-old black male who arrives in the ER stating he'd had chest pain for about a half hour prior to arrival, but right now the pain is gone. See his EKG in Figure 14–19.

4. What do you see in Leads II, III, and aVF that would be consistent with myocardial ischemia? _____

   _____

   The ER physician orders lab work and the nurse keeps a close eye on Mr. Jones. Thirty minutes later, Mr. Jones calls his nurse, complaining of crushing chest pain and shortness of breath. His blood pressure has dropped and his skin is ashen, cool, and clammy. The nurse calls for the physician and repeats an EKG. See Figure 14–20.

5. What is happening? _____

   _____

   The physician orders medication for the pain and sends Mr. Jones to the cath lab for PCI. Within the hour, Mr. Jones feels much better and his EKG is much improved. He is sent to the coronary care unit for a few days and does well.

PEARSON
myhealthprofessionskit™

Use this address to access the Companion Website created for this textbook. Simply select "Basic Health Science" from the choice of disciplines. Find this book and log in using your username and password to access video clips, animations, assessment questions, and more.

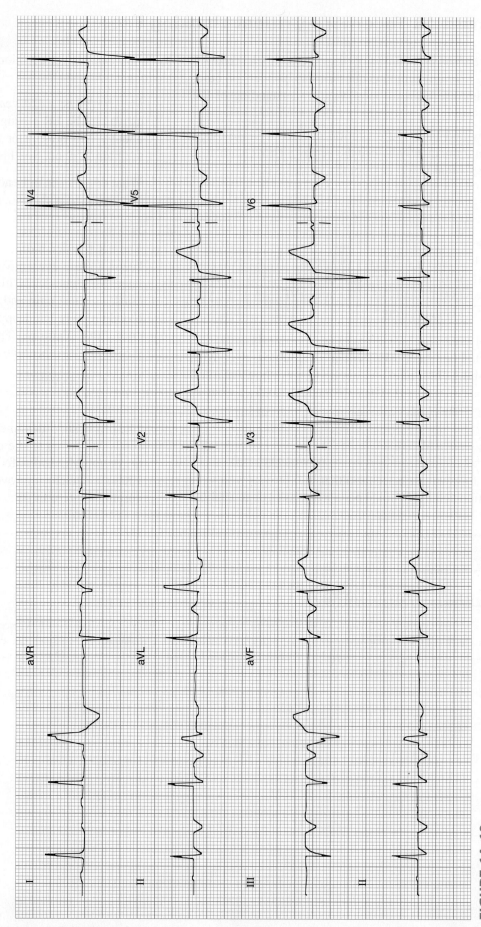

FIGURE 14–19

Mr. Jones's first EKG.

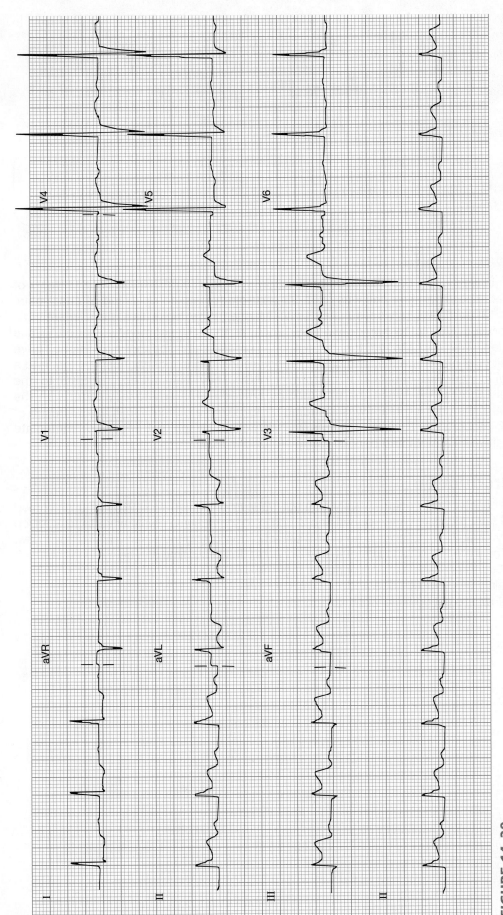

FIGURE 14-20

Mr Jones's second EKG.

15 12-Lead EKG Practice

What It's All About

Mamie was a new paramedic on orientation with Jake, a paramedic with 12 years of experience. Their first call was for a 65-year-old female complaining of chest pain. The 12-lead EKG looked suspicious to Mamie. "She looks like she's infarcting," whispered Mamie to her co-worker, "Look at that ST segment elevation." Jake agreed. The duo started the patient on oxygen, assessed her vital signs, gave sublingual nitroglycerine, and called in their report to the closest hospital that had a cardiac cath lab capable of performing PCI. They transmitted the EKG to the receiving hospital. When the paramedics arrived at the emergency room with the patient, the cath lab team was standing by to take the patient for PCI. As a result of their recognition that an MI was in progress, the patient received immediate definitive treatment and her MI was minimized in size.

Introduction

This chapter pulls together everything you've learned so far about rhythm and 12-lead EKG interpretation. First, you will find a comprehensive summary of what to look for on every EKG, then a checklist. Refer to these when evaluating the 12-lead EKGs that follow.

There are 20 EKGs to interpret in this chapter. Take your time and be methodical. Don't hesitate to go back and review portions of this text if you find that you're a little weak in certain areas. Practice does indeed make perfect.

Now let's get down to work.

12-Lead EKG Interpretation in a Nutshell

You've seen all the criteria for 12-lead EKG interpretation. Let's put it all in condensed form. Look for the following on every 12-lead EKG:

The Basics	Rhythm, Rate, Intervals (PR, QRS, QT)
Axis quadrant	Normal, LAD, RAD, or indeterminate?
BBB/Hemiblock	RBBB = RSR′ in V_1, QRS $\geq$ 0.12 seconds
	LBBB = QS or RS in V_1, QRS $\geq$ 0.12 seconds
	LAHB = small Q in I, small R in III, left axis deviation
	LPHB = small R in I, small Q in III, right axis deviation
Hypertrophy	RVH = R $\geq$ S in V_1, right axis deviation; inverted T may or may not be present
	LVH = S in V_1 + R in V_5 or V_6 $\geq$ 35
Miscellaneous	Digitalis effect = Sagging ST segments, prolonged PR interval
	Hyperkalemia = Tall, pointy, narrow T waves
	Severe hyperkalemia = Wide QRS complex
	Hypokalemia = Prominent U waves, flattened T waves
	Hypercalcemia = Shortened ST segment causing short QT interval
	Hypocalcemia = Prolonged ST segment causing prolonged QT
Infarction	Anterior MI = ST elevation and/or significant Q in V_2 to V_4
	Inferior MI = ST elevation and/or significant Q in II, III, aVF
	Lateral MI = ST elevation and/or significant Q in I, aVL, V_5 to V_6
	Anteroseptal MI = ST elevation and/or significant Q in V_1 plus any anterior lead(s)
	Extensive anterior (extensive anterior-lateral) = ST elevation and/or significant Q in I, aVL, V_1 to V_6
	Posterior MI = Large R + upright T in V_1 to V_2; may also have ST depression
	Non-ST elevation MI = Widespread ST depression and T wave inversion in many leads
	Ischemia = Inverted T waves in any lead, as long as not BBB-related

12-Lead EKG Interpretation Checklist

The Basics

- Rhythm _____
- Rate _____
- Intervals: PR _____ QRS _____ QT _____

Axis

Circle one:

- Normal
- Abnormal (what quadrant?) _____

Bundle Branch Blocks/Hemiblocks

Circle if present:

■ RBBB	■ LBBB
■ LAHB	■ LPHB

Hypertrophy

Circle if present:

- RVH
- LVH

Infarction/Ischemia

Circle if present:

- Infarction
- Ischemia

Which walls of the heart? _____

Miscellaneous Effects

Circle if present:

■ Digitalis effect	■ Hyperkalemia
■ Severe hyperkalemia	■ Hypokalemia
■ Hypercalcemia	■ Hypocalcemia

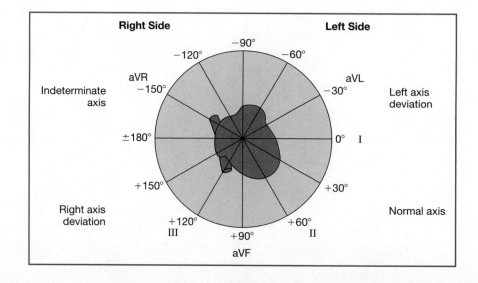

Practice EKGS

1. Rhythm and rate _Sinus rhythm with 1st degree AV block_ 63

Axis _Normal_   PR _.20 - .24_   QRS _.016_   QT _0.44-.48_

Hypertrophy _None_   BBB/HB _LBBB_

Miscellaneous effects _None with QRs from LBBB_

Infarction _None_

2. Rhythm and rate Sinus Arrhythmia PR 0.18 QRS 0.12 QT 0.34

Axis Normal PR 0.18 QRS 0.12 QT 0.24

Hypertrophy RVH BBB/HB

Miscellaneous effects None

Infarction None

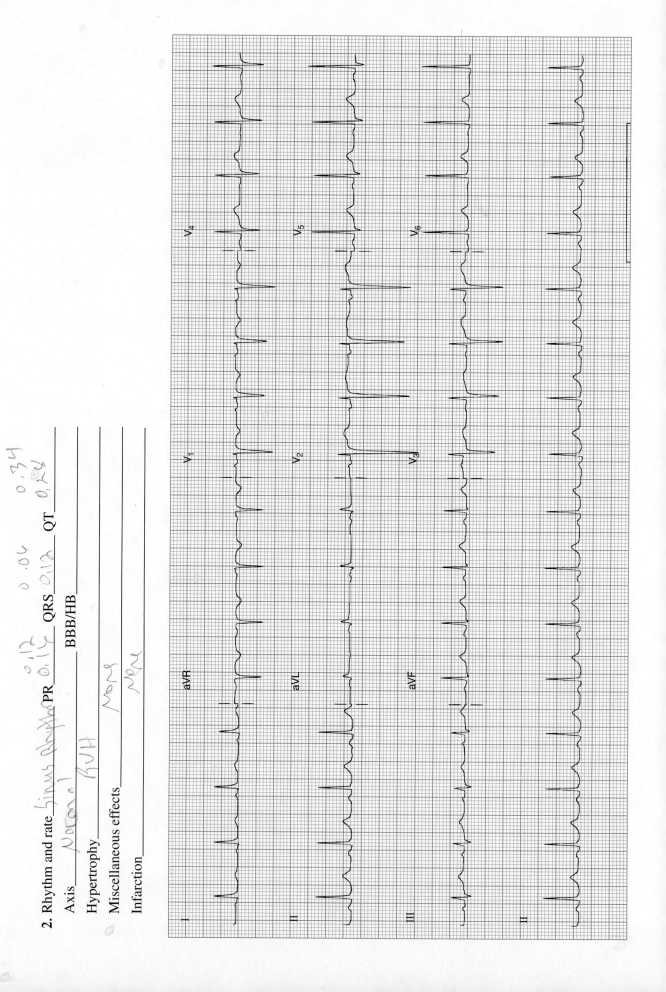

3. Rhythm and rate ___94/min Sinus Rhythm___ **PR** _0.16_ **QRS** _____ **QT** _0.40_

Axis _____ **BBB/HB** _____

Hypertrophy _____

Miscellaneous effects _____

Infarction _____

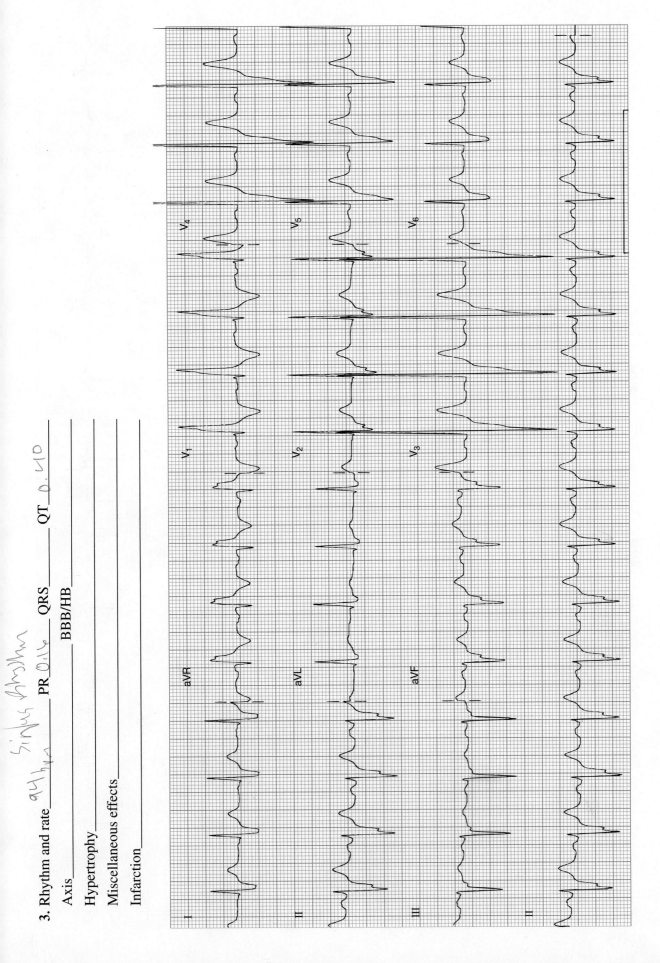

4. Rhythm and rate _____ PR _____ QRS _____ QT _____

Axis _____ BBB/HB _____

Hypertrophy _____

Miscellaneous effects _____

Infarction _____

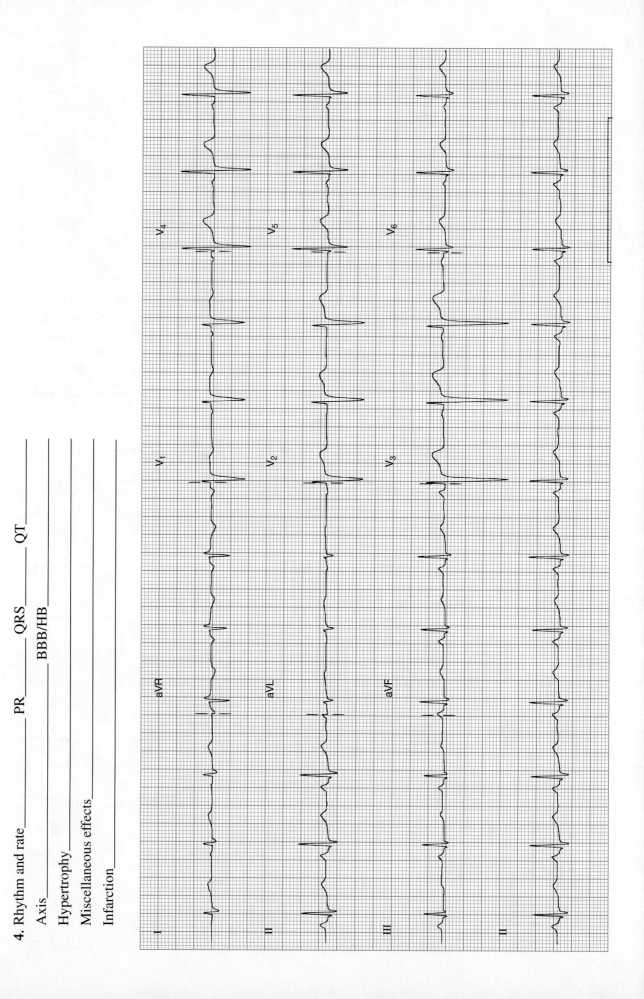

5. Rhythm and rate _____ PR _____ QRS _____ QT _____

Axis _____ BBB/HB _____

Hypertrophy _____

Miscellaneous effects _____

Infarction _____

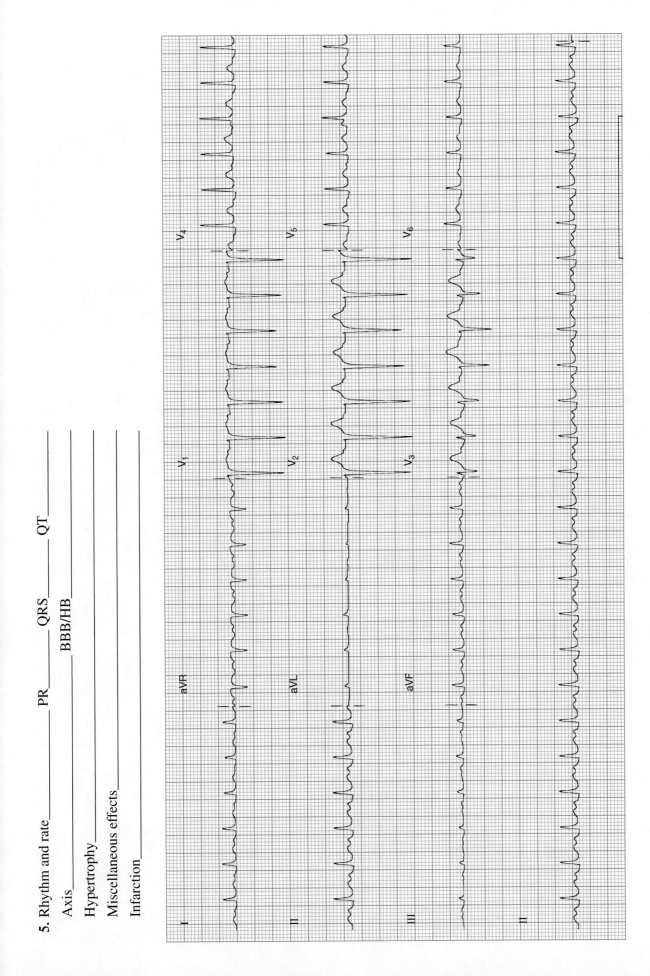

6. Rhythm and rate _____

Axis _____ PR _____ QRS _____ QT _____

Hypertrophy _____ BBB/HB _____

Miscellaneous effects _____

Infarction _____

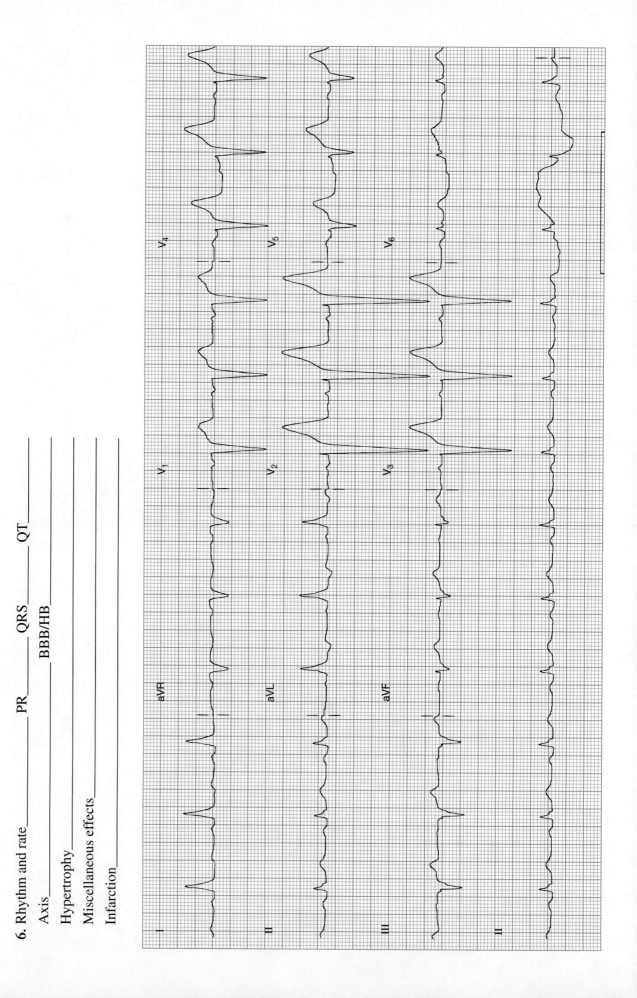

7. Rhythm and rate _____ PR _____ QRS _____ QT _____

Axis _____ BBB/HB _____

Hypertrophy _____

Miscellaneous effects _____

Infarction _____

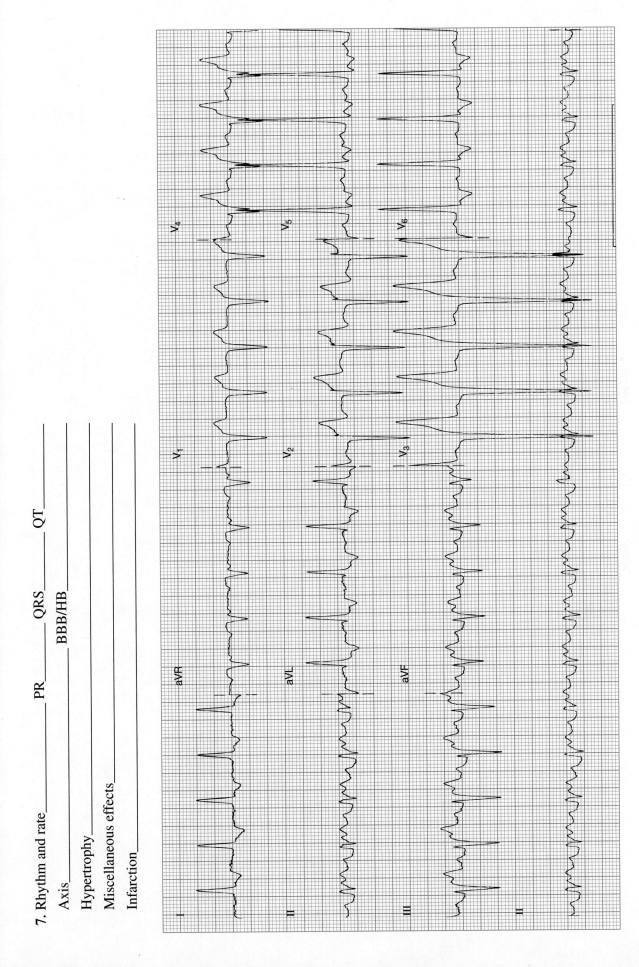

345

8. Rhythm and rate _____ PR _____ QRS _____ QT _____

Axis _____ BBB/HB _____

Hypertrophy _____

Miscellaneous effects _____

Infarction _____

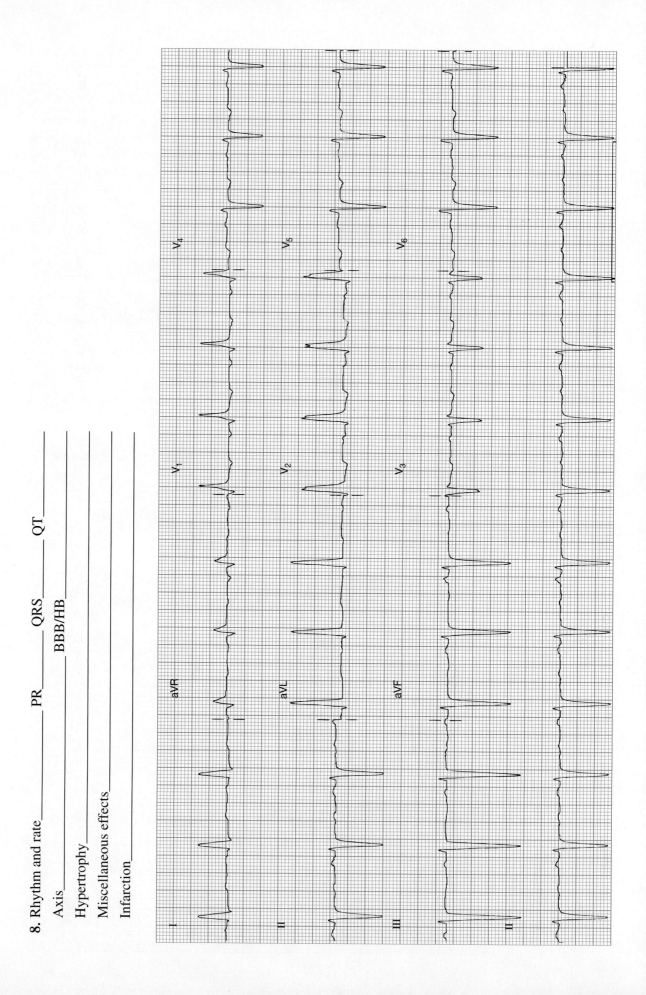

9. Rhythm and rate _____ PR _____ QRS _____ QT _____

Axis _____ BBB/HB _____

Hypertrophy _____

Miscellaneous effects _____

Infarction _____

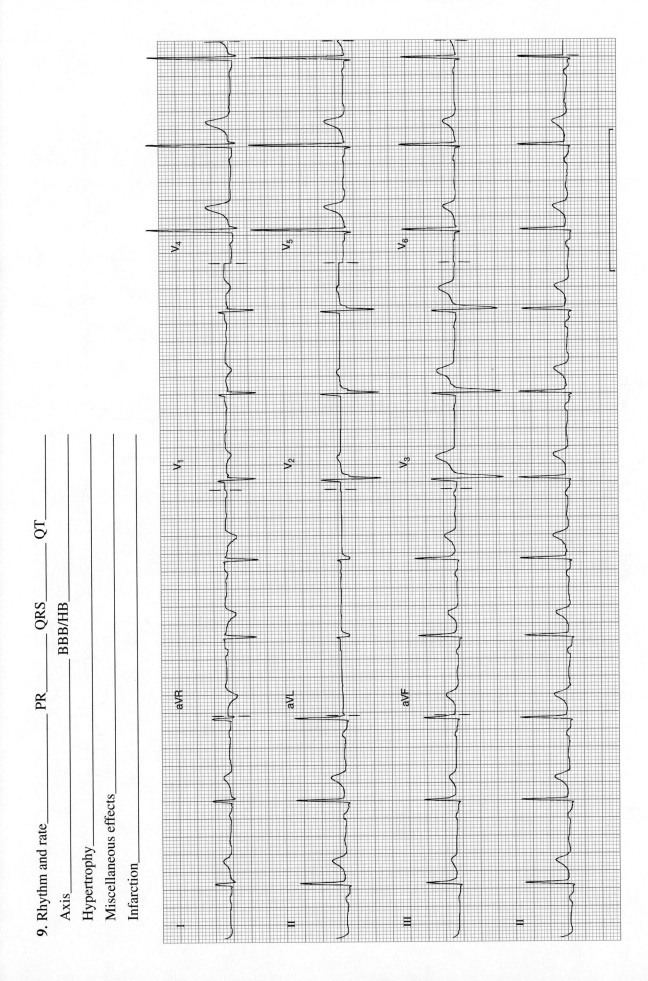

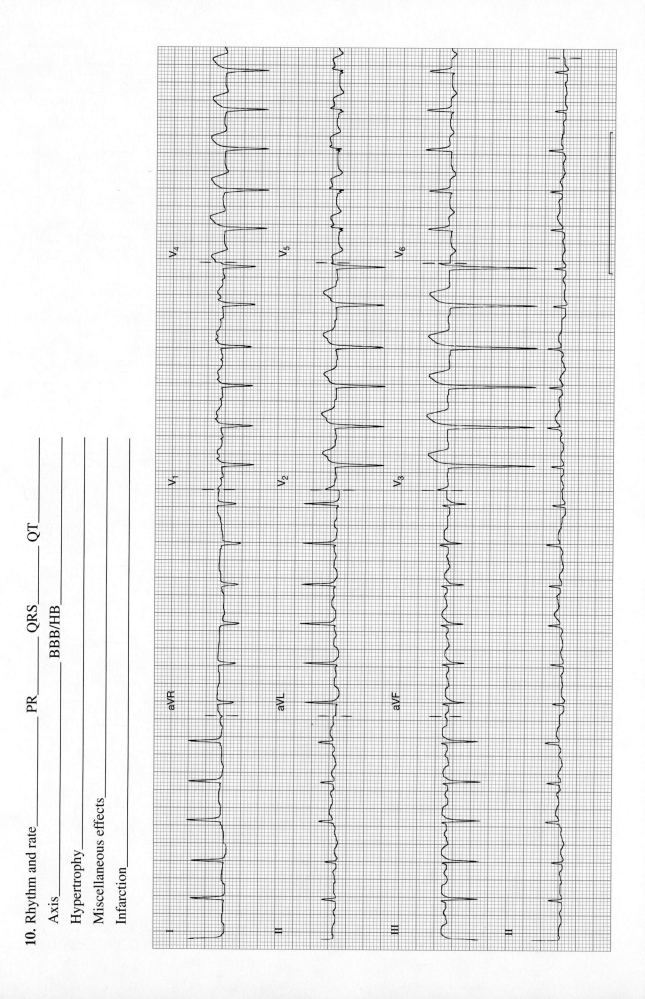

10. Rhythm and rate _____

Axis _____ PR _____ QRS _____ QT _____

Hypertrophy _____ BBB/HB _____

Miscellaneous effects _____

Infarction _____

11.

Rhythm and rate _____ PR _____ QRS _____ QT _____

Axis _____ BBB/HB _____

Hypertrophy _____

Miscellaneous effects _____

Infarction _____

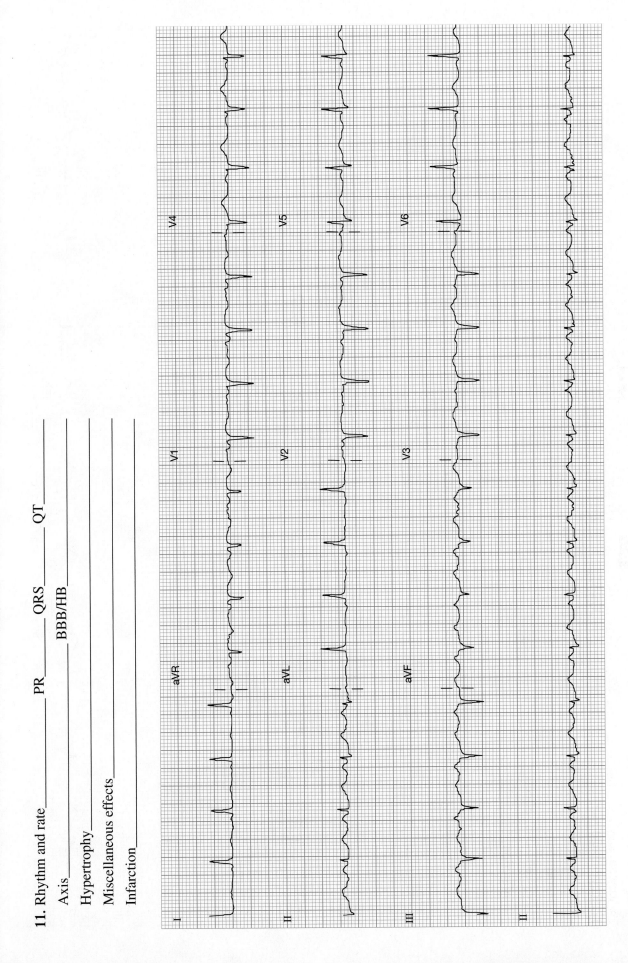

349

12. Rhythm and rate _____ PR _____ QRS _____ QT _____

Axis _____ BBB/HB _____

Hypertrophy _____

Miscellaneous effects _____

Infarction _____

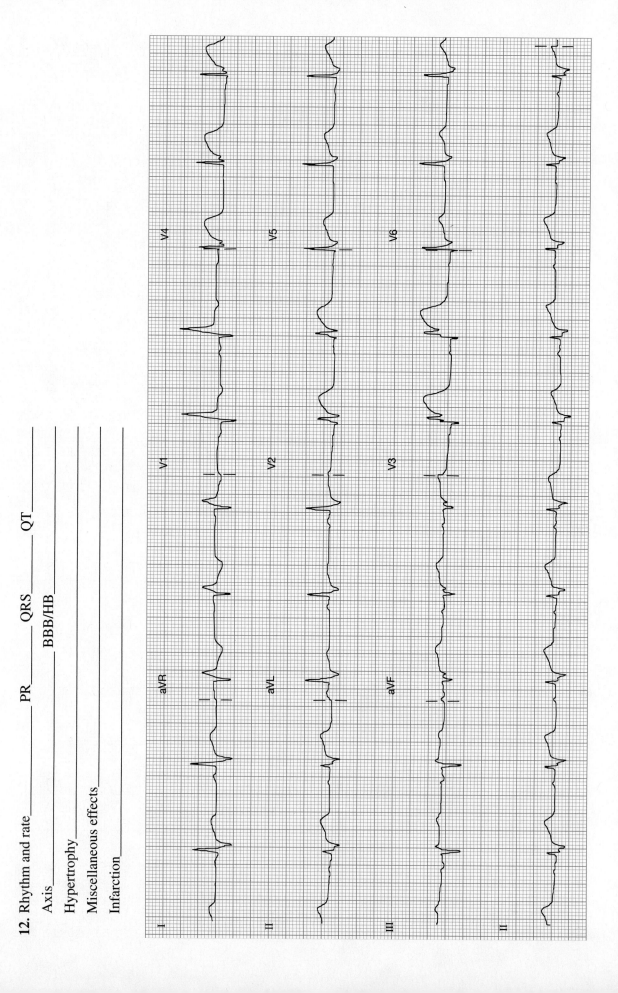

13. Rhythm and rate_____ PR_____ QRS_____ QT_____

Axis_____ BBB/HB_____

Hypertrophy_____

Miscellaneous effects_____

Infarction_____

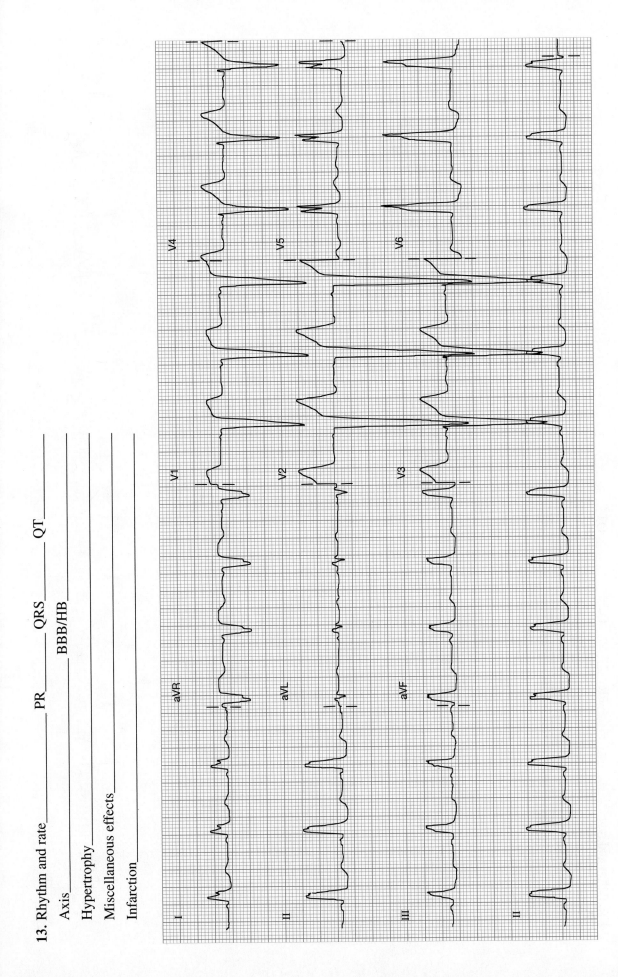

14. Rhythm and rate _____

Axis _____ PR _____ QRS _____ QT _____

Hypertrophy _____ BBB/HB _____

Miscellaneous effects _____

Infarction _____

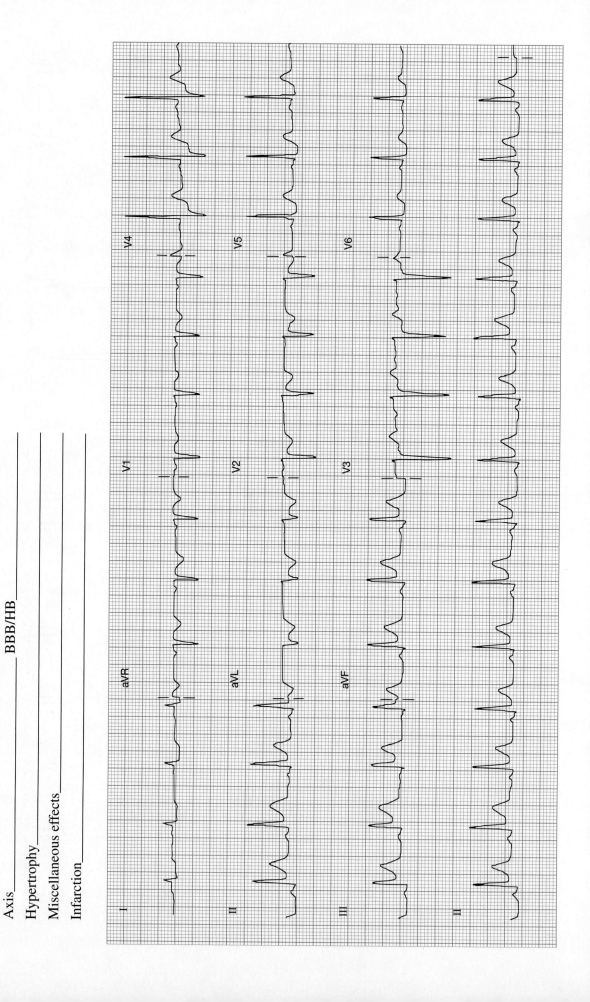

15. Rhythm and rate _____ PR _____ QRS _____ QT _____

Axis _____ BBB/HB _____

Hypertrophy _____

Miscellaneous effects _____

Infarction _____

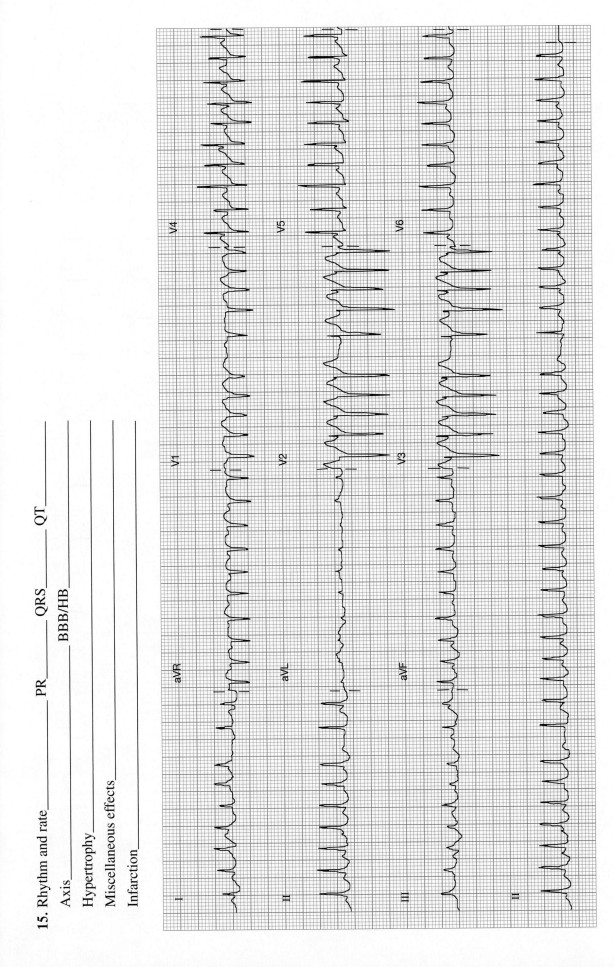

16. Rhythm and rate _____ PR _____ QRS _____ QT _____

Axis _____ BBB/HB _____

Hypertrophy _____

Miscellaneous effects _____

Infarction _____

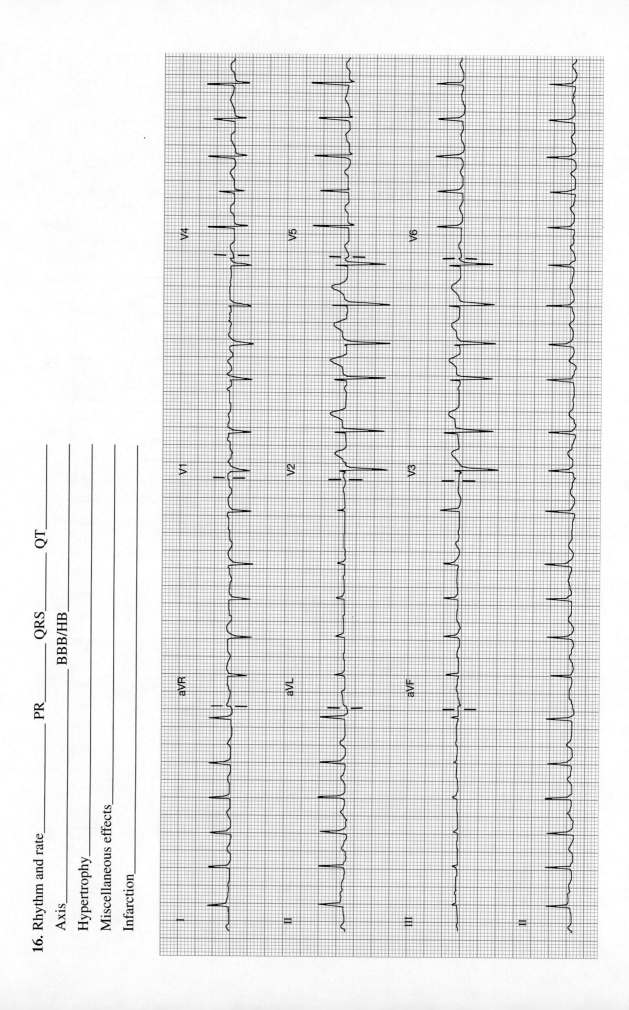

17. Rhythm and rate _____ PR _____ QRS _____ QT _____

Axis _____ BBB/HB _____

Hypertrophy _____

Miscellaneous effects _____

Infarction _____

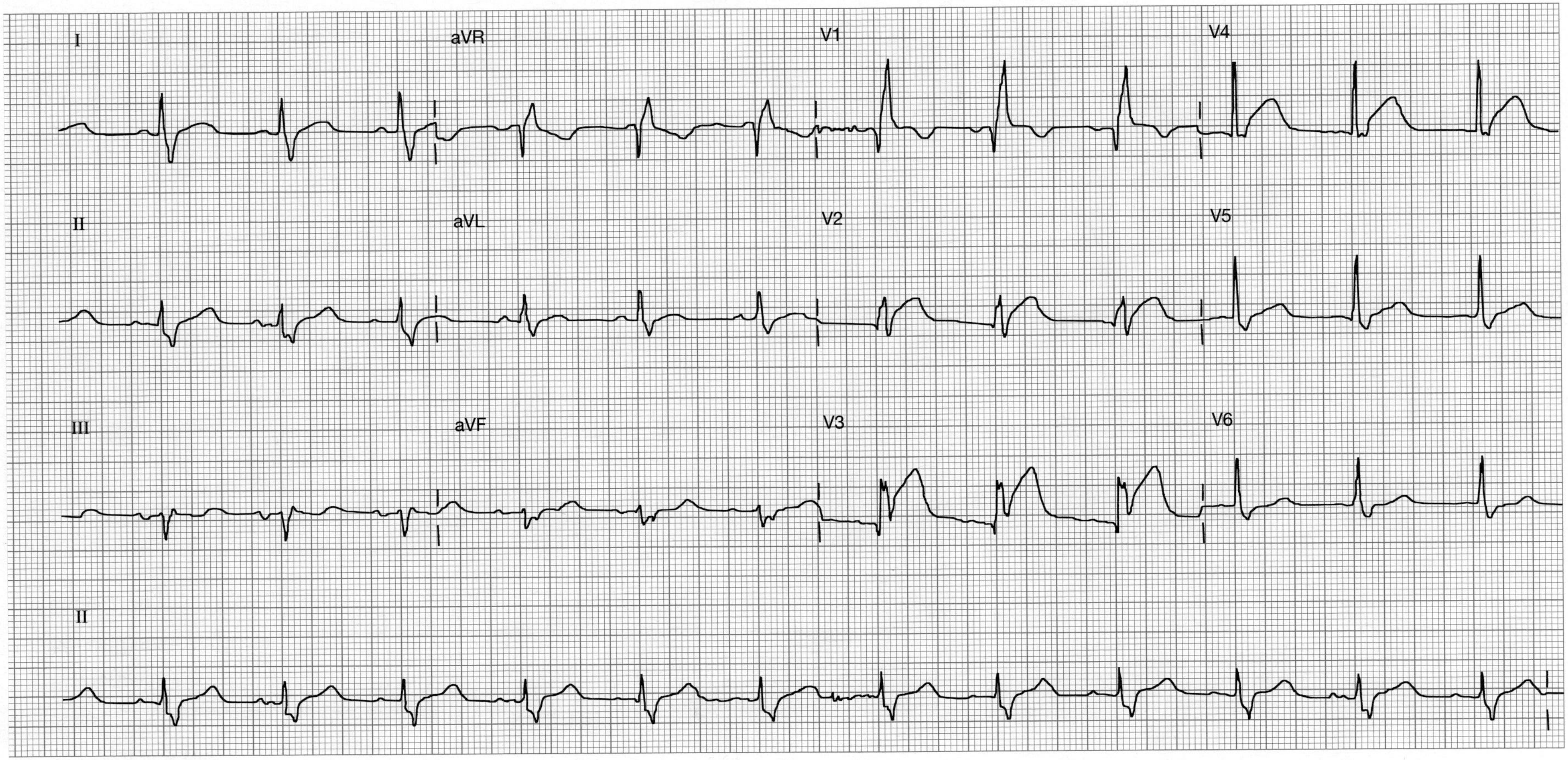

18. Rhythm and rate _____ PR _____ QRS _____ QT _____

Axis _____ BBB/HB _____

Hypertrophy _____

Miscellaneous effects _____

Infarction _____

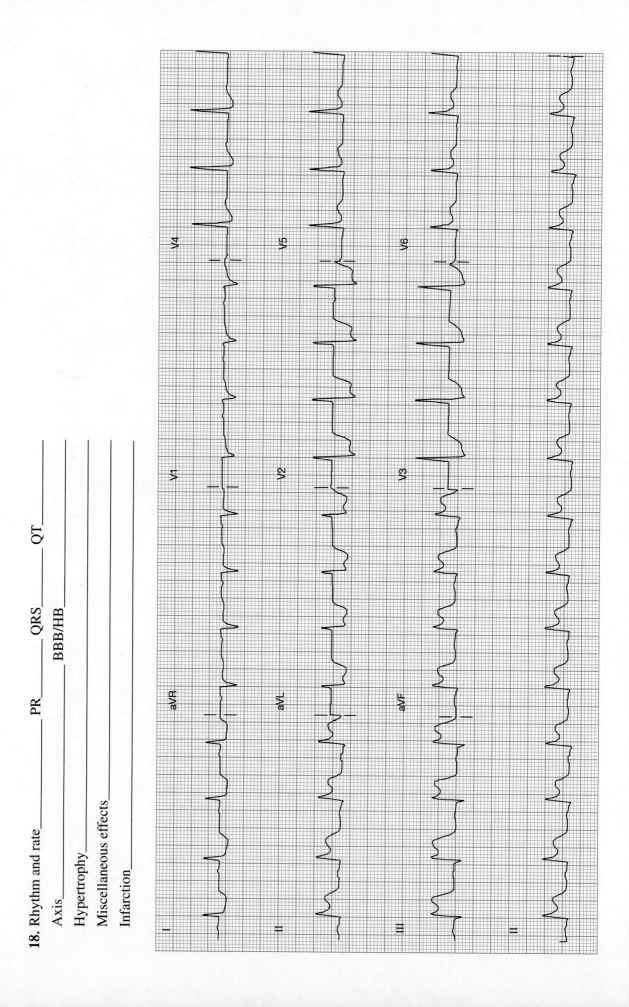

19. Rhythm and rate _____ PR _____ QRS _____ QT _____

Axis _____ BBB/HB _____

Hypertrophy _____

Miscellaneous effects _____

Infarction _____

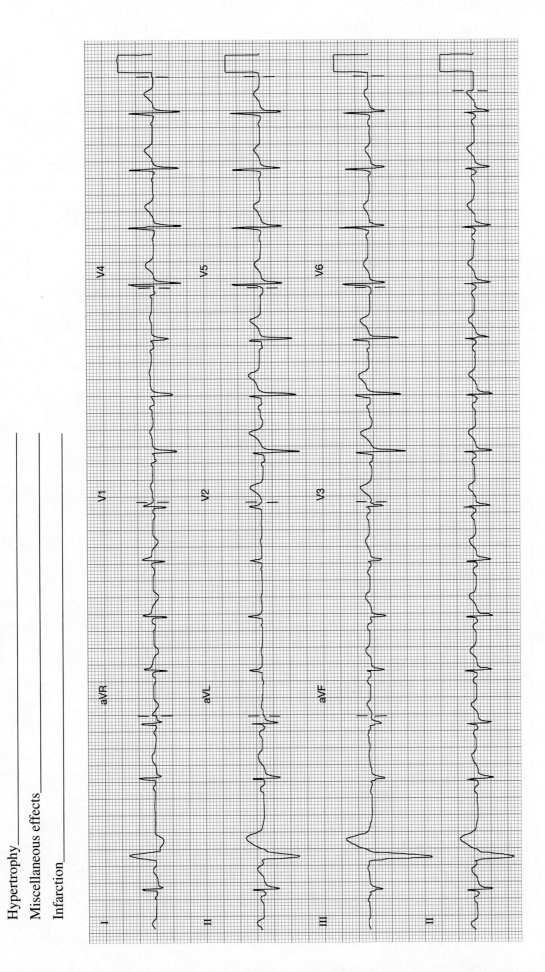

20. Rhythm and rate _____ PR _____ QRS _____ QT _____

     Axis _____ BBB/HB _____

     Hypertrophy _____

     Miscellaneous effects _____

     Infarction _____

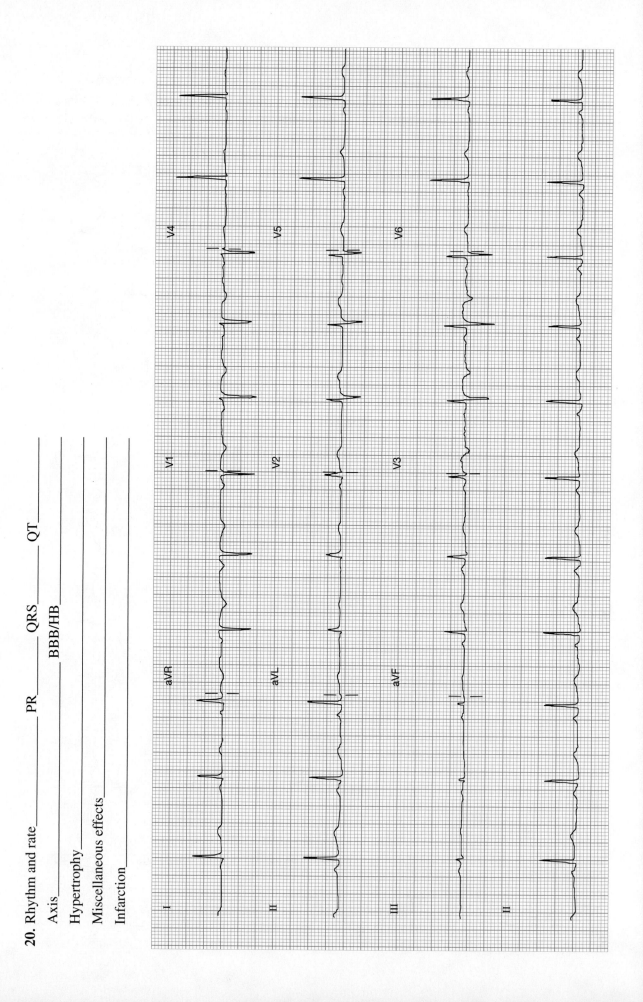

PEARSON

myhealthprofessionskit

Use this address to access the Companion Website created for this textbook. Simply select "Basic Health Science" from the choice of disciplines. Find this book and log in using your username and password to access video clips, animations, assessment questions, and more.

16 Medications and Electrical Therapy

What It's All About

The monitor alarmed and the ICU nurses shot up from their chairs and ran into Mr. Roman's room. He was in V-tach and had no pulse. "Get the code cart!" yelled nurse Sherdeane as she pushed the code button to summon help. Tanya started chest compressions and Jean began artificial respirations using a special oxygen mask. In no time, the nurses had defibrillated the patient, done two more minutes of CPR, and rechecked the rhythm. It was now a junctional bradycardia with a heart rate of 38. The patient did have a pulse but his blood pressure was very low. "Give atropine and let's get the transcutaneous pacemaker on him at a rate of 60," ordered the physician. The pacemaker did not show capture so the nurse turned up the voltage. That worked. The patient was now showing a beautiful paced rhythm. Within a few minutes, the atropine was kicking in—the patient's heart rate increased and soon he was in sinus rhythm with a heart rate of 83. The pacemaker sensed the patient's inherent rhythm and was no longer firing. When Mr. Roman woke up later and asked what happened, his wife, the physician, and Sherdeane explained his condition. An angiogram done a few days later showed several narrowed coronary arteries. Mr. Roman had bypass surgery and no further complications.

Introduction

Treatment of arrhythmias can involve medications, electrical shock to the heart, or an electrical stimulus to pace the heart. Let's look at these now.

Medications

Cardiac medications are used to treat arrhythmias or abnormalities in cardiac function. Other medications are used to treat other conditions or diseases, but can have EKG effects. Let's look at the various classifications of medications.

Antiarrhythmics

These medications are used to treat and/or prevent arrhythmias. They all affect the action potential. See Figure 16–1 for the effects of each class on the action potential. There are four classes of antiarrhythmic medications. Let's look at the four classes.

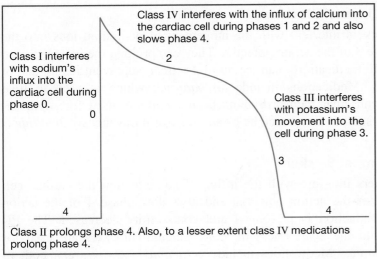

Class IV interferes with the influx of calcium into the cardiac cell during phases 1 and 2 and also slows phase 4.

Class I interferes with sodium's influx into the cardiac cell during phase 0.

Class III interferes with potassium's movement into the cell during phase 3.

Class II prolongs phase 4. Also, to a lesser extent class IV medications prolong phase 4.

FIGURE 16–1

Effects of each class of antiarrhythmic medications on the action potential.

Class I: Sodium Channel Blockers

Class I medications block the influx of sodium ions into the cardiac cell during depolarization. This results in decreased excitability of the cardiac cell and decreased myocardial contractility. Class I antiarrhythmic medications affect phase 0 of the action potential. There are three categories of class I antiarrhythmics:

- *Class Ia.* These medications include *quinidine* and *procainamide,* and they cause prolonged QT intervals as well as decreased cardiac contractility. They can also cause hypotension. Quinidine is especially notorious for causing wide T waves. Most class Ia antiarrhythmics can be used to treat supraventricular as well as ventricular arrhythmias. Quinidine is usually given orally. In rare instances it may be given intravenously. Procainamide can be given orally or intravenously. Both medications have lost favor in current practice, since other meds have proved safer and more therapeutic.

- *Class Ib.* These medications include *lidocaine* and *tocainide,* both of which have a local anesthetic effect. They are used for treatment of ventricular arrhythmias only. They suppress the ventricles' irritability and raise the fibrillatory threshold, making it less likely that the ventricles will fibrillate. Class Ib medications have minimal, if any, effect on conductivity. Lidocaine is given intravenously. Tocainide is given orally.

- *Class Ic.* These medications slow impulse conduction and are useful in treating SVT and ventricular arrhythmias. Unfortunately, they are also prone to causing arrhythmias and are therefore used only in life-threatening situations. These medications include *flecainide* and *propafenone,* both of which are given orally.

Class II: Beta-Blockers

Beta-blockers slow the heart rate by blocking the sympathetic nervous system's **beta-receptors**. There are two kinds of beta-receptors: *Beta-1 receptors* increase heart rate, conductivity, and contractility. *Beta-2 receptors* relax smooth muscle in arteries and bronchi. Blocking these receptors decreases or blocks these actions. Beta-blockers decrease the automaticity of the sinus node, slow AV conduction, and slow the process of depolarization.

They are used to treat supraventricular tachyarrhythmias (tachycardias that originate above the ventricle). They depress phase 4 of the action potential. Beta-blockers include medications such as *propranolol* and *atenolol.* Propranolol can be given orally or intravenously. Atenolol is given orally. Beta-blockers should be used with caution in patients with asthma or heart failure, as the effects could be life threatening.

Class III: Potassium Channel Blockers

Potassium channel blockers interfere with the movement of potassium ions into the cardiac cell during phase 3 of the action potential. They can prolong the PR, QRS, and QT intervals. Class III medications can be used to treat supraventricular and/or ventricular arrhythmias. Medications include *amiodarone,* which is used to treat ventricular and supraventricular tachyarrhythmias, and *ibutilide,* used for supraventricular tachyarrhythmias. Amiodarone can be given orally or intravenously. *Ibutilide* is given intravenously.

Class IV: Calcium Channel Blockers

Calcium channel blockers interfere with the influx of calcium into the cardiac cell during phases 1 and 2 of the action potential and also slow phase 4 of the action potential. Thus, AV conduction is prolonged and contractility decreased. The PR interval will prolong and the heart rate will slow. Calcium blockers are used for supraventricular arrhythmias. Medications include *verapamil* and *diltiazem,* both of which can be given orally or intravenously. Overdose of calcium channel-blockers is treated by administration of calcium.

There are other antiarrhythmic medications that do not fall into any of the four classes. These include but are not limited to *adenosine,* which is used to treat SVT, and *digitalis,* classified as a cardiac glycoside, which is used to treat heart failure and supraventricular arrhythmias.

Let's summarize the antiarrhythmic medications. See Table 16–1.

TABLE 16–1 Antiarrhythmic Medications Summary

Class	Known as	Mode of Action	Examples	Kind of Arrhythmias Treated
I	Sodium channel blockers	Block sodium's influx into the cardiac cell, decrease myocardial excitability and contractility	*Ia.* Quinidine, procainamide *Ib.* Lidocaine, tocainide *Ic.* Flecainide, propafenone	*Ia.* Supraventricular and ventricular *Ib.* Ventricular only *Ic.* Supraventricular and ventricular
II	Beta-blockers	Block the sympathetic nervous system's beta-receptors, slow the heart rate	Propranolol, atenolol	Supraventricular
III	Potassium channel blockers	Decrease potassium's movement into the cardiac cell, prolong PR, QRS, and QT intervals	Amiodarone, bretylium, ibutilide	Ventricular *or* supraventricular
IV	Calcium channel blockers	Decrease calcium's influx into the cardiac cell, slow AV, conduction, decrease contractility	Verapamil, diltiazem	Supraventricular

Emergency Cardiac Medications

Emergency cardiac medications are used during cardiac arrest or in situations in which the patient's condition is rapidly deteriorating because of an arrhythmia.

- *Atropine.*   Atropine is used to increase the heart rate during asystole or bradycardias. It reverses any vagal influence that could slow or stop the heart. It is given intravenously or intraosseous (IO involves a large-bore needle inserted into the marrow of a large bone such as the femur [thigh bone]).
- *Epinephrine.*   Epinephrine causes vasoconstriction (narrowing of the arteries), thus increasing the blood pressure, and beta-receptor stimulation, thus restoring the heartbeat and increasing heart rate in cardiac arrest. It is given IV or IO and is used for asystole, V-fib, pulseless V-tach, pulseless electrical activity, and as an infusion for profound bradycardias.
- *Vasopressin.*   Vasopressin can be used in place of the first or second dose of epinephrine during cardiac arrest to increase heart rate and restore heartbeat.
- *Dopamine.*   Dopamine increases heart rate and renal blood flow. It can be used as an infusion in bradycardias.
- *Amiodarone.*   A class III antiarrhythmic, amiodarone has become the first-line medication for treatment of ventricular fibrillation and pulseless ventricular tachycardia. Additionally, it can be used to treat supraventricular arrhythmias as well. It is given IV or IO during an emergency and can later be given by mouth to prevent arrhythmia recurrences.
- *Adenosine.*   Adenosine is used in emergency situations to convert supraventricular tachycardias back to sinus or to slow the heart rate to a more tolerable level if conversion is not possible. It is given IV and can have the unnerving side effect of causing transient asystole of 6 or 7 seconds before the rhythm converts to sinus.
- *Sodium bicarbonate.*   This medication used to be a front-line medication routinely given during cardiac arrest, but its use has fallen out of favor in recent years due to research that has shown it to be potentially damaging if given when not indicated by blood gas studies. Sodium bicarb combats the blood's acidity that develops in the oxygen-deprived setting of cardiac arrest. Combating this acidity can help convert arrhythmias back to normal in a cardiac arrest. Nowadays, sodium bicarb is given most often in prolonged cardiac arrest situations or in those complicated by hyperkalemia. It is given IV.
- *Oxygen.* Although most people do not think of oxygen as a medication, when it is used to treat disease or a medical condition, it is indeed a medication. Oxygen is used to provide the tissues with the oxygen they are lacking. This alone can help convert arrhythmias back to normal. Oxygen can be given by mask, nasal cannula (small prongs in the nose), endotracheal tube (a tube inserted into the trachea by way of the mouth), and **tracheotomy** (surgically inserting a tube through the neck into the trachea).

Let's summarize the emergency medications. See Table 16–2.

Other Medications with EKG Effects

The following medications are given for non-EKG-related purposes, but they have effects on the heart rhythm or heart rate.

- Diuretics   Are medications given to increase the urine output in patients with heart failure, renal disease, or hypertension. Examples of diuretics include but are not limited to *furosemide, bumetanide, ethacrynic acid,* and *mannitol.* Since diuretics cause increased urination, they can result in dehydration and electrolyte disturbances such as hypokalemia. Hypokalemia, you'll recall, is low blood

TABLE 16–2　Emergency Medications Summary

Medication	Mode of Action	Indication
Atropine	Increases heart rate	Bradycardias, asystole
Epinephrine	Stimulates contractility, increases heart rate and BP	Cardiac arrest, bradycardias
Vasopressin	Increases heart rate and BP, stimulates contractility	Bradycardias, cardiac arrest
Dopamine	Increases heart rate	Bradycardias
Amiodarone	Helps convert rapid ventricular and supraventricular arrhythmias back to sinus	Rapid ventricular arrhythmias, PVCs, supraventricular arrhythmias
Adenosine	Decreases heart rate	Supraventricular tachycardias
Sodium bicarbonate	Decreases blood's acidity	Cardiac arrest with acidosis; hyperkalemia
Oxygen	Increases tissue oxygenation	Symptomatic arrhythmias, cardiac arrest

potassium level, and it can cause ventricular irritability and ventricular arrhythmias such as V-tach. Dehydration decreases cardiac output and can result in tachycardias.

- **Bronchodilators**　Are medications that dilate narrowed airways in patients with asthma or chronic lung disease. Examples of bronchodilators include *albuterol, levalbuterol, perbuterol, salmeterol,* and *formoterol*. Bronchodilators often cause tachycardia—sometimes with heart rates up to the 140s to 150s. And this tachycardia can cause decreased cardiac output, cardiac ischemia, and chest pain.
- **Antihypertensives**　Are medications given to treat high blood pressure. They can include diuretics (which we've already discussed), **beta-blockers**, and **vasodilators**. Beta-blockers treat hypertension by decreasing the workload of the heart and by dilating arterial walls; however, because of their slowing action on the AV node, they can also result in AV blocks or other kinds of bradycardia. Examples of beta-blockers are *esmolol, propranolol, metoprolol,* and *labetalol*. Vasodilators relax the walls of arteries and/or veins and thereby lower the blood pressure. This can also decrease cardiac output and result in a tachycardia. Examples of vasodilators include *hydralazine, nitroglycerine,* and *diltiazem*.
- **Nitrates**　Are medications given to dilate the coronary arteries and improve coronary blood flow, thus reducing or eliminating chest pain. The typical example is *nitroglycerine tablets*. Nitrates can cause a drop in blood pressure, inducing tachycardias and, if severe enough for long enough, ischemia (ST depression) or MI.
- **Glaucoma medications**　Are eye drops used to decrease the intraocular (eyeball) pressure. There are many kinds of glaucoma meds, but one kind is a beta-blocker, which as you know can cause bradycardias. An example of beta-blocker eyedrops is *timolol*.
- **Erectile dysfunction medications**　Such as *sildenafil* and *tadalafil* can cause a profound drop in blood pressure as well as cardiac ischemia, MI, and tachycardias, especially if these medications are taken by patients who use prescription nitrates such as nitroglycerine for chest pain.
- **Tricyclic antidepressants (TCA)**　Such as *amitriptyline* and *dosulepin* are used to treat clinical depression. Unfortunately, they are also used with some frequency in suicide attempts by overdose. At toxic levels, TCAs can cause bradycardias including AV blocks, as well as sinus tachycardia, unstable

ventricular arrhythmias, asystole, widened QRS, and prolonged PR and QT intervals.

- ■ *Illegal drugs (cocaine, amphetamines, ecstasy).* Are used for their buzz. They have wide-ranging cardiac effects, including but not limited to prolonged QT intervals predisposing to torsades de pointes, hypotension, hypertension, tachycardias, AV blocks, myocardial ischemia and/or MI, and coronary artery spasm.
- ■ Thrombolytics Such as *alteplase* and *tenecteplase* are used to dissolve the blood clot causing a heart attack or stroke. They can result in bleeding that can increase heart rate. If thrombolytics are successful at aborting a STEMI in progress, the elevated ST segment should return to normal or near-normal.
- ■ Anticoagulants Are used to prevent blood clots and are routinely used in patients with atrial fibrillation, MI, and other conditions that can predispose patients to blood clots. Since anticoagulants are blood thinners, bleeding can result and lead to tachycardias.

As you can see, although all of these medications/drugs are used for non-EKG-related purposes, they have EKG effects. Always look at *all* your patient's medications to determine if any of them may be causing his or her rhythm or rate disturbances. Also consider that your patient's various medications may be *interacting* and causing rhythm and rate problems. And don't forget to ask about illegal/recreational drugs. Check out Table 16–3.

TABLE 16–3 Other Medications with EKG Effects Summary

Type of Medication	Examples	Used for	Cardiac Effects
Diuretics	Furosemide, bumetanide, mannitol, ethacrynic acid	Heart failure, renal failure, hypertension	Ventricular irritability, ventricular arrhythmias, tachycardias
Bronchodilators	Albuterol, salmeterol, formoterol	Asthma, COPD	Tachycardias, cardiac ischemia, chest pain
Antihypertensives (beta-blockers)	Esmolol, metoprolol, labetolol	Hypertension	Bradycardias, AV blocks, hypotension
Antihypertensives (vasodilators)	Hydralazine, diltiazem, nitroglycerine	Hypertension	Hypotension, tachycardias
Nitrates	Nitroglycerine tablets	Chest pain	Tachycardias, cardiac ischemia or MI
Glaucoma medication eyedrops	Timolol eyedrops	Glaucoma	Bradycardias
Erectile dysfunction medications	Sildenafil, tadalafil	Erectile dysfunction	Profound hypotension if used when already on nitrates for chest pain; tachycardias, cardiac ischemia and/or MI
Tricyclic antidepressants	Amitriptyline, dosulepin	Clinical depression	Bradycardias including AV blocks, sinus tachycardia, prolonged PR and QT intervals, ventricular arrhythmias, asystole
Illegal drugs	Cocaine, amphetamines, ecstasy	Recreation	Prolonged QT intervals predisposing to torsades de pointes; hypotension, hypertension, tachycardias, AV blocks, myocardial ischemia and/or MI, and coronary artery spasm
Thrombolytics	Tenecteplase, alteplase	Acute STEMI	Tachycardias secondary to bleeding, ST segment normalization
Anticoagulants	Warfarin	Atrial fibrillation, MI, other conditions	Tachycardias secondary to bleeding

Electrical Therapy

Electrical therapy involves utilizing electrical stimuli to either speed up (or in some cases slow) the heart rate or to shock the heart out of a dangerous or unstable rhythm. There are two kinds of electrical therapy—artificial pacemakers and cardioversion/defibrillation.

Artificial Pacemakers

> **Quick Tip**
>
> Pacemakers do not force the heart to beat. They simply send out an electrical signal, just as the heart's normal pacemakers do. If the heart is healthy enough, it should respond to that stimulus by depolarizing.

The primary function of an artificial pacemaker is to prevent the heart rate from becoming too slow. Pacemakers provide an electrical stimulus when the heart is unable to generate its own or when its own is too slow to provide adequate cardiac output. You'll recall from Chapter 10 that pacemakers can pace the atrium, the ventricle, or both.

Another use for pacemakers is antitachycardia pacing (also called overdrive pacing). This special programming function on some pacemakers allows the pacemaker to interrupt a tachycardia by interjecting a series of paced beats in the middle of the tachycardia, thus interrupting the rapid circuit and allowing the sinus node to resume control. On other pacemakers without the antitachycardia pacing function, the physician can simply stand at the patient's bedside and increase the pacemaker's heart rate until it exceeds the tachycardia. This puts the pacemaker in control and abolishes the tachycardia. The pacemaker's heart rate can then be decreased back down to a normal rate.

Indications

Indications for a pacemaker may include the following:

- Symptomatic sinus bradycardia
- Junctional rhythms
- Idioventricular rhythm
- Dying heart
- Asystole
- 2:1 AV block
- Mobitz II second-degree AV block
- Third degree AV block
- Antitachycardia pacing

Permanent versus Temporary Pacemakers

A **permanent pacemaker** is inserted when the arrhythmia that necessitates it is thought to be permanent. It has two components—a *pulse generator* (a battery pack), inserted surgically into a pocket made just under the right or left clavicle, and a *pacing catheter,* which is inserted via the subclavian vein into the superior vena cava and down into the right atrium and/or ventricle. Permanent pacemaker batteries are made of lithium and usually last between 5 and 15 years. See Figure 16–2.

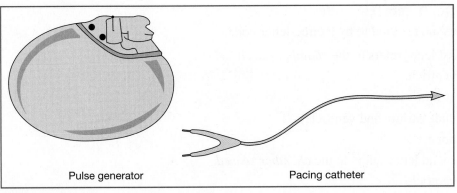

FIGURE 16-2

Pulse generator and pacing catheter of a permanent pacemaker.

Temporary pacemakers are used to help the patient "get over the hump" after an MI or other problem temporarily causes symptomatic bradycardia. Temporary pacemakers have various types, the two most common being the transvenous, in which a pacing catheter is inserted into a large vein and threaded into the right atrium and down into the right ventricle, and the transcutaneous, which involves large pacing electrodes attached to the chest and back that pace the heart through the chest wall. Both of these temporary pacer methods require a pulse generator at the patient's bedside. See Figures 16–3 and 16–4.

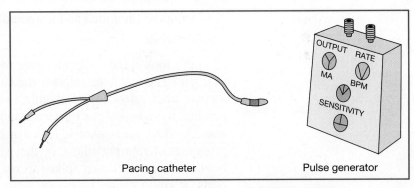

FIGURE 16-3

Transvenous pacemaker components.

Pacemaker Terminology

Firing refers to the pacemaker's generation of an electrical stimulus. It is noted on the EKG by the presence of a *pacemaker spike*.

Capture refers to the presence of a P wave or a QRS complex (or both) after the pacemaker spike. This indicates that the tissue in the chamber being paced has depolarized. The pacemaker is then said to have "captured" that chamber. Paced QRS complexes are wide and bizarre and resemble PVCs.

Sensing refers to the pacemaker's ability to recognize the patient's own intrinsic rhythm or beats in order to decide if it needs to fire. Most pacemakers function on a *demand mode*, meaning they fire only when needed (only on demand).

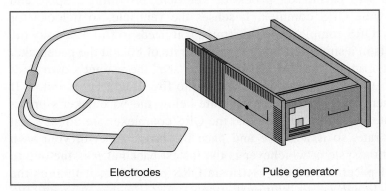

FIGURE 16-4

Transcutaneous pacemaker components.

Three-Letter Pacemaker Code

Pacemakers are referred to by a three-letter code:

- The first letter refers to the *chamber paced.*

  V = ventricle

  A = atrium

  D = dual (atrium and ventricle)

  O = none

- The second letter refers to the *chamber sensed.*

  V = ventricle

  A = atrium

  D = dual (atrium and ventricle)

  O = none

- The third letter refers to the *response to sensed events.*

  I = inhibited (pacemaker watches and waits, does not pace until needed)

  T = triggered (pacemaker sends out a signal in response to a sensed event)

  D = dual (inhibited and triggered)

  O = none

Let's look at the codes in a little more depth. What would a VOO pacemaker do, for example? The first letter refers to the chamber paced, so the VOO paces the ventricle. The second letter refers to the chamber sensed, so it senses nothing. And since it senses nothing, it obviously can't have a response to sensed events, so the last letter has to be O also. A VOO pacemaker is called a **fixed-rate pacemaker** because it will fire at its programmed rate regardless of the patient's own rate at the time. This is dangerous, because if the pacemaker spike hits on top of the T wave of the patient's own (**intrinsic**) beats, it could cause V-tach or V-fib. Fixed-rate pacemakers are not used today. All pacemakers in use today are *demand pacemakers.* They have a sensor that tells the pacemaker when to fire.

VVI Pacemakers

The most common kinds of pacemakers in use today are the VVI and the DDD. The **VVI pacemaker,** also known as a **ventricular demand pacemaker,** was at one time the most commonly used permanent pacer. It's now in second place. The VVI pacer consists of a catheter with both pacing and sensing capabilities and is inserted into the right ventricle. See Figure 16–5.

The VVI pacemaker paces the ventricle, providing a spike and then a wide QRS complex. It senses the ventricle, so it looks for intrinsic QRS complexes to determine if it needs to fire. Let's say the patient is in a sinus rhythm with a heart rate of 80 and the pacemaker is set at a rate of 60. The sensor would "see" the patient's own QRS complexes and realize it does not need to fire. It will be inhibited. If the patient's heart rate falls to a rate below the pacemaker's preset heart rate, the pacer will see that the QRS complexes are not at a fast enough rate, so it will fire and pace the heart. As with your own conduction system, whichever is the fastest pacemaker is the one in control. Since the VVI pacer senses only intrinsic QRS complexes, it ignores the P waves. Therefore, *there will be no relationship between P waves and paced QRS complexes.*

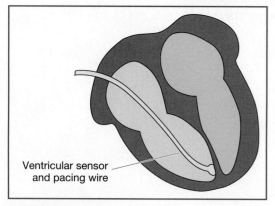

Ventricular sensor and pacing wire

FIGURE 16–5

VVI pacemaker inserted into the right ventricle.

VVI pacemakers provide two options:

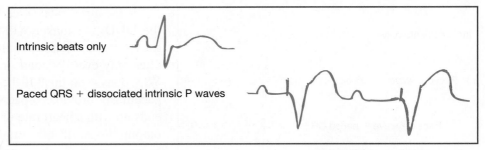

- *Intrinsic beats only.* The pacemaker does not pace because it doesn't need to. The rhythm is fast enough, so the pacemaker is inhibited. There will be no pacemaker spikes. The rhythm is produced completely by the patient.

FIGURE 16–6

VVI pacemaker options.

- *Paced QRS, dissociated intrinsic P waves.* The pacemaker senses and paces only the ventricle. There will be pacemaker spikes preceding only the QRS complexes. Intrinsic P waves, if present, will be ignored by the pacemaker. See Figure 16–6.

DDD Pacemakers

The **DDD pacemaker** is the most modern and the most physiologic. It is known as a **universal pacemaker** and is now the most commonly inserted permanent pacemaker. It paces and senses both atrium and ventricle. See Figure 16–7.

The DDD pacemaker senses intrinsic atrial activity and takes advantage of the patient's own P waves. If the DDD pacemaker senses the patient's P waves within its preset rate, it will not need to give another P wave, so its atrial pacer will be inhibited. The ventricle, however, will then be triggered to give a QRS if the patient does not have his or her own QRS in the preset length of time after the P wave. *DDD pacemakers provide a constant relationship between P waves and QRS complexes.* If the pacemaker senses intrinsic P waves and QRS complexes within the appropriate time interval, it will be inhibited; it will just watch and wait until it's needed. If there are no Ps or QRS complexes in the preset time interval, the pacemaker will pace both chambers, providing a paced P and a paced QRS. Basically, the DDD provides whatever the patient cannot do on his or her own.

DDD pacemakers are usually **rate-responsive,** meaning that they will provide a paced QRS to follow the patient's intrinsic P waves within preset heart rate limits. These limits are usually 60 to 125. Within this range, the DDD pacemaker will provide a paced QRS for every intrinsic P wave. Below these limits, the pacemaker will provide paced P waves also, as the intrinsic atrial rate is too slow. Above these limits, the DDD pacemaker will not provide a paced QRS for each intrinsic P wave because that would result in a tachycardia dangerous to the patient.

Let's break that down a bit. Say the patient has an underlying third-degree AV block, which means a lot of P waves compared to QRS complexes. If the atrial rate (the rate of the P waves, you'll recall) is between 60 and 125, the DDD pacemaker will "track the P waves." This means the pacemaker will provide a paced QRS complex as needed to follow each intrinsic P wave. It will not provide paced P waves, as it won't need to; the patient has his or her own Ps at a fast enough rate.

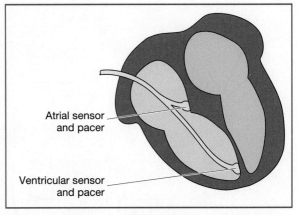

Atrial sensor and pacer

Ventricular sensor and pacer

FIGURE 16–7

DDD pacemaker and sensor wires in right atrium and ventricle.

If the atrial rate drops below 60, the rate of the P waves is too slow; the DDD pacemaker will then provide paced P waves as well as QRS complexes as needed to keep the heart rate within the range of 60 to 125.

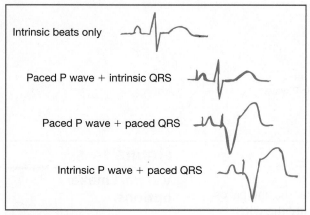

FIGURE 16–8

DDD pacemaker options.

If the atrial rate exceeds 125, the P waves are now too fast; the DDD pacemaker will ignore some of those P waves and track others. Therefore, there may be paced QRS complexes after only every second or third intrinsic P wave, and so forth. Why does it do this? If the atrial rate is faster than 125, and the pacemaker provides a paced QRS after each P wave, the patient ends up with a heart rate of 125. That may be so fast that cardiac output drops. If the atrial rate exceeds the upper limit, the pacemaker senses the atrial rate and decides to obey only some, rather than all, of the intrinsic P waves.

DDD pacemakers provide four options:

- *Intrinsic beats only.* The pacemaker does not fire because it does not need to. The intrinsic rate is fast enough. There will be no pacemaker spikes.

- *Paced P wave, intrinsic QRS.* The pacemaker paces the atrium, providing a pacemaker spike and a paced P wave. Following this, the patient's own QRS occurs. There is therefore a spike only before the P wave.

- *Paced P wave, paced QRS.* The pacemaker paces both chambers, providing a spike before the P wave and a spike before the QRS.

- *Intrinsic P wave, paced QRS.* The patient has his or her own P waves, so the pacemaker tracks them and provides a paced QRS to follow. There is a pacemaker spike only before the QRS. See Figure 16–8.

DDD versus VVI Practice

On the following strips, tell whether the pacemaker is DDD or VVI (or undeterminable).

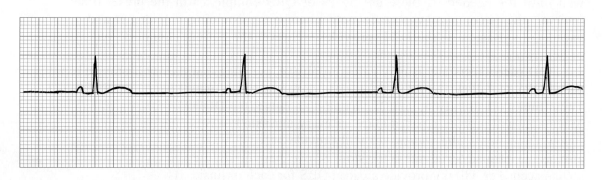

1. _____

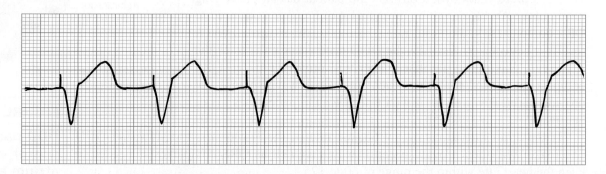

2. _____

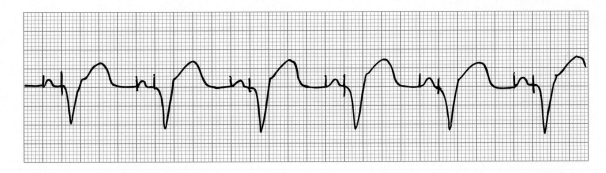

3. _____

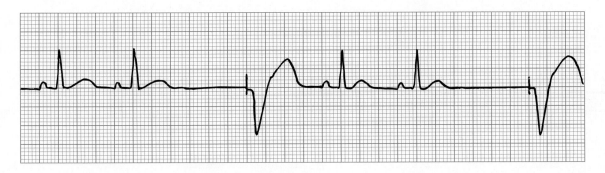

4. _____

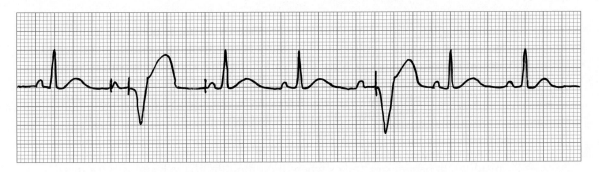

5. _____

Pacemaker Malfunctions

Like any gadget, pacemakers sometimes malfunction. The typical malfunctions:

- *Failure to Fire.* Here the pacemaker fails to send out its electrical stimulus when it should. This can mean the pacemaker battery is dead or the connecting wires are interrupted. Or it can mean the pacemaker has oversensed something like extraneous muscle artifact and thinks it's not supposed to fire. Failure to fire is evidenced by the lack of pacemaker spikes where they should have been. It usually results in a pause. Figure16–9 is an example of failure to fire.

  In Figure 16–9, assume the patient's pacemaker rate is set at 60. There are no pacemaker spikes anywhere. The rhythm is a slow sinus bradycardia with a heart rate of about 28. The pacemaker should have prevented the heart rate from going this slowly, but it didn't fire.

- *Loss of Capture.* There is no P or QRS after the pacemaker spike in loss of capture. This is often simply a matter of turning up the pacemaker's voltage so that it sends out more "juice" to tell the heart what to do. Maybe the signal it sent out was too weak to get a response from the chamber. Another possibility is that the pacing catheter has lost contact with the wall of the chamber it's in and cannot

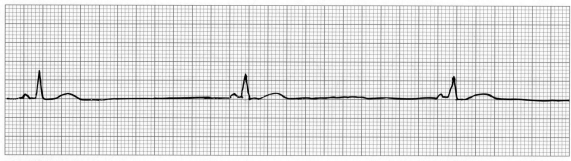

FIGURE 16–9

Failure to fire.

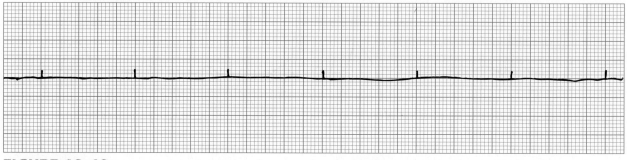

FIGURE 16–10

Loss of capture.

cause depolarization. That could be corrected by a simple position change of the patient, or it could necessitate minor surgery to adjust the catheter placement. Loss of capture can also occur when the heart is too damaged to respond to the pacer's stimulus. See Figure 16–10 for an example of loss of capture.

Figure 16–10 shows asystole with pacemaker spikes but no Ps or QRS complexes after the spikes. The pacemaker has fired, as evidenced by the spikes, but it has not captured the chamber it's in.

■ *Undersensing.* Here the pacemaker fires too soon after an intrinsic beat, often resulting in pacemaker spikes where they shouldn't have been, such as in a T wave, an ST segment, or right on top of another QRS. This happens when the pacemaker just doesn't see that other beat. The pacemaker's sensor needs adjusting. Another possibility is a fractured sensing wire or battery failure. In Figure 16–11 we have undersensing.

In Figure 16–11, note the spikes at times when the pacer should not have fired. How do you detect undersensing? Look at the distance between two consecutive pacemaker spikes. That's the normal pacing interval, which will correspond to a certain paced heart rate. *There should be exactly that same distance between the*

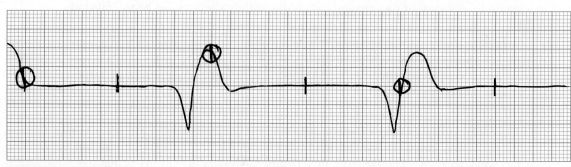

FIGURE 16–11

Undersensing.

patient's own intrinsic beats and the next paced beat. If the distance is less than that, there is undersensing. In Figure 16–11, the circled pacemaker spikes indicate undersensing.

But this strip also shows another malfunction. Do you know what it is? Look it over carefully before continuing.

There is loss of capture in addition to the undersensing. All the uncircled spikes plus the first circled one did not result in a P wave or QRS complex at a time when they should have. The second and third circled spikes would not be considered loss of capture even though they also don't result in a P or QRS. Why? Remember the refractory periods? From the beginning of the QRS to the upstroke of the T wave is the absolute refractory period. A spike that occurs during that time cannot possibly capture. That's not a pacemaker malfunction; it's just physiology.

For a summary of pacemaker malfunctions, see Table 16–4.

TABLE 16–4   Pacemaker Malfunctions Summary

Pacemaker Malfunctions	EKG Evidence
Failure to fire	Lack of pacemaker spikes where they should have been. Usually results in a pause.
Loss of capture	Pacemaker spikes not followed by P waves or QRS complexes.
Undersensing	Paced beats or spikes too close to previous beats. Often results in spikes inside T waves, ST segments, or QRS complexes.

Pacemaker Malfunctions Practice

On the strips that follow, indicate the pacer malfunction(s), if any.

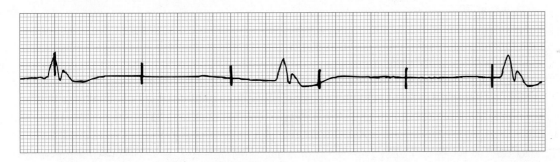

Situation: This patient passed out at home. The paramedics found him with a barely palpable, very slow pulse. His VVI pacemaker is set at 60.

1.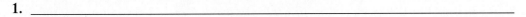

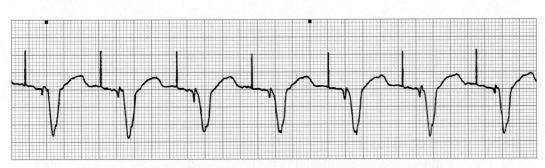

Situation: This patient had a DDD pacemaker inserted 3 years ago and now appears in the ER complaining of sudden onset of dizziness and syncope. The pacemaker rate is set at 68.

2. _____

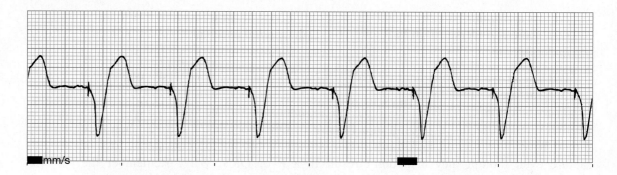

■■mm/s

Situation: This patient has a DDD pacemaker set at 72. She's seen in her doctor's office for a routine checkup. She feels fine.

3. _____

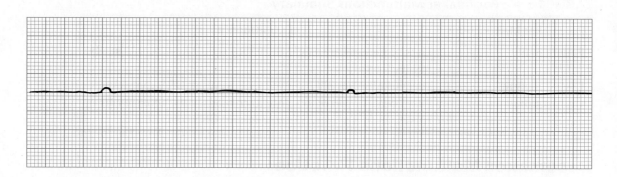

Situation: This patient is seen in the ER in cardiac arrest. His DDD pacemaker is set at 70.

4. _____

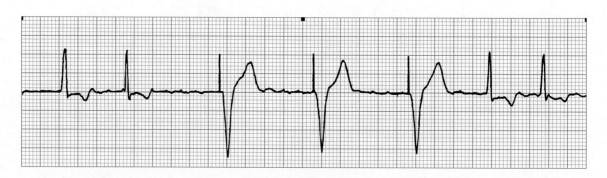

Situation: This patient had a VVI pacemaker inserted recently because of slow atrial fibrillation. It's set at 60. She feels fine.

5. _____

Let's move on now to other kinds of electrical therapy: electrical cardioversion and defibrillation.

Electrical Cardioversion

The word cardioversion means changing the heart (see website for a video on the topic of cardioversion). Electrical cardioversion is a small electrical shock to the heart and is usually performed to convert supraventricular tachycardias back to sinus, but it can also be used for ventricular tachycardia, provided the patient has a pulse. (Pulseless V-tach requires defibrillation, not cardioversion.) The goal here is to interrupt an abnormal electrical circuit within the heart that is allowing an arrhythmia to continue. Electrical cardioversion is performed using a defibrillator that can be set to "synchronous" mode. *Synchronizing is what differentiates cardioversion from defibrillation.* Once the synchronizer button is activated on the defibrillator, the machine delays delivery of the shock until it has synchronized with the patient's QRS complexes. The shock must be delivered at a critical point in the cardiac cycle. *If a shock is delivered at the wrong point in the cardiac cycle, it can put the patient into ventricular fibrillation*—not a good thing if the patient was just in SVT. Perhaps the most critical thing to know about cardioversion is *when not to use it:* Do not try to cardiovert V-fib—this rhythm requires defibrillation. *Turn the synchronizer button off when defibrillating or the shock will not be delivered!*

Defibrillation

Defibrillation differs from cardioversion in that the shock is delivered immediately upon pressing the button (see website for a video on the topic of defibrillation). There is no synchronizing in defibrillation. And the electrical current delivered tends to be much larger, causing the entire myocardium to depolarize at once. This interrupts the abnormal rhythm and causes a brief asystole, after which the heart's normal automaticity should allow it to restart with normal conduction. *Defibrillation is the treatment for ventricular fibrillation and pulseless ventricular tachycardia.* There are several kinds of defibrillators: the monitor/defibrillator used in hospitals, AICDs (automated implantable cardioverter-defibrillators), and AEDs (automated external defibrillators). See Figure 16–12 for photos of each. Let's look at these now:

> **Quick Tip**
>
> If the rhythm is *V-fib* you must *defib!*

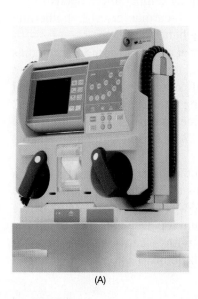

(A)

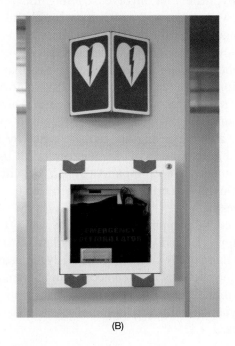

(B)

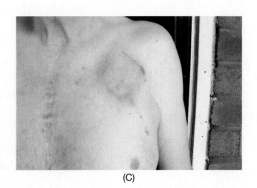

(C)

FIGURE 16–12

(A) Monitor-defibrillator, (B) AED, and (C) AICD in patient's left chest.

Source: (A) Beerkoff/Shutterstock (B) Eric Gevaert/Shutterstock (C) © Michael F. O'Keefe

- *Monitor/defibrillator.*   Is a combination of a cardiac monitor with a 3- or 5-lead cable plus a cardioverter-defibrillator. It is attached to the patient, and then health care personnel analyze the rhythm and activate the buttons to either cardiovert or defibrillate the patient. Use of this device requires knowledge of rhythms and their appropriate treatment by the user. Defibrillators come in *monophasic* and *biphasic* types. They deliver their energy/shock in different doses, so it's important to know which type defibrillator is used at your facility.
- *AICD.*   Is an implanted device that is programmed to analyze abnormal rhythms and deliver a small internal electrical shock to abort an abnormal rhythm such as V-tach or V-fib. It is completely contained within the body. The AICD also has a pacemaker that allows it to pace the heart if the shock causes asystole. Antitachycardia pacing is also an option with AICDs.
- *AED.*   Is a defibrillator meant for use by the lay public. It can be found in airports, shopping malls, and on airplanes. Extremely simple to use, the device is attached to the patient and automatically analyzes the rhythm. It can then either tell the rescuer what to do (as in "push the button to defibrillate") or do everything automatically without rescuer intervention. In either case, the AED requires no medical or technical knowledge by the rescuer. The machine, once plugged in, tells the rescuer step by step what to do next.

So what happens to our cardiac arrest patient who has a return of spontaneous circulation (ROSC) after we've defibrillated him or her and given our emergency medications? Let's talk a moment about therapeutic hypothermia.

Therapeutic Hypothermia (TH)

Therapeutic hypothermia involves cooling the post–cardiac arrest patient's body temperature down to about 90 to 93 degrees Fahrenheit in order to reduce the risk of ischemic damage (particularly brain damage) caused by the period of decreased or absent blood flow. It has long been known that lower body temperatures decrease the body's metabolic demands. Research has shown that post–cardiac arrest hypothermia protects brain function and can help the patient achieve a better outcome.

Here's how it works: Say a man suffers a cardiac arrest at a football game. Paramedics successfully resuscitate the man, who then regains a spontaneous pulse. Paramedics can begin TH in the ambulance en route to the hospital by infusing ice-cold saline IV, or TH can be provided in the intensive care unit or the ER using either chilled water blankets or gel pads in contact with the patient's skin, or with iced saline fluids IV through a large central vein. Hypothermia is maintained for about 12 to 24 hours and then gradual rewarming is begun.

During the cool-down phase, the PR, QRS, and QT intervals can prolong and there is increased risk for atrial and ventricular arrhythmias. Sinus tachycardia is common at the start of TH, but this usually slows to sinus bradycardia as cooling continues. Hypokalemia is common during cool-down, often necessitating potassium replacement.

The rewarming period is the most dangerous, with electrolyte disturbances (particularly hyperkalemia) very common. Watch for tall pointy T waves and widening QRS complexes.

Cardiac medications and electrical therapy are being constantly updated and improved, and therapeutic hypothermia can help maximize your patients' chance of a good post–cardiac arrest outcome. Keeping up with these advances is critical in caring for your patients.

chapter sixteen notes TO SUM IT ALL UP . . .

- **Classes of antiarrhythmic medications:**
  - *I—Sodium channel blockers*—Decrease myocardial contractility and excitability
    - Ia—Causes prolonged QT interval, decreases contractility, lowers blood pressure
    - Ib—Used for ventricular arrhythmias only
    - Ic—Decreases impulse conduction
  - *II—Beta-blockers*—Decrease sinus node automaticity, slow AV conduction, decrease heart rate
  - *III—Potassium channel blockers*—Prolong PR, QRS, and QT intervals
  - *IV—Calcium channel blockers*—Slow AV conduction, decrease contractility, increase PR interval, slow heart rate

- **Emergency cardiac medications:**
  - *Atropine*—Treats bradycardias and asystole—speeds up heart rate
  - *Epinephrine*—Treats bradycardias, asystole, V-fib, pulseless V-tach, PEA—increases heart rate and blood pressure
  - *Vasopressin*—Can replace first or second dose of epinephrine in cardiac arrest situation—treats asystole, PEA, pulseless V-tach and V-fib. Not used for bradycardias.
  - *Dopamine*—Used as an infusion for bradycardias—increases heart rate and blood pressure
  - *Amiodarone*—Treats supraventricular and ventricular arrhythmias—helps abolish those rhythms
  - *Adenosine*—Treats SVT—can cause brief asystole before rhythm converts back to sinus
  - *Sodium bicarbonate*—Treats acidosis—used when indicated by blood gas studies
  - *Oxygen*—Used in all emergencies—increases tissue oxygenation and can combat arrhythmias

- **Other medications with EKG effects:**
  - *Diuretics*—Used to increase urine output—can cause dehydration and lead to electrolyte disturbances that can in turn cause ventricular irritability
  - *Bronchodilators*—Used to open narrowed air passages in patients with asthma or chronic lung disease—can cause tachycardias
  - *Antihypertensive medications*—Used to treat hypertension—can cause tachycardias or bradycardias, AV blocks, hypotension
  - *Nitrates*—Used to dilate coronary arteries and decrease/eliminate chest pain—can cause hypotension, tachycardias
  - *Glaucoma medications*—Used to decrease eyeball pressure—can cause bradycardias
  - *Erectile dysfunction medications*—Used to enable males to obtain/maintain an erection—can cause profound decrease in blood pressure, which can cause chest pain, myocardial ischemia, or MI

- *Thrombolytics*—Used to abort a STEMI in progress—dissolves the blood clot causing the MI—can cause tachycardias if bleeding results—should cause elevated ST segment to return to normal
- *Anticoagulants*—Blood thinners—used to prevent blood clots—can cause tachycardias if bleeding results

- **Pacemakers**—Used to speed up (or in some cases slow down) the heart rate
- **Permanent pacemakers are implanted into the body.**
- **Temporary pacemakers can be temporarily inserted into or externally attached to the body.**
- **Pacemaker terminology:**
  - *Firing*—Pacemaker's generation of an impulse—results in pacemaker spike on EKG
  - *Capture*—Chamber responds to pacemaker signal by depolarizing—results in P wave and /or QRS following pacer spike
  - *Sensing*—Pacemaker's ability to sense patient's underlying rhythm to determine if it needs to fire—results in appropriate delay before next paced beat on EKG

- **Pacemaker code:**
  - *First letter*—Chamber paced
  - *Second letter*—Chamber sensed
  - *Third letter*—Response to sensed events

- **VVI pacemaker**—Paces and senses the ventricle
- **DDD pacemaker**—Paces and senses atrium and ventricle
- **Pacemaker malfunctions:**
  - *Failure to fire*—No pacer spikes noted
  - *Loss of capture*—Spikes present, but no P or QRS following them
  - *Undersensing*—Pacer spikes inside QRS complexes or T waves

- **Electrical cardioversion**—Electrical shock using synchronizer button—shock is synchronized with cardiac cycle
- **Defibrillation**—Electric shock delivered immediately upon pressing button—normal treatment for V-fib and pulseless V-tach; not synchronized
- **Monitor-defibrillator**—Used in hospitals—can monitor different leads and can cardiovert/defib patient
- **AICD**—Implanted defibrillator—programmed to shock certain arrhythmias
- **AED**—Defibrillator found in public areas such as airports—for use by lay public
- **Therapeutic hypothermia**—Cooling the post–cardiac arrest patient down to 90 to 93 degrees Fahrenheit—helps improve neurologic function and provides better outcomes. During cool-down period: atrial and ventricular arrhythmias common. Sinus tach common at first, slowing to sinus brady as temperature drops further. During warm-up phase: watch for hyperkalemia—tall pointy T waves and widening QRS complexes

Practice Quiz

1. Digitalis is classified as which kind of medication?

   _____

2. Class I antiarrhythmic medications have which effect on the action potential? _____

   _____

3. What effect does atropine have on the heart rate?

   _____

4. What effect does vasoconstriction have on the blood pressure? _____

   _____

5. True or false: An AED is meant for use by lay people.

6. What effect do class III antiarrhythmic medications have on the action potential? _____

   _____

7. Explain the use of therapeutic hypothermia. _____

   _____

8. Explain what the three letters of the pacemaker code refer to. _____

   _____

9. How does cardioversion differ from defibrillation?

   _____

   _____

10. Describe antitachycardia pacing and how it differs from routine pacing for bradycardias. _____

   _____

Putting It All Together—Critical Thinking Exercises

These exercises may consist of diagrams to label, scenarios to analyze, brain-stumping questions to ponder, or other exercises to help boost your understanding of the chapter material.

1. For the following "shockable" rhythms, state whether the rhythm should be cardioverted or defibrillated:

   a. Atrial fibrillation _____

   b. Ventricular tachycardia with a pulse _____

   c. Ventricular fibrillation _____

   d. Ventricular tachycardia without a pulse _____

   e. SVT _____

2. The following scenario will provide you with information about a fictional patient and ask you to analyze the situation, answer questions, and decide on appropriate actions.

   Mr. Johnson had a temporary transvenous VVI pacemaker inserted yesterday because of slow atrial fibrillation. It's set at a rate of 60. This morning he calls you to his room complaining of feeling faint. His blood pressure has dropped and his rhythm is as seen on the strip that follows. See Figure 16–13.

   a. What is this rhythm and heart rate? _____

   b. What is the pacemaker doing? _____

   c. Describe how to utilize the pacemaker to abolish this rhythm. _____

   _____

   _____

   _____

   Within a few minutes, Mr. Johnson's rhythm has changed. See Figure 16–14. His blood pressure remains low and he still feels faint.

   d. What is this rhythm and heart rate? _____

   e. What is the pacemaker doing? _____

   f. Is there a pacer malfunction? Explain. _____

   _____

   _____

   g. What corrective measures can help remedy the pacer malfunction? _____

   _____

   _____

h. Explain the physiological reason that he had low blood pressure and a feeling of faintness with both rhythms seen on his rhythm strips.

_____

_____

After corrective measures, the pacemaker now works properly, and Mr. Johnson is in paced rhythm with a good blood pressure. He feels much better.

3. How'd you do with these questions? Let's do one more scenario.

Mr. Lohtrip is a 65-year-old male with a history of diabetes and erectile dysfunction. His medications are sildenafil and insulin. Tonight, as usual, he experienced mild chest pressure after sexual intercourse with his wife, but this time it didn't go away spontaneously as it usually did, so he took one of his wife's nitroglycerine tablets. Shortly after taking the nitro, Mr. Lohtrip collapsed. His wife called 911 and the ambulance took him to the hospital where his heart rate is noted to be 135, BP low at 68/30, and his 12-lead EKG shows he is having an MI.

a. What do you suspect is causing his tachycardia, low BP, and MI? _____

_____

_____

b. What would you teach Mr. Lohtrip in the future about his medications? _____

_____

_____

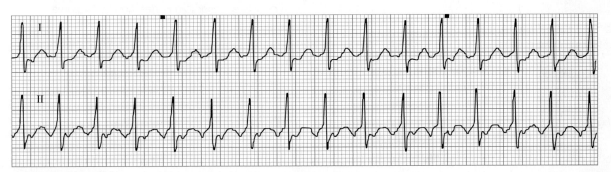

FIGURE 16–13

Mr. Johnson's first rhythm strip.

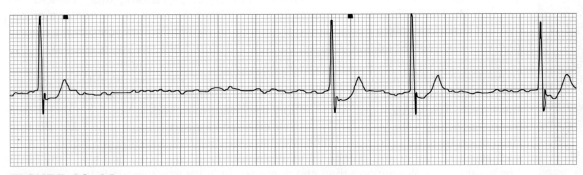

FIGURE 16–14

Mr. Johnson's second strip.

CHAPTER 17 OBJECTIVES

Upon completion of this chapter, the student will be able to:

- Define *stress testing.*
- State the goal of stress testing.
- Define *MET.*
- Describe the indications for stress testing.
- Describe the relative and absolute contraindications for stress testing.
- State how to calculate target heart rate.
- Describe how a stress test is done.
- Describe how a pharmacologic stress test is done.
- Name the three most commonly used protocols for treadmill exercise testing.
- Describe the reasons to terminate the test.
- Describe normal signs and symptoms during the stress test.
- Describe the normal EKG changes that occur during stress testing.
- Describe the EKG changes that indicate a positive stress test.
- Explain Bayes's theorem as it relates to the reliability of stress testing.
- Define *specificity* and *sensitivity.*
- Describe the indications for Holter monitoring.
- Explain why an event monitor might be superior to a Holter monitor for some patients.
- State what a positive Holter or event monitor is.

What It's All About

Mr. Walter had been experiencing dizziness for a few weeks and went to the doctor to see what was wrong. "I feel like I'm going to faint half the time," he complained. "I'm scared to drive a car because I'm afraid I'll pass out at the wheel." Dr. Friedman did a 12-lead EKG and saw no abnormality. "Let's put you on a Holter monitor to see if we can see any heart rhythm abnormality that could be causing this," he told the anxious Mr. Walter. Twenty-four hours later, Mr. Walter returned to the doctor's office. "Well, it looks like you're having some short runs of ventricular tachycardia. It's a heart rhythm that, if sustained, can cause your heart to stop. Let's get you started on some medication to treat this, and we'll send you over to the lab to have some blood work done. I also want you to see the cardiologist to see if you need an AICD. That's an implantable defibrillator that can provide a small internal shock to the heart to abolish the V-tach. The cardiologist will probably also want to schedule you for a stress test soon, especially with your family history of heart disease." "Holy cow," Mr. Walters thought as he left the doctor's office with his daughter. "It's amazing what they can do with little EKG wires and patches and implantable devices. They can see if my heart has an abnormal rhythm and then shock me out of it. It's like science fiction."

Introduction

Diagnostic electrocardiography involves an EKG done to rule out disease. It can involve a resting EKG, a stress test, or ambulatory monitoring such as Holter monitoring. We've talked about resting EKGs in depth. Let's look at the other two now.

Stress Testing

Stress testing is a diagnostic procedure done to determine the likelihood of coronary artery disease (CAD). The heart is stressed by physical exertion, usually on a bicycle or a treadmill, or by administration of medication that causes increased heart rate and thus stresses the heart. The patient's symptoms and EKG during the stress test give vital information regarding the **patency** (openness) of his or her coronary arteries.

Goal of Stress Testing

The goal of stress testing, whether exercise or pharmacologic, is to increase the heart rate to a maximal level that increases myocardial oxygen demand and to evaluate the EKG and subjective responses of the patient. Decreased flow through narrowed coronary arteries will usually become evident as the test progresses. In other words, are there EKG changes that signal ischemia or infarction? Does the patient experience chest pain or arrhythmias with this stress? The test is concluded when the patient's symptoms (chest pain, fatigue, or ST segment changes) preclude continuing or, for submaximal tests, when a target heart rate is reached.

Indications for Stress Testing

Stress testing is usually done to search for coronary artery disease in a patient having suspicious symptoms. But there are other indications as well. Here are a few:

- **Post-CABG or postangioplasty evaluation**   The patient has had bypass surgery or a balloon procedure to open up blocked coronary arteries. The stress test is a way to determine if those procedures have improved coronary flow.
- *Diagnosis or treatment of exercise-induced arrhythmias.*   Some patients have arrhythmias only on exertion. The stress test is a safe way to induce those arrhythmias in a controlled environment so that they can be identified and treated.
- *Follow-up to cardiac rehab.*   The post-MI patient has gradually worked up to more normal exercise levels. The stress test helps determine if his or her heart is tolerating this increased exertion.
- *Family history of heart disease.*   The individual with a family history of heart disease and two or more of the recognized heart disease risk factors is advised to have a stress test at age 40 and periodically thereafter. If CAD is detected, treatment can begin early.

Absolute Contraindications

Who is *not* a candidate for stress testing under any circumstances? For people with the following conditions, the risks of the test greatly outweigh the potential benefits. Testing these people could have serious or fatal consequences.

- *Acute MI less than 48 hours old.*   The heart is too unstable to tolerate exertion. Stress testing could cause the infarcted area to extend.
- *Uncontrolled symptomatic heart failure.*   The heart cannot tolerate the extra stress.
- **Unstable angina** *not previously stabilized on medications.*   Patients with unstable angina will not tolerate stress. It could cause them to infarct.
- *Uncontrolled cardiac arrhythmias accompanied by signs of decreased cardiac output.*   The rhythm could deteriorate to V-fib.
- *Symptomatic severe* **aortic stenosis**   As a result of a narrowed aortic valve opening, cardiac output is low, and stressing these patients could cause them to faint or suffer cardiac arrest.
- **Dissecting aneurysm**   This is a ballooning out of the wall of an artery. Stress causes an increase in blood pressure, which could cause the aneurysm to blow.
- *Acute pulmonary embolus (PE).*   This is a blood clot in a lung artery. PEs result in low blood oxygen levels and require the patient to be on bed rest for a time. Exertion could move the embolus farther into the artery, causing more damage.

Relative Contraindications

Some individuals should have a stress test *only* if the benefits outweigh the risks. In other words, it must be determined that the information to be gained from the stress test is so valuable that it outweighs the risks involved to individuals with the following conditions:

- *Left main coronary artery stenosis.*   The patient could have a massive MI.
- *Mental/physical issues that render the patient unable to exercise adequately.*
- *Uncontrolled tachyarrhythmias (fast arrhythmias) or* bradyarrhythmias *(slow arrhythmias).*   With the heart rate already too fast or too slow prior to the stress test, it won't take much to make the cardiac output fall.
- *Severe* hypertension *(systolic >200, diastolic > 110).*   Stress testing could result in stroke.
- *High degree AV block (second and third degree).*   Stressing the patient can lead to worsening AV block and the need for an emergent pacemaker.
- *Electrolyte abnormalities.*   This could lead to arrhythmias such as V-tach or V-fib.
- *Moderate stenotic heart valve disease.*   A heart valve is not able to open completely, so flow through it is impeded. This can decrease cardiac output.
- Hypertrophic cardiomyopathy *(overgrown septum) or other forms of outflow obstruction.*   This causes decreased cardiac output.

Preparation Techniques

The single most important piece of equipment in performing a stress test is a 12-lead EKG machine. The electrode patches should adhere securely to the skin, and they may be taped if necessary. Female patients are advised to wear a bra in order to decrease artifact. To prevent nausea, patients are advised not to eat a large meal for at least 4 hours prior to the test. They should wear comfortable, loose clothing and walking shoes or other appropriate footwear. They should take their routine medications as usual unless specifically instructed not to by the physician. Certain medications, such as beta-blockers and calcium channel blockers, may be held for a period of time before the test, as they can prevent the heart rate from reaching target levels. Also, nitrates might be held, as they could prevent symptoms of coronary artery disease, such as chest pain, and could thus result in a false-negative test. Likewise, caffeinated beverages might be withheld, as they can increase the heart rate and blood pressure.

How Is It Done?

Before all stress tests, a resting EKG is done. A history is obtained, with special emphasis on a description of any symptoms the patient has been having that prompted the test (chest pain, shortness of breath, etc.). Baseline vital signs (heart rate, blood pressure, respiratory rate) are checked with the patient lying down and standing. An EKG may be done with the patient standing up hyperventilating (breathing very rapidly). ST segment and T wave changes can be caused by hyperventilation, and during the stress test it's important to know if any ST-T changes are from ischemia or simply from hyperventilating.

For the **exercise test,** the patient then exercises on a treadmill or bicycle, or uses a special arm bicycle called an arm ergometer, while a continuous EKG is run. A nurse or technician checks the patient's blood pressure at frequent intervals and inquires about any symptoms the patient may be developing. The stress test is continued until at least 85% of the target heart rate is achieved or the patient develops EKG changes or symptoms that require termination of the test. *The target heart rate is 220 minus the patient's age.* A 60-year-old patient would thus have a target heart rate of $220 - 60 = 160$. For the test to be valid for interpretation, a heart rate of 85% of 160, or 136, would be required. For a submaximal test following an MI, the test is concluded when 70% of the target heart rate is achieved, assuming the patient is asymptomatic. If myocardial **perfusion** (adequacy of blood flow to the heart muscle) is to be studied, radioisotopes such as **thallium-201** can be injected during the last minute of exercise and then special X-rays done. Thallium follows potassium ions into the heart and diffuses into the tissues. Poor myocardial uptake of the thallium produces a "cold spot" on the X-ray (compared to the "hot spots" from adequate thallium uptake) and indicates impaired myocardial blood flow in the artery supplying that area. *Multiple gated acquisition* (MUGA) scans can also be done after the exercise test to check myocardial perfusion. MUGA scans are nuclear scans that use an injected radioisotope to point out areas of poor myocardial blood flow.

The **pharmacologic stress test** does not involve exercise. This kind of testing is appropriate for individuals with physical limitations that preclude exercise, such as amputations, or for the elderly who could not do enough exercise to reach the target heart rate. For this test, an IV line is started, and the patient is given an intravenous dose of medication that causes the heart rate to climb to the target level. This increased heart rate stresses the heart and should provide the same symptoms and EKG changes as an exercise test. As with the exercise test, a continuous EKG is run, vital signs are checked, and symptoms are assessed. After at least 85% of the target heart rate is achieved, the test is concluded. The most common medications used in pharmacologic stress tests are *cardiolyte, dobutamine, dipyridamole,* and *adenosine.*

Exercise Protocols

Three main protocols are used in treadmill exercise stress tests—the Bruce, modified Bruce, and Naughton protocols. Speed and incline of the treadmill, as well as the frequency of the changes in the protocol's stages, are determined by the protocol used. The intensity of exercise is measured in metabolic equivalents (**METs**), which are reflections of oxygen consumption. One MET is the oxygen consumption of a person sitting down resting. Most average adults can reach a MET level of 13 with exertion. Those with coronary artery disease may have symptoms of ischemia at low MET levels, such as 4 METs. Sometimes a *double product* is calculated in order to determine the level of exercise achieved. Double product is calculated as the heart rate times the systolic blood pressure (HR × SBP = DP). A double product greater than 25,000 indicates that an acceptable level of exercise has been achieved during stress testing. Let's look at the different protocols.

- *Bruce.* This is the most commonly used protocol for maximal testing. The treadmill's speed and incline are increased every 3 minutes up to a total of 21 minutes. Let's look at the stages of the Bruce protocol. See Table 17–1.
  As you can see in Table 17–1, the speed starts out at a comfortable walking pace at a low incline; then every 3 minutes it accelerates until by stage VII the patient is running uphill at a 22° incline. An advantage of the Bruce protocol is the relatively short duration needed to produce maximal effort in the patient. On the downside,

TABLE 17–1 Bruce Protocol Stages

Stage	Speed	Incline
I	1.7 mph	10°
II	2.5 mph	12°
III	3.4 mph	14°
IV	4.2 mph	16°
V	5.0 mph	18°
VI	5.5 mph	20°
VII	6.0 mph	22°

this protocol can be very demanding and may be too ambitious for the sedentary individual.

■ *Modified Bruce.* Many institutions have modified the Bruce protocol so that the initial work is less strenuous, and the stage change is in smaller increments. This is appropriate for patients who might not tolerate the standard Bruce protocol.

■ *Naughton.* This is a slower-moving submaximal test in which the settings are changed every 2 minutes. Although the settings change more quickly than in the Bruce protocol, they are more gradual and allow the individual to adjust more easily. The Naughton protocol is used most often for testing post-MI patients just before or shortly after hospital discharge.

---

chapter CHECKUP

We're about halfway through this chapter. To evaluate your understanding of the material thus far, answer the following questions. If you have trouble with them, review the material again before continuing.

Sixty-year-old Mr. Scotty has reached a heart rate of 150 during his stress test. The physician wants a maximal test done.

1. Has Mr. Scotty reached his target heart rate for a maximal test?
2. What is his target heart rate?
3. How would Mr. Scotty's beta-blocker medication that he took this morning affect his ability to reach his target heart rate?

Termination of the Test

The stress test should be immediately stopped if any of the following occur:

■ *ST segment elevation.* This indicates severe myocardial ischemia and injury. The sudden development of ST segment elevation is an ominous sign. Continuing the test could result in irreversible cardiac damage.

■ *Sustained ventricular tachycardia.* Cardiac arrest could result if the test is not stopped.

■ *Moderate to severe chest pain, especially if accompanied by ST segment depression or elevation.* Mild chest pain unaccompanied by ST segment changes may not be indicative of significant coronary artery disease. More severe chest pain, especially that accompanied by ST segment changes, is more reflective of significant disease.

■ *Drop in blood pressure more than 10 mm Hg along with other evidence of ischemia such as chest pain or ST segment depression or elevation.* The blood pressure usually rises in response to exercise. A drop in BP can indicate pump failure.

■ *Technical problems with the monitoring systems or the treadmill.*

■ *Patient requests to stop.* Before stopping, ask why the patient wants to stop the test. There may be an occasional unmotivated patient who requests to stop the test before achieving target levels. In this case, the physician might gently encourage the patient to continue, since the test that is stopped at too early a stage will be inadequate at ruling out CAD.

■ *Patient becomes dizzy, begins to stumble, or feels faint.* The patient is showing neurologic symptoms of decreased cardiac output.

■ *Patient becomes cold and clammy.* These are signs of decreased cardiac output. The patient is not tolerating the test.

Test Interpretation

The following EKG changes are normal on the stress test:

- *Shortened PR interval.*   AV conduction and heart rate usually accelerate with exertion.
- *Tall P waves.*   This is often a result of increased lung capacity.
- *Lower-voltage QRS complexes.*   This may be due to increased volume of air in the lungs muffling the cardiac impulse as it heads toward the skin.
- *Increased heart rate (shorter R-R intervals).*   The ability of the heart rate to increase with exercise is known as the chronotropic reserve. Heart rate that does not increase with stress is chronotropic incompetence.

Normal Signs and Symptoms

The following patient signs and symptoms are normal during a stress test:

- *Decreased systemic vascular resistance due to vasodilation.*   Exercise causes blood vessels to dilate, lowering the resistance to the outflow of blood from the heart and increasing cardiac output.
- *Increased respiratory rate.*   Exercise causes increased oxygen demand, so the respiratory rate increases to allow more oxygen intake.
- *Sweating.*
- *Fatigue.*
- *Muscle cramping in calves or sides.*   This is a common phenomenon in exercise and does not imply poor myocardial function.
- *Increased blood pressure.*   The ability of the blood pressure to rise with exercise is known as inotropic reserve. Blood pressure that does not rise with exercise can imply inotropic incompetence.
- *J point depression.*   The J point is the point at which the QRS joins the ST segment. J point depression means the ST segment takes off before the QRS complex has gotten back up to the baseline. Note the J point in Figure 17–1. It is below the baseline. This is J point depression.

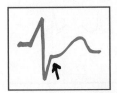

FIGURE 17–1

J point depression.

Positive Stress Test

The following indicate a positive (abnormal) stress test:

- *ST segment depression greater than or equal to 1.0 to 1.5 mm that does not return to the baseline within 0.08 seconds (two little blocks) after the J point.*   ST depression can be of 3 different types: upsloping, horizontal, and downsloping. In terms of cardiac implications, upsloping is the least indicative of coronary artery disease, horizontal is intermediate, and downsloping is the most indicative of CAD. See Figure 17–2.

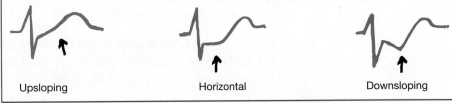

Upsloping   Horizontal   Downsloping

FIGURE 17–2

Types of ST segment depression.

Let's compare ST segments on a pre-exercise resting EKG and a stress test EKG. See Figures 17–3 and 17–4. Ignore the QRS width on these examples. In Figure 17–3, note the

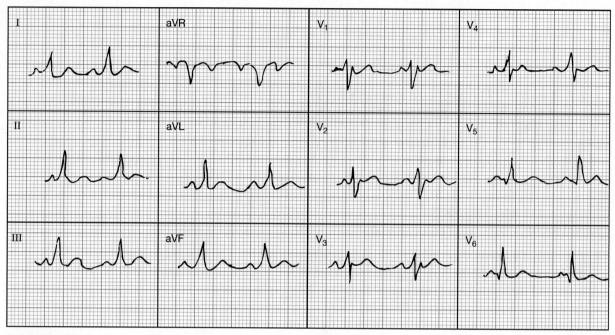

FIGURE 17–3

Pre-exercise resting EKG.

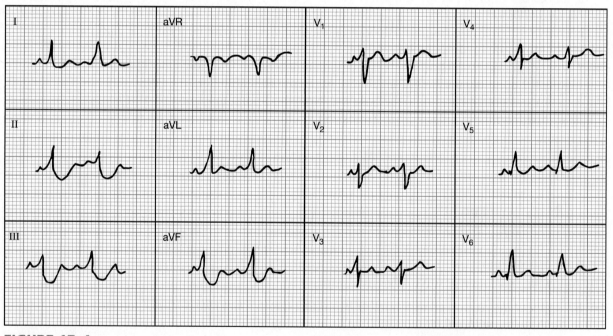

FIGURE 17–4

Stress test EKG.

normal ST segments and the relatively slow heart rate. Now see Figure 17–4 for the stress test EKG. Note the normal increase in heart rate along with significant downsloping ST segment depressions in Leads II, III, and aVF. This is a positive stress test.

- *U wave inversion or new appearance of U waves.* Although a much less common phenomenon than ST segment changes, U wave inversion—or indeed the sudden appearance of U waves during the exercise test—is indicative of coronary ischemia. See Figure 17–5, and note the inverted U waves following the upright T waves.

- *ST segment elevation.*   Elevation of the ST segment is an indication of considerable transmural myocardial ischemia progressing to the injury phase. The stress test should be stopped immediately to prevent permanent tissue damage.

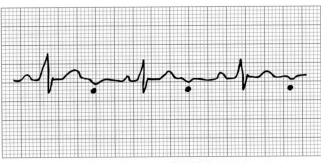

FIGURE 17–5

Inverted U waves.

Reliability of Stress Tests

How reliable are stress tests in diagnosing coronary artery disease? Like any medical testing, the stress test is not infallible. There can be false positives and false negatives. The validity of stress test results can be absolutely determined only by angiogram, a procedure in which dye is injected into the coronary arteries to determine if there is indeed coronary artery disease. For the stress EKG to show any diagnostic changes that indicate CAD, the coronary artery in question must be at least 75% narrowed. And conditions other than CAD can result in a positive test. To better understand the reliability of the test results, it is necessary to understand the terms *sensitivity* and *specificity.*

Sensitivity refers to the percentage of patients who have a positive stress test and CAD as proven by angiogram. In other words, is the stress test sensitive enough to pick up those individuals who truly have coronary artery disease?

Specificity refers to the percentage of patients who have negative (normal) stress tests and normal coronary arteries as proven by angiogram. Is the stress test specific enough to exclude individuals who do not have CAD?

Thus the term *positive* refers to the test's sensitivity and *negative* refers to its specificity.

Categories of Stress Tests

Stress test results fall in four categories:

- *True positive.*   The stress test is positive (indicating coronary artery disease) and the angiogram is also positive, confirming CAD.
- *False positive.*   The stress test is positive for CAD, but the angiogram is negative, revealing normal coronary arteries.
- *True negative.*   The stress test and angiogram are both negative for CAD.
- *False negative.*   The stress test is negative, but the angiogram is positive for CAD.

Bayes's theorem suggests that the true predictive value of any test is not just in the accuracy (sensitivity and specificity) of the test itself, but also in the patient's probability of disease, as determined before the test was done. In other words, before the stress test is done, there should be a risk assessment, based on the patient's history, heredity, and physical exam, to predict the likelihood of that patient having CAD. If this pretest risk of CAD is low, but his or her stress test turns out to be positive, it is likely that the stress test result is a false positive. If the pretest risk is high but the stress test is negative, it's likely that the stress test is a false negative.

After the Stress Test

What happens after the stress test? If the stress test is positive, the patient will likely be either treated with medications or scheduled for an angiogram for further diagnostic evaluation. If the test is negative, there may be no treatment indicated.

Stress Test Assessment Practice

Let's look at a few EKGs from stress tests. On the first five, *assess the EKG and decide if the test should continue or be terminated.* Assume that each person's rhythm was sinus rhythm with a heart rate of 70 and the EKG was otherwise completely normal at the start of the stress test. Assume this EKG was done 3 minutes into the Bruce protocol.

Quick Tip

The question to be answered is: Is the stress test result true or false (as proven by the angiogram results)? There are 2 steps to determining true or false, positive or negative:

- First, determine the stress test result. Is it positive or negative? Write down the word "positive" or "negative."
- Second, what is the angiogram result—positive or negative? If the stress test and angiogram results differ—if one is positive and the other is negative, for example—the stress test result will be considered false. Write "false" in front of the stress test result. If stress test and angiogram agree (both positive or both negative), the stress test result is true. Write "true" in front of the stress test result.

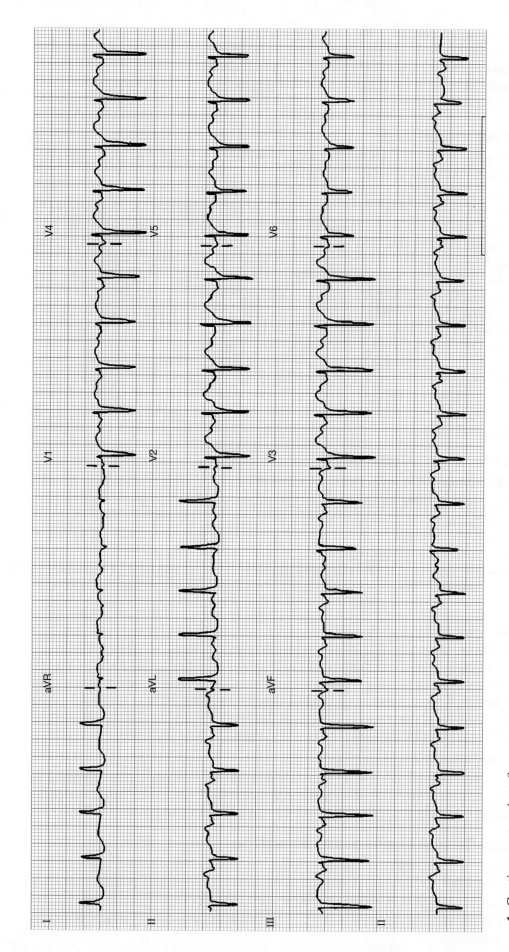

1. Continue or terminate?

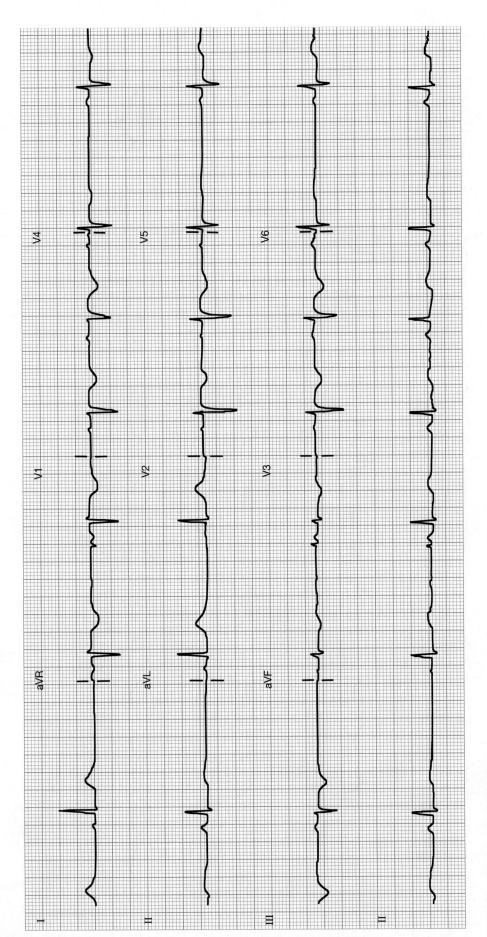

2. Continue or terminate? _____

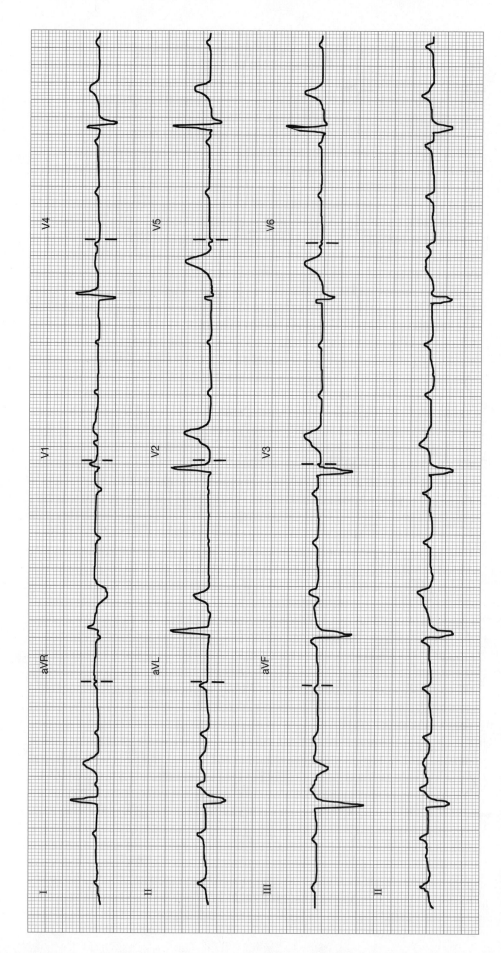

3. Continue or terminate?

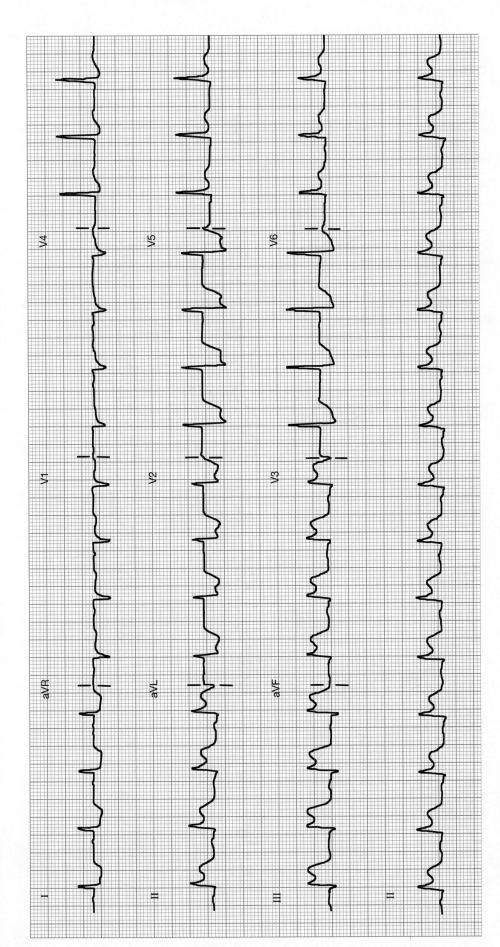

4. Continue or terminate? _____

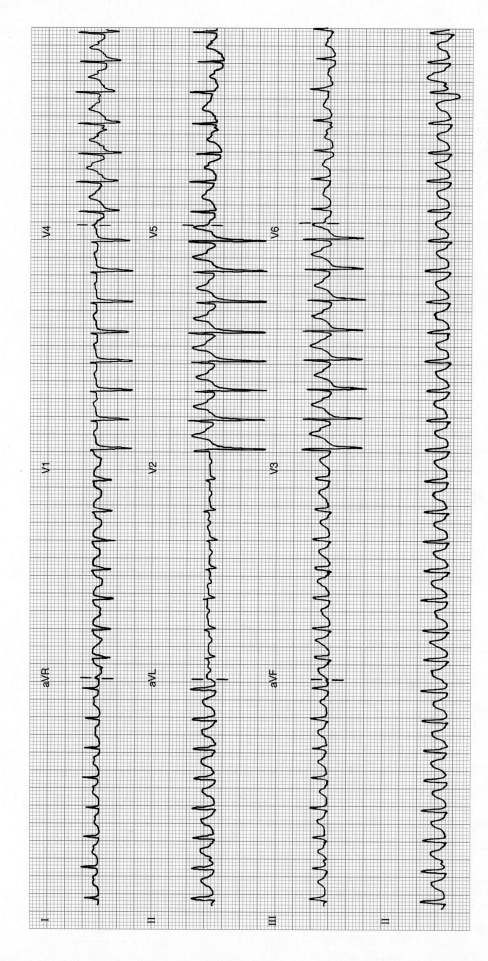

5. Continue or terminate?

On these final five, assess the EKG and determine if the stress test is positive or negative for CAD. Then *state whether the stress test is positive, false positive, true negative, or false negative* based on the indicated angiogram results. Again, assume all pretest EKGs were normal.

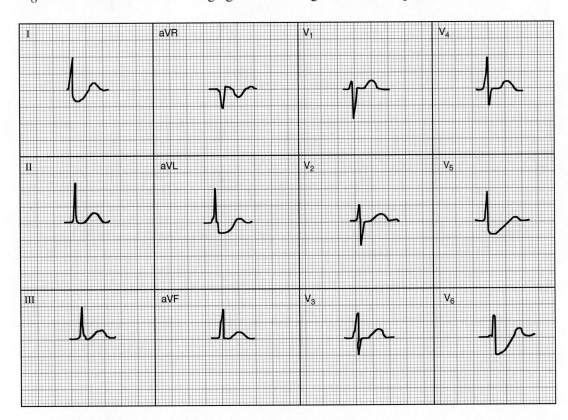

6. If the angiogram is negative, this stress test result is _____

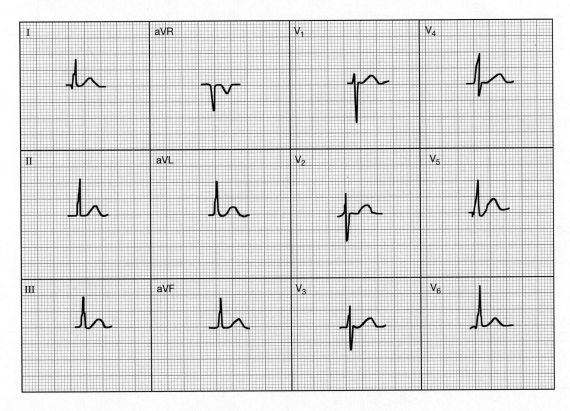

7. If the angiogram is positive, this stress test result is _____

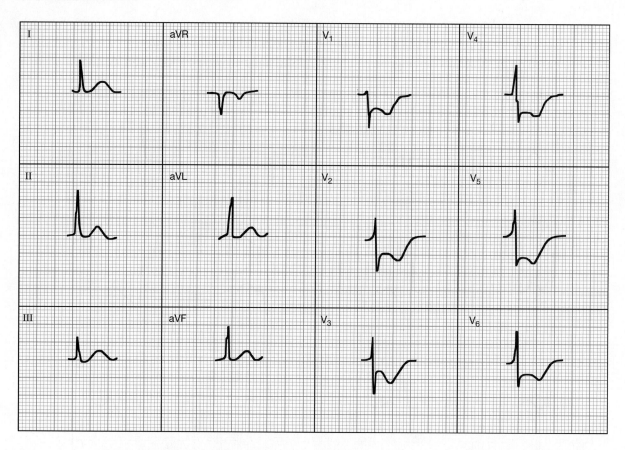

8. If the angiogram is negative, this stress test result is _____

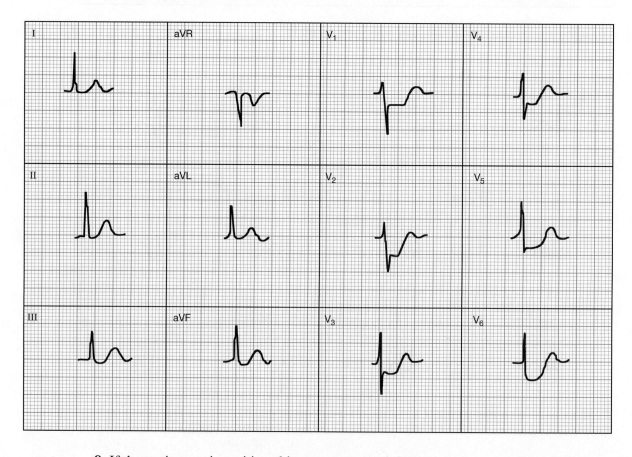

9. If the angiogram is positive, this stress test result is _____

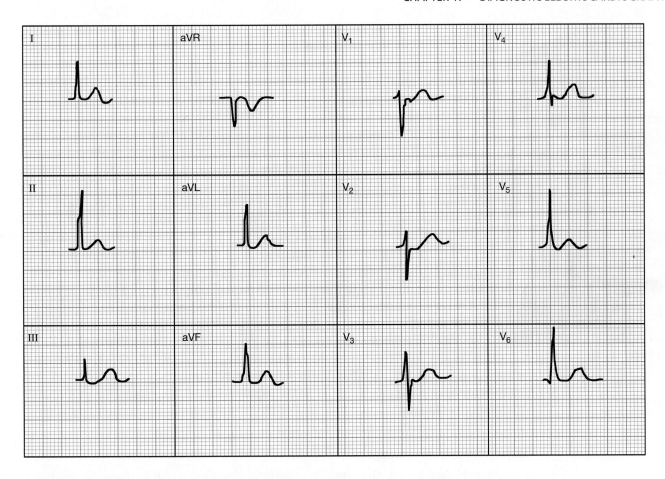

10. If the angiogram is negative, this stress test result is _____

Holter Monitoring

The Holter monitor is an ambulatory EKG device used to rule out intermittent arrhythmias or cardiac ischemia that might be missed on a routine EKG. The Holter monitor consists of electrodes and a small battery-powered digital flash-memory device onto which the rhythm is recorded. The data are later uploaded into a computer that analyzes the rhythm. Technicians then review the analysis for further study. The device is small enough to be worn in a pocket or on a strap over the shoulder. It may be used as an inpatient or outpatient, although most often it is used on an outpatient basis.

Indications for Holter Monitor Use

- *Syncope or near-syncopal episodes.*   Fainting spells could be caused by arrhythmias, which could be evident on Holter monitoring.
- *Intermittent chest pain or shortness of breath.*   These could be signs of myocardial ischemia, which could be detected with a Holter monitor.
- *Suspicion of arrhythmias.*   The patient who complains of palpitations, dizzy spells, or skipped beats may have arrhythmias that the Holter monitor would show.
- *Determination of arrhythmia treatment effectiveness.*   Holter monitoring can reveal if the rhythm being treated is still occurring and can demonstrate if a newly implanted pacemaker is functioning properly.

Preparation Techniques

The patient is attached to five or more electrodes that are put on the trunk instead of the arms and legs in order to prevent muscle artifact. See Figure 17–6. Male patients with considerable chest hair might need the electrode sites to be clipped to allow the electrode patches to adhere properly. Female patients should have chest leads positioned

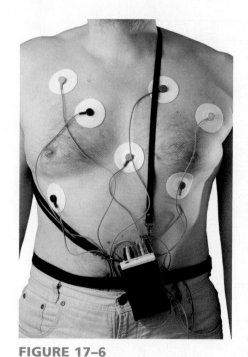

FIGURE 17–6

Man with Holter monitor.

Source: Vadim Kozlovsky

beneath, not on top of, the breast. The skin is prepped prior to attaching the electrodes. This skin prep involves abrading the thin outer layer of skin so the electrodes adhere to the skin without losing contact. The electrodes are then taped to the skin to prevent dislodgment, since they will be on for 24 hours or longer. Typically, at least two leads are simultaneously recorded—either Leads V_1 and V_5 or Leads V_1 and II.

After being attached to the Holter monitor, the patient is given instructions, including not to remove the electrodes and not to take a bath or shower during the time the Holter is in use, as this could cause the electrodes to become dislodged. A careful sponge bath is OK. The patient is otherwise instructed to go about normal daily activities. This includes work, hobbies, sex, and so on. The patient should not curtail activities just because the Holter is in use. The whole purpose of the Holter monitor is to catch abnormalities that show up in the course of daily activities. Curtailing those activities defeats the purpose.

The patient is advised to document any symptoms experienced while on the Holter monitor in a small diary provided for that purpose. By pressing the marker button on the Holter monitor, the patient marks the point in the EKG at which he or she feels symptoms so that this part of the EKG can be more closely examined for changes that could cause the symptoms. For example, if at 4 P.M., the patient feels dizzy, and the Holter reveals a short run of V-tach at that time, the arrhythmia would explain the dizziness. Treatment could then be started to prevent further ventricular arrhythmias. After the prescribed duration of Holter monitoring, the patient returns the Holter to the hospital or physician's office, whereupon it is entered into a computer and scanned for abnormalities.

What Is a Positive Holter?

A positive Holter is one that reveals *abnormalities that could explain the patient's symptoms.* These abnormalities might include one or more of the following:

- Tachycardias
- Bradycardias
- Pauses
- ST segment elevation or depression

A negative Holter has no significant arrhythmias or ST changes.

Event Monitoring

For patients whose symptoms are sporadic, a Holter monitor might not be the best answer, as the symptoms may not occur while the Holter is in use. An **event monitor** is a small device (often the size of a credit card) that the patient carries that can be programmed to record abnormalities in rhythm or ST segments or that can be activated by the patient whenever symptoms appear. Special types of event monitors can even be implanted under the skin on the chest for patients who need an even longer monitoring period.

There are two kinds of event monitors. One monitors the rhythm continuously, but only prints out abnormalities it has been preprogrammed to find. In addition, the patient can activate this recorder whenever symptoms occur. The device then records the patient's rhythm at that time and also, by way of a built-in memory, the rhythm that was present up to 5 minutes before the event. The rhythm can then be transmitted via telephone or the device turned in to the physician's office for immediate interpretation.

The second type of event monitor is not programmed to recognize abnormalities, nor does it monitor the rhythm continuously. It must be activated by the patient whenever symptoms occur. It will then record the rhythm present at that time as well as just before the event.

Unlike a Holter monitor, which is usually worn for only 24 hours, event monitors can be carried or worn for extended periods of time and are thus more likely to pick up abnormalities that are only sporadic. Like the Holter monitor, the event monitor is said to be *negative* if arrhythmias or ST-T changes are not found.

chapter seventeen notes TO SUM IT ALL UP . . .

- **Diagnostic electrocardiography**—Involves an EKG done to rule out disease.
- **Stress testing**—Involves utilizing exercise or medications to increase the heart rate and stress the heart—helps determine patency of coronary arteries.
- **Indications for stress testing:**
  - Post-cardiac surgery or post-PCI evaluation.
  - Diagnose/treat exercise-induced arrhythmias.
  - Follow-up to cardiac rehab.
  - Family history of heart disease.
- **Absolute contraindications to doing stress test:**
  - MI less than 48 hours old.
  - Uncontrolled symptomatic heart failure.
  - Unstable angina not stabilized medically.
  - Uncontrolled symptomatic cardiac arrhythmias.
  - Symptomatic severe aortic stenosis.
  - Dissecting aneurysm.
  - Acute pulmonary embolus.
- **Relative contraindications to doing stress test:**
  - Left main coronary artery stenosis (narrowing).
  - Uncontrolled tachyarrhythmias or bradyarrhythmias.
  - Mental or physical issues that prevent adequate exercise.
  - Severe hypertension (systolic <200, diastolic <110).
  - Electrolyte abnormalities.
  - High degree AV block (second or third degree).
  - Moderate stenotic heart valve disease.
  - Hypertrophic cardiomyopathy or other forms of outflow obstruction.
- **Target heart rate**—for stress testing is calculated as 220 minus age.
- **Maximal test**—Must reach 85% of target heart rate.
- **Submaximal test**—Must reach 70% of target heart rate.
- **MET**—Metabolic equivalent—a measurement of oxygen consumption.
- **Stress testing protocols:**
  - *Bruce*—Most commonly used—treadmill speed and incline changes every 3 minutes.
  - *Modified Bruce*—Changes occur in smaller increments.
  - *Naughton*—Slower-moving submaximal test—for MI patients prior to discharge from hospital.
- **Terminate stress test when any of the following occur:**
  - ST segment elevation.
  - Sustained ventricular tachycardia.
  - Drop in systolic blood pressure >10 mm Hg.
  - Moderate to severe angina.
  - Dizziness, stumbling, feeling faint.
  - Patient's desire to stop.
  - Technical problems doing the stress test.
  - Cold and clammy skin.

- **Normal EKG changes during stress test:**
  - Shortened PR interval.
  - Tall P waves.
  - Low-voltage QRS complexes.
  - Faster heart rate.
- **Normal signs and symptoms during stress test:**
  - Decreased systemic vascular resistance.
  - Increased respiratory rate.
  - Sweating.
  - Fatigue.
  - Muscle cramping in calves or sides.
  - Increased blood pressure.
  - Increased heart rate.
  - J-point depression.
- **Positive stress test:**
  - ST depression greater than 1–1.5 mms at 0.08 secs following the J point or
  - U wave inversion or new U wave or
  - ST segment elevation.
- **Sensitivity**—Percentage of patients with positive stress test and coronary artery disease proven by angiogram.
- **Specificity**—Percentage of patients with negative stress test and no coronary artery disease as proven by angiogram.
- **Categories of stress tests:**
  - True positive—Stress test positive, angiogram positive.
  - False positive—Stress test positive, angiogram negative.
  - True negative—Stress test negative, angiogram negative.
  - False negative—Stress test negative, angiogram positive.
- **Bayes's theorem**—The predictive value of any test is based not just on its accuracy but also on the patient's probability of disease.
- **Holter monitor**—Ambulatory EKG—to rule out arrhythmias or ischemic changes that could be causing the patient's symptoms.
- **Indications for Holter monitoring:**
  - Syncope or near-syncope.
  - Chest pain and/or shortness of breath.
  - Suspicion of arrhythmias.
  - Determine the effectiveness of treatment for arrhythmias.
- **Event monitor**—ambulatory EKG—to rule out very sporadic ischemia and/or arrhythmias that are unlikely to be noted on a Holter monitor—allows much longer monitoring periods; device can be implanted or carried.
- **Two kinds of event monitors:**
  - Continuously monitoring, pre-programmed to retain certain data.
  - Patient-activated—monitors only when activated by patient.
- **Indications for event monitor use**—same as for Holter.

Practice Quiz

1. The type of monitor that is worn for 24 hours to uncover any arrhythmias or ST segment changes that might be causing the patient's symptoms is the

   _____

2. List three indications for stress testing. _____

3. What does Bayes's theorem have to say about the validity of test results? _____

   _____

4. Is ST segment elevation of 5 mm indicative of a positive stress test or a negative stress test? _____

   _____

   _____

5. True or false: Patients on medications such as beta-blockers and nitrates might be advised to avoid taking these medications for a period of time before the stress test.

6. Target heart rate is calculated as_____

7. Event monitoring differs from Holter monitoring in what ways? _____

   _____

8. The most commonly used protocol for treadmill stress testing is the _____

   _____

9. The protocol used most often for post-MI patients just before or following hospital discharge is the

   _____

10. What is a MET? _____

Putting It All Together—Critical Thinking Exercises

These exercises may consist of diagrams to label, scenarios to analyze, brain-stumping questions to ponder, or other challenging exercises to boost your knowledge of the chapter material.

The following scenario will provide you with information about a fictional patient and ask you to analyze the situation, answer questions, and decide on appropriate actions.

Mr. Cameron, a 46-year-old male, is having a stress test required by his new insurance company. He is 5 feet 9 inches tall and weighs 325 pounds. He smokes two packs of cigarettes daily. Aside from an occasional twinge in his chest when he mows the lawn (the only exercise he gets), he has had no chest pain. Blood pressure is 160/90 (high), respiratory rate is 22 (slightly fast). The plan is to do a maximal test using the Bruce protocol.

You explain the stress test procedure and attach Mr. Cameron to the EKG. His resting EKG is shown in Figure 17–7.

1. Do you see anything in this EKG that is of concern?

   _____

   _____

You start the Bruce protocol and all is going well, although Mr. Cameron does seem to be getting winded (slightly short of breath) quickly.

2. What in his history tells you this is nothing to be surprised about? _____

   _____

   _____

By stage II of the Bruce protocol, Mr. Cameron's heart rate is 148 and his PR intervals have shortened.

3. Should the test continue or be terminated at this point? _____

The test continues and at 7 minutes into the test, Mr. Cameron complains of fatigue and dizziness. Blood pressure is now 82/64 and his skin is cool and clammy. He looks pale but denies chest pain. You continue the test and 2 minutes later, he loses consciousness. Mr. Cameron's rhythm is seen in Figure 17–8.

4. What is this rhythm? _____

5. What is the appropriate course of action? _____

   _____

6. After appropriate treatment, Mr. Cameron is sent to the coronary care unit. Looking back on the test, what should you have done differently? _____

   _____

   _____

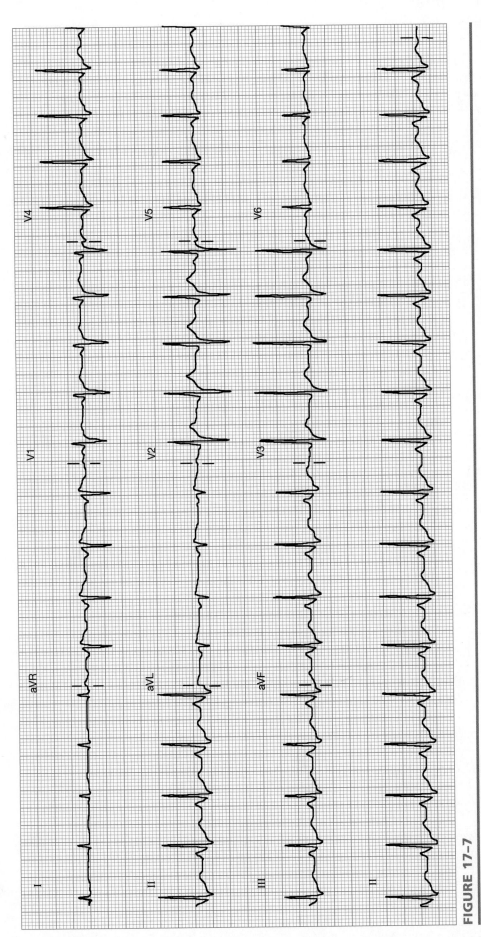

FIGURE 17–7

Mr. Cameron's resting EKG.

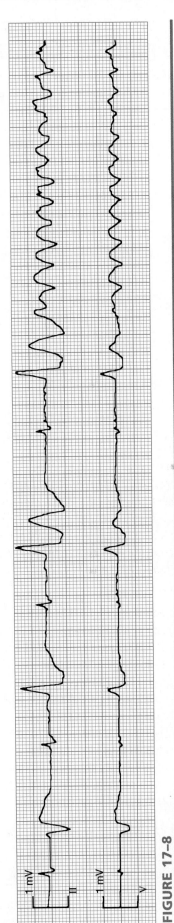

FIGURE 17–8

Mr. Cameron's rhythm when he loses consciousness.

PEARSON
myhealthprofessionskit™

Use this address to access the Companion Website created for this textbook. Simply select "Basic Health Science" from the choice of disciplines. Find this book and log in using your username and password to access video clips, animations, assessment questions, and more.

CHAPTER 18 OBJECTIVES

Upon completion of this chapter, the student will be able to:

- Correlate certain rhythms and 12-lead EKGs with their treatment.
- Display critical thinking skills.

What It's All About

Mr. Coleman was having an inferior MI. Emergency department tech Patrick determined that because he could see the ST segment elevation in Leads II, III, and aVF on the 12-lead EKG he'd just done. Plus Mr. Coleman was having typical symptoms of an MI—chest heaviness, shortness of breath, nausea, cool clammy skin. But Mr. Coleman's blood pressure was also very low—not typical of an uncomplicated inferior MI. Patrick suspected the patient might also be having a right ventricular infarction. He did a right-sided EKG and confirmed his suspicions—Mr. Coleman was having an inferior wall MI with right ventricular infarction. Patrick notified ER nurse Daniel, who alerted the ER physician, and all hurried to the bedside of the stricken Mr. Coleman. By the time the cardiologist arrived from home, Daniel had already notified the cardiac cath lab staff to come to the hospital and had, per hospital protocol, started Mr. Coleman on oxygen and given him an aspirin tablet to chew. Mr. Coleman was soon taken to the cardiac cath lab where he underwent a PCI procedure. He recovered uneventfully.

Introduction

Throughout the previous chapters, you've been working with practice skills and critical thinking exercises to boost your understanding of the chapter material. It's time now to put everything you've learned together in a big way. In the following scenarios, you will use every skill you've learned. You will analyze rhythms and 12-lead EKGs and decide on a course of action. What's going on? Why is it happening? What was done about it in the scenario? What *should have* been done? Is there an MI? What's the rhythm? What medication and/or electrical therapy is indicated? This is the pinnacle of the learning experience—not just mindlessly memorizing material, but using it in a practical way. Let's get started.

Scenario A: Mr. Johnson

Mr. Johnson, age 52, was admitted to the hospital's telemetry floor complaining of mild chest discomfort that lasted 2 hours and was unrelieved by antacids. Both of his parents had a history of heart disease, so Mr. Johnson was afraid he might be having a heart attack. His initial EKG in the emergency department was completely normal, and his pain was relieved with one sublingual nitroglycerin tablet. Medical history included a two-pack-a-day cigarette habit, as well as major surgery the previous week to remove a small colon cancer. Mr. Johnson had been asleep in his room for about an hour when the nurse observed the strip shown in Figure 18–1 on his cardiac monitor.

1. What do you see of concern on the rhythm strip in Figure 18–1? _____

   _____ *ST Segment elevation* _____

The nurse went to check on Mr. Johnson and found him just awakening and complaining of a dull ache in his chest. Per unit protocol, the nurse did a 12-lead EKG, shown in Figure 18–2.

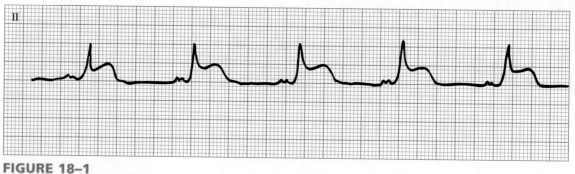

FIGURE 18–1

Mr. Johnson's rhythm.

2. What conclusion do you draw from the EKG in Figure 18–2? _inferior MI_
   ST Segment elevation in leads II, III, aVF

3. Mr. Johnson was moved to the coronary care unit and was started on a
   nitroglycerin infusion. For what purpose was this infusion started? _dialute_
   Coronary arteries ʒ increase bld. flow

4. Mr. Johnson was also started on oxygen by nasal prongs. What beneficial effect
   would the oxygen be expected to have? _↑ tissue concentration of work O₂_
   too ʒ ↓ ♡ work load

5. The physician considered starting thrombolytic therapy (their small community
   hospital didn't have a cardiac cath lab to do PCI), but due to Mr. Johnson's recent
   surgery decided he was not a candidate for thrombolytics. What is the mode of
   action of thrombolytic medications? _dissolve bld clots_

6. What is the danger of giving thrombolytics to someone who had recent
   surgery? _bleeding out_

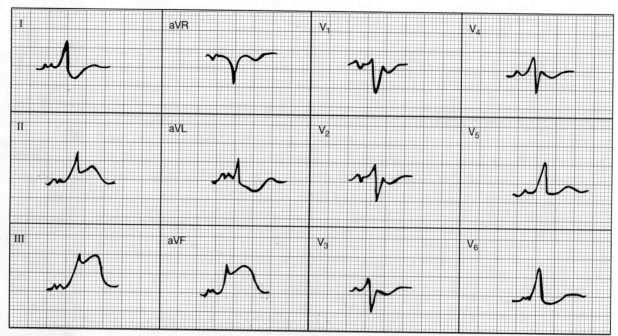

FIGURE 18–2

Mr. Johnson's 12-lead EKG done during chest pain.

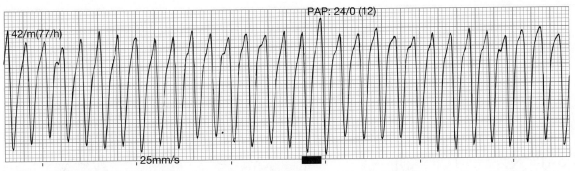

FIGURE 18–3

Mr. Johnson's second rhythm strip.

Shortly after arrival in the CCU, Mr. Johnson called his nurse and told her he felt "funny." He denied pain but stated he felt "full in the head." The nurse noticed the rhythm in Figure 18–3 on the monitor in Mr. Johnson's room.

7. What is the rhythm shown in Figure 18–3? ___V tach___

8. Mr. Johnson's arrhythmia spontaneously converted back to sinus rhythm without treatment. The nurse notified the physician, who ordered labs to be drawn. What electrolyte abnormality can cause this rhythm? ___hypokalemia___

9. What other blood abnormality can cause this rhythm? ___Hypoxia___

10. What medications could have been used to treat this arrhythmia if it had continued? ___lidocaine or amiodarone___

Mr. Johnson's lab work revealed a very low potassium level. He was given supplemental potassium intravenously, and his arrhythmia did not recur. His blood oxygen level was normal.

Shortly after breakfast the next morning, Mr. Johnson developed midsternal chest pain (pain under the center of the breastbone) radiating to his left arm. The pain was severe, and he broke out in a cold sweat and complained of mild nausea. His nurse gave him a sublingual nitroglycerin tablet and increased the rate of his nitroglycerin infusion.

11. What is another medication that could be given to treat Mr. Johnson's chest pain? ___Morphine___

12. A 12-lead EKG was done stat (immediately) and is seen in Figure 18–4. What conclusion do you draw from this EKG? ___ST elevation spreading to lateral wall___

Within 15 minutes, Mr. Johnson's pain was gone but his blood pressure was low and his rhythm had changed. See Figure 18–5 for his next rhythm.

13. What is the rhythm in Figure 18–5? ___2:1 AV block___

14. What effect does this rhythm have on cardiac output? ___↓ CO___

15. What is the appropriate treatment for this rhythm? ___Atropine___

16. Where are the possible sites of the block? ___AV ~~node~~ node or bundle branch___

17. If the block were at the bundle branches, what effect would atropine have? _____
    ___wouldn't work___

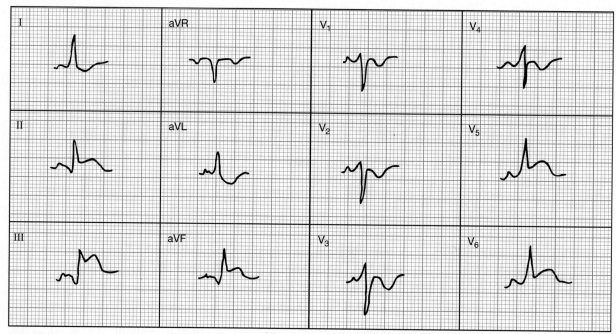

FIGURE 18–4

Mr. Johnson's second 12-lead EKG.

After the appropriate treatment was given, Mr. Johnson's blood pressure returned to normal, and his rhythm was as seen in Figure 18–6.

18. What rhythm is shown in Figure 18–6? _Sinus rhythm_

19. What symptoms, if any, would you expect Mr. Johnson to have with this rhythm? _No symptoms; should feel better_

Concerned about the implications of the most recent EKG and his arrhythmias, Mr. Johnson's physician conferred with cardiologists at a large teaching hospital 60 miles away. Soon Mr. Johnson was transferred by helicopter to that hospital and taken straight to its cardiac catheterization lab, where an emergency angiogram was done. It revealed significant blockage in two of his coronary arteries.

20. Based on the two EKGs in Figures 18–2 and 18–4, which two coronary arteries do you suspect might be blocked? _RCA & Cx_

PCI was attempted but was unsuccessful, so Mr. Johnson was taken to the operating room to have bypass surgery. He recovered uneventfully.

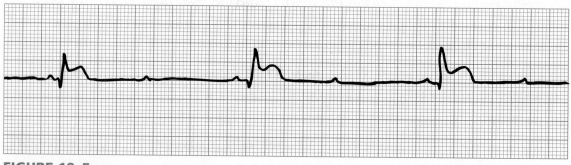

FIGURE 18–5

Mr. Johnson's third rhythm strip.

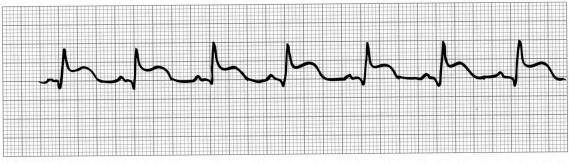

FIGURE 18–6

Mr. Johnson's fourth rhythm strip.

Scenario B: Ms. Capitano

Ms. Capitano was a 23-year-old woman who presented to the ER with complaints of fatigue and dizziness. She had a negative medical history and did not smoke. Aside from birth control pills, she took no medication and denied illegal drug use. She did drink five or six soft drinks daily and had two to three cups of coffee every morning. Cardiac monitor revealed the rhythm seen in Figure 18–7.

1. What is the rhythm shown in Figure 18–7? _SVT   150 bpm_

2. What is the likely cause of this rhythm in Ms. Capitano's case? _too much_
   caffiene

3. The physician ordered adenosine to be given intravenously. The rhythm strip shown in Figure 18–8 was the result. What happened? _slowed to a_
   junctional bradycardia

After a few seconds of the slow heart rate, Ms. Capitano's heart rate sped back up—to the 250s this time—and she complained of feeling faint. Her blood pressure, which had been normal at 110/60, plummeted to 68/50, and she was now pale and drenched in a cold sweat.

4. What effect was the tachycardia having on her cardiac output? _↓ CO_

Ms. Capitano's condition had worsened—she was now in shock. The ER physician elected to perform synchronized electrical cardioversion. After a low-voltage shock, Ms. Capitano's rhythm converted to sinus rhythm with a heart rate in the 90s and her blood pressure improved. Soon her color was back to normal and her skin was dry. She was admitted to the coronary care unit for close observation and was started on calcium channel blockers to prevent recurrences of her tachycardia. The physician advised her to curtail her caffeine intake. After a day in CCU, Ms. Capitano was transferred to the telemetry floor. She was sent home a day later, doing well.

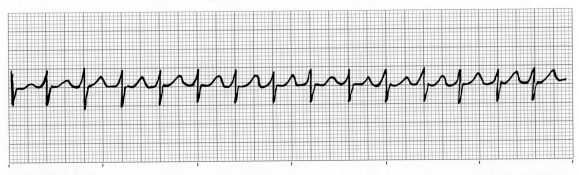

FIGURE 18–7

Ms. Capitano's initial rhythm in the ER.

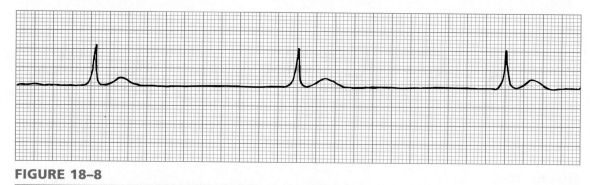

FIGURE 18–8

Ms. Capitano's rhythm after adenosine administration.

Scenario C: Mr. Farley

A few years ago, Mr. Farley had been diagnosed with chronic atrial fibrillation and was started on digitalis. He'd done well, with a heart rate running in the 70s and 80s since then. For the past few days, however, Mr. Farley had felt lousy—nothing specific, just "not right," as he would later describe it. He didn't think it was important enough to bother his physician, although his wife had fussed at him to do so. Believing his problem to be related to his atrial fibrillation, Mr. Farley doubled up on his digitalis dose. If one pill a day was good, two a day had to be better, he reasoned. After five days of this, he began suffering from violent nausea and vomiting episodes. His wife dragged the reluctant Mr. Farley to the hospital. His initial rhythm strip is shown in Figure 18–9.

1. What is the rhythm in Figure 18–9? <u>Slow atril fibrilation</u>

2. What effect does this rhythm have on the atrial kick? <u>There is no atrial</u> <u>kick in a fib</u>

3. Lab tests revealed that the level of digitalis in Mr. Farley's bloodstream was at toxic levels. Name three rhythms that can be caused by digitalis toxicity. <u>almost any</u> <u>arrhythmia;</u>

The physician contemplated sending Mr. Farley to the CCU, but since his blood pressure was good and he looked OK, he was sent to the telemetry floor instead. His nausea was treated with medication and he was taken off digitalis. Three hours after arriving on the telemetry floor, Mr. Farley passed out in the bathroom. His wife ran to get the nurse just as the nurses, having seen his rhythm on the monitor, were running toward his room. His new rhythm is shown in Figure 18–10.

4. What is the rhythm in Figure 18–10? <u>asystole</u>

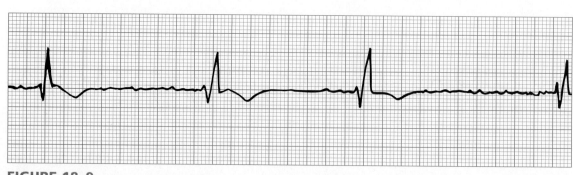

FIGURE 18–9

Mr. Farley's initial rhythm strip.

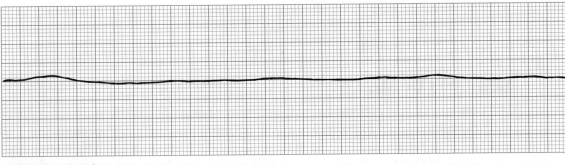

FIGURE 18–10

Mr. Farley's second rhythm strip.

5. The emergency team was called and CPR was initiated. What two medications would be appropriate to give at this time? _Atropine & epinephrine_

6. After successful resuscitation, Mr. Farley was transferred to the CCU, where a temporary transvenous pacemaker was inserted. What beneficial effect would the pacemaker have? _preventing his heart from going to slow_

7. A few hours after the pacemaker was inserted, the nurse noticed evidence of loss of capture on the monitor. On the monitor strip in Figure 18–11, what would tell her there was loss of capture? _pacemaker spikes not followed by a QRS_

8. What can be done to restore capture? _repositioning, change batteries_

   Capture was restored, and Mr. Johnson rested well for the next few hours. Suddenly, he went into V-tach with a heart rate of 200. The nurses could tell by the deflection of the QRS complexes that the V-tach was originating in the left ventricle, so they knew it was not induced by irritation from the pacemaker wire in the right ventricle.

9. With a pacemaker in place, what can be done to terminate the tachycardia? _____
   Dial it up to over ride the tachy rhythm

10. With the V-tach now resolved, Mr. Farley was started on an amiodarone infusion to prevent a recurrence of the V-tach. What is amiodarone's effect on the ventricle? _↓ irritability of the vent & makes it less responsive to impulse_

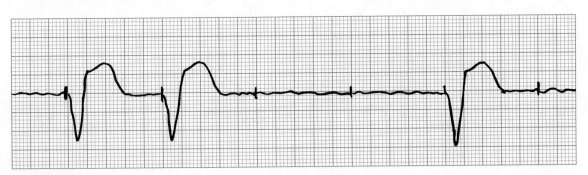

FIGURE 18–11

Mr. Farley's third rhythm strip.

11. The rest of Mr. Farley's hospital stay was uneventful. Since his problem began with his inappropriate self-dosing of digitalis, what would you tell Mr. Farley regarding his digitalis dose in the future? _____

Scenario D: Mr. Lew

Mr. Lew, age 78, had outlived his wife and most of their friends. He had never been in the hospital and had not seen his physician in 7 years. By all accounts, he was unusually healthy for his age. He was not alarmed by the occasional tightness in his chest—and in fact took it as a sign that he was out of shape and needed to exercise more. One summer day, while he was mowing the lawn, his chest tightness came back, but this time it was much more intense, and Mr. Lew became concerned. He called his son to take him to the hospital. On the way, Mr. Lew passed out in the car and slumped over onto his son, causing an accident. Ambulances rushed the duo to the closest ER. Stephen, the son, was treated for a fractured arm and was discharged in a cast. Although not injured in the accident, Mr. Lew was in much worse shape. See his EKG in Figure 18–12.

1. What conclusion do you draw from the EKG in Figure 18–12? _____
extensive anterior MI

Mr. Lew's condition was precarious. His blood pressure was low and he was in danger of cardiac arrest. Thrombolytic therapy was started (PCI was not possible at this small local hospital) and within one hour Mr. Lew's blood pressure had improved. Soon he was in the rhythm shown in Figure 18–13.

2. What is the rhythm in Figure 18–13? *accelerated idioventricular rhythm AIVR*

3. What, if any, treatment does this rhythm require in this case? *none*

4. What in the past was thought to be the significance of this rhythm? *reperfusion*

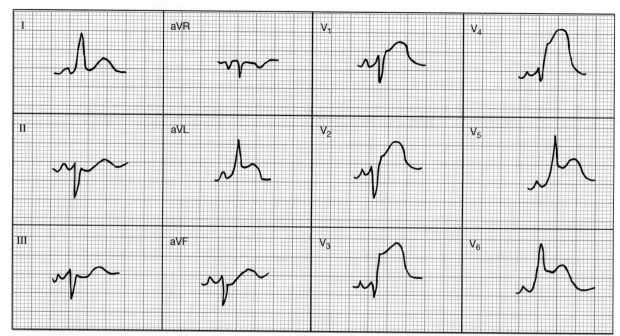

FIGURE 18–12

Mr. Lew's initial 12-lead EKG.

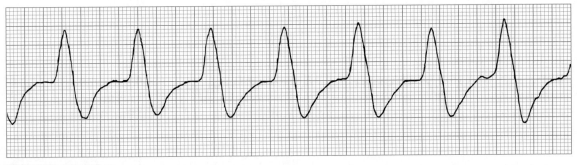

FIGURE 18–13

Mr. Lew's rhythm strip after thrombolytic therapy.

This rhythm converted back to sinus rhythm within 30 minutes. Mr. Lew's condition improved over the next hour, and he was transferred to the coronary care unit, where he stabilized.

When Stephen came by to see his dad the next day, Mr. Lew whispered to him that he was having mild chest pain again, but that it wasn't bad enough to bother the nurses. Stephen alerted the nurse, who did an EKG while the pain was in progress. See the EKG in Figure 18–14.

5. What conclusion do you draw from the EKG in Figure 18–14?_____
   _MI extended to inferior wall_____

Mr. Lew's nitroglycerin infusion was adjusted and he was taken for an emergency angiogram. An occlusion of the left main coronary artery was noted, along with blockage in another coronary artery.

6. Based on the two EKGs in Figures 18–12 and 18–14, which other coronary artery is involved?___RCA_____

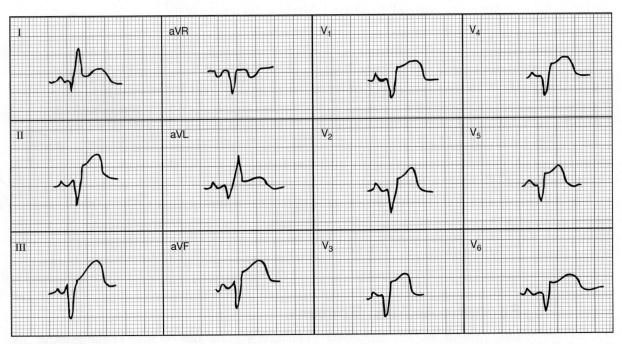

FIGURE 18–14

Mr. Lew's EKG done during chest pain.

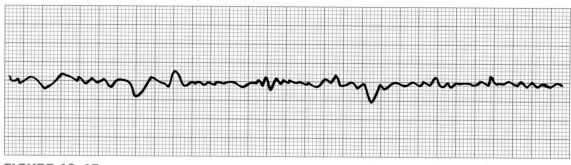

FIGURE 18–15

Mr. Lew's rhythm during cardiac arrest.

7. What is the cause of the ST segment depression noted on Mr. Lew's first EKG? _____
   _____*reciprocal change*_____

Mr. Lew was taken to the operating room for emergency bypass surgery. Following cardiac arrest in the operating room, he returned to the CCU in critical condition. Before the surgical nurses could get back to the OR after bringing Mr. Lew to CCU, they heard the emergency page on the loudspeaker. Mr. Lew was in cardiac arrest again. They rushed back to CCU to help. The cardiac surgeon had opened the chest sutures and was doing manual chest compressions by squeezing Mr. Lew's heart in his hands. Mr. Lew's rhythm strip is shown in Figure 18–15.

8. What is the rhythm in Figure 18–15? _*V. fib*_

Internal defibrillator paddles were inserted into the open chest cavity and placed on either side of Mr. Lew's heart. A small volt was discharged, and Mr. Lew's rhythm changed to the one shown in Figure 18–16.

9. What is the rhythm in Figure 18–16? _*agonal rhythm*_

CPR was started again, and the staff administered various medications as well as temporary pacing—all to no avail. Mr. Lew did not make it.

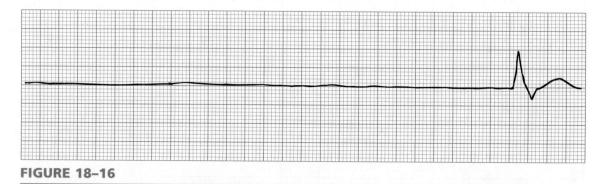

FIGURE 18–16

Mr. Lew's rhythm after defibrillation.

Scenario E: Mrs. Epstein

Mrs. Epstein had her pacemaker implanted 4 years ago because of third-degree AV block. She'd been doing well until this morning, when she began to feel dizzy. She took her pulse as she'd been taught to do and found it to be 38. Her rate-responsive DDD

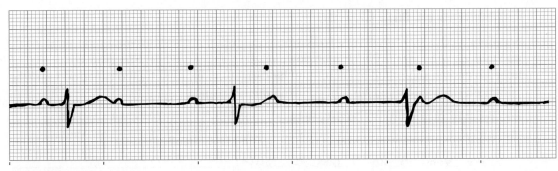

FIGURE 18–17

Mrs. Epstein's rhythm during a dizzy spell in the hospital.

pacemaker was set at a rate of 60 to 125. At the physician's office, the cardiologist found that the pacemaker needed a new battery. Because her heart rate was now in the 60s, he thought the battery change could wait until the next morning. He sent Mrs. Epstein to the hospital, where she was admitted to the telemetry floor.

A few hours after arrival, Mrs. Epstein complained again of dizziness, this time much worse. Her rhythm is shown in Figure 18–17.

1. What is the rhythm in Figure 18–17? ___3rd degree AV Block___

2. What is her pacemaker doing? ___Nothing / not firing___

3. What is the likely cause of this problem? ___dead battery___

The nurse, following hospital protocol, gave atropine and called for her coworkers to bring in the transcutaneous pacemaker. The pacemaker was attached and set on demand mode at a rate of 60.

After notifying the cardiologist of the situation, the nurse rushed Mrs. Epstein to the cardiac catheterization lab, where an emergency pacemaker battery change was done. After her return to the telemetry floor, the nurse noted her rhythm as shown in Figure 18–18.

4. What is the rhythm in Figure 18–18? ___dual chamber pacing___

5. Is the pacemaker functioning properly? If not, what is the problem? ___functioning properly___

Mrs. Epstein was discharged the following day in good condition.

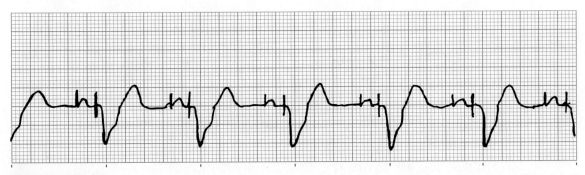

FIGURE 18–18

Mrs. Epstein's rhythm on return from her pacemaker battery change.

Scenario F: Mr. Calico

Mr. Calico, age 76, was taking a walk when he developed chest heaviness. He went inside and told his wife he was going to lie down on the sofa for a while. She grew concerned an hour later when she called his name and he didn't answer. Mrs. Calico called 911 and the paramedics arrived to find Mr. Calico in the rhythm seen in Figure 18–19.

1. What is this rhythm? _asystole_

2. What symptoms would you expect to see in Mr. Calico? _____
   No vital signs & cool to touch

3. Mr. Calico was unconscious and had no pulse and no breathing. What should the paramedics do to resuscitate Mr. Calico? _CPR, Atropine & epinephrine_

After appropriate initial treatment, Mr. Calico's pulse returned and he began to awaken. The paramedics ran another rhythm strip. See Figure 18–20.

4. What is this rhythm? _SVT_

Paramedics rushed Mr. Calico to the nearest hospital, where a 12-lead EKG was done. His 12-lead EKG is seen in Figure 18–21.

5. What conclusion do you draw from this EKG? _Anterioseptal MI_

6. Thrombolytic medication was started and the EKG was repeated. See Figure 18–22. What has changed since the last EKG? _MI aborted_

7. Mr. Calico went into ventricular fibrillation a few minutes later. The nurse prepared to cardiovert the rhythm, but when he depressed the buttons to deliver the shock, nothing happened. Why and what corrective action is needed for this problem?
   needs to defibrilate

After correctly defibrillating Mr. Calico, the ER staff sent him to the CCU, where he spent a week recovering. He went home and did well with no further problems.

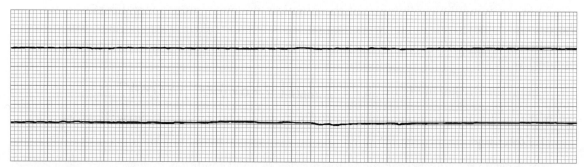

FIGURE 18–19

Mr. Calico's initial rhythm.

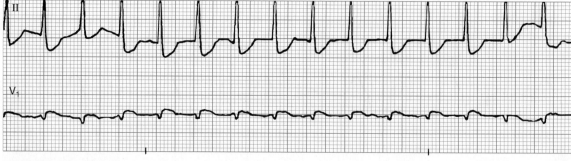

FIGURE 18–20

Mr. Calico's rhythm after initial treatment.

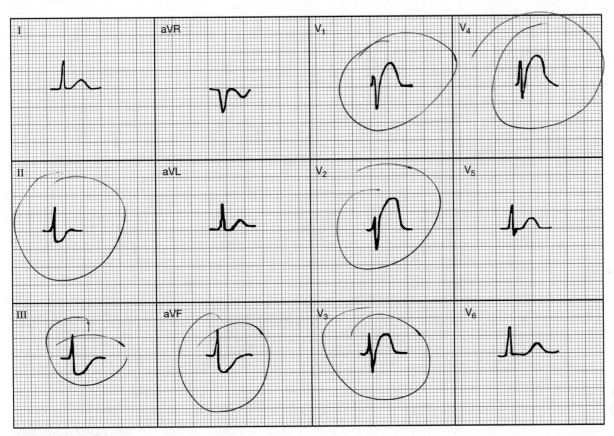

FIGURE 18–21

Mr. Calico's initial 12-lead EKG.

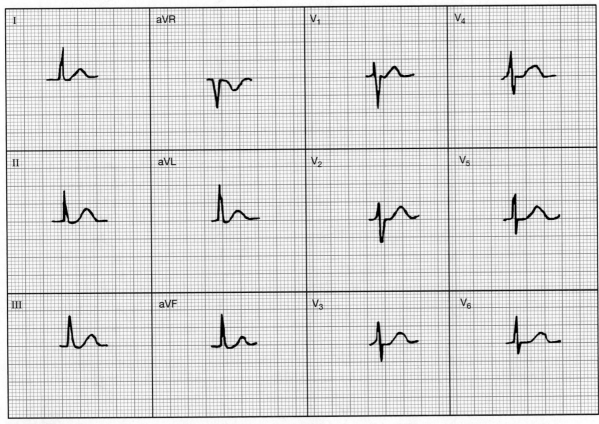

FIGURE 18–22

Mr. Calico's EKG after thrombolytic medication.

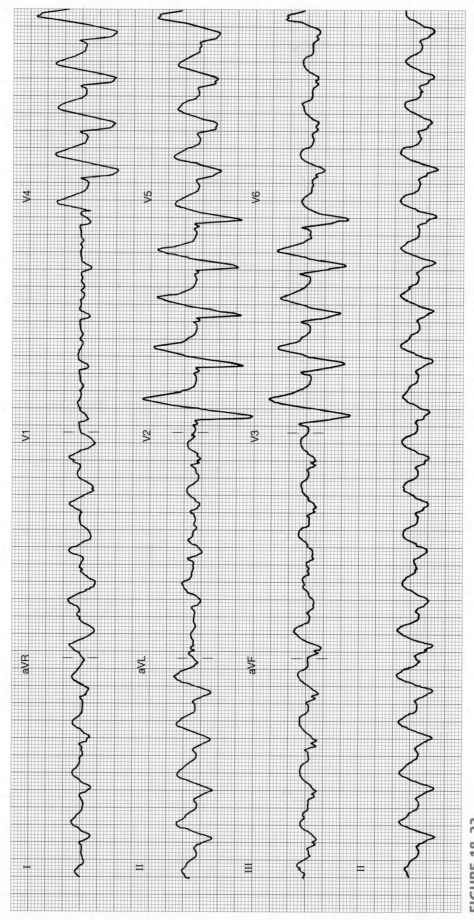

FIGURE 18-23

Mrs. Taylor's first EKG.

Scenario G: Mrs. Taylor

Mrs. Taylor hated dialysis (a method of removing waste from the bloodstream when the kidneys are unable to do so). Being attached to a machine for 3 days a week, 4 hours each time, was, in her words, "not my idea of living." At age 45, she'd been in kidney failure for 15 years and had required dialysis for most of that time. Because of other health problems (diabetes, heart disease, asthma), she was not a candidate for a kidney transplant. At her local hospital, Mrs. Taylor was notorious for coming in critically ill after skipping two or three dialysis treatments. She'd be admitted to the intensive care unit, treated, and released a week or so later, with a warning not to skip dialysis any more. But a few months later she'd be back again.

Tonight Mrs. Taylor comes in yet again. Her potassium level, which should be 5.0 at the most, is 8.9, dangerously high. Her EKG is shown in Figure 18–23.

1. In Chapter 13, you learned that elevated potassium levels can cause two main effects on the EKG. What are they and which one or ones do you see on this EKG? _____
   HyperKalemia , Tall Pointy T waves (eventually wide QRS too)

Almost immediately after arrival in the ER, Mrs. Taylor loses consciousness and suffers cardiac arrest. The nurse records the following rhythm strip as she begins CPR. See Figure 18–24.

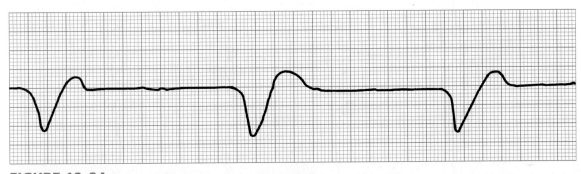

FIGURE 18–24

Mrs. Taylor's rhythm strip during cardiac arrest.

2. What is this rhythm? _____

The physician orders calcium to be given intravenously. Calcium decreases the potassium level in the bloodstream. After giving the calcium, the nurse runs the following EKG. See Figure 18–25.

3. What change do you see in the QRS complex? _idioventricular rhythm_

Mrs. Taylor's pulse and breathing resume after the calcium. She is sent to the intensive care unit, where she undergoes dialysis. Four days later, she is well enough to go home. Once again she is warned that the next time she skips dialysis, it could be fatal. She smiles at the nurses and says, "I know, I know."

Scenario H: Mr. Foster

Mr. Foster was a 28-year-old male who'd been abusing cocaine for years. Tonight he and some friends had been "partying" with various substances—cocaine, ecstasy, and other assorted drugs—when Mr. Foster began to complain of chest pain. His friends were alarmed when Mr. Foster clutched his chest and curled into a ball on the ground, moaning in pain. They pulled him up and brought him to the hospital, then abandoned him outside the ER door. A security guard saw the distraught Mr. Foster and alerted the ER staff, who brought the patient into the ER.

A 12-lead EKG was done and is shown in Figure 18–26.

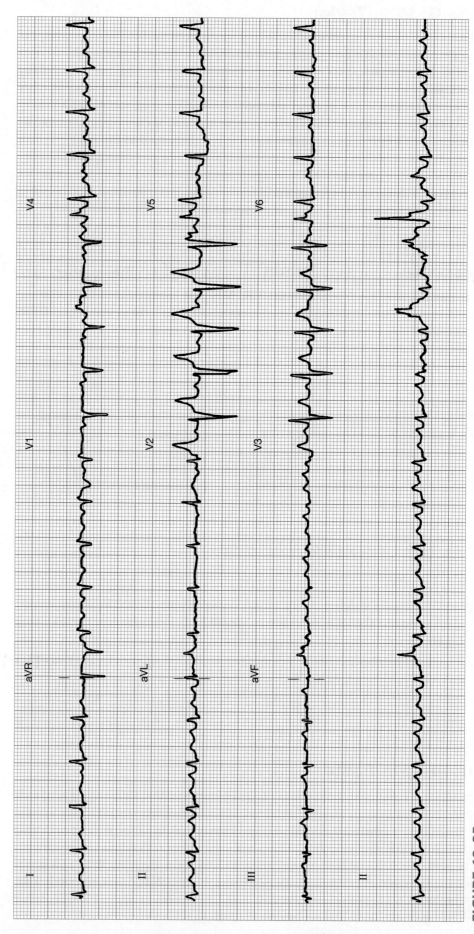

FIGURE 18–25

Mrs. Taylor's EKG after calcium.

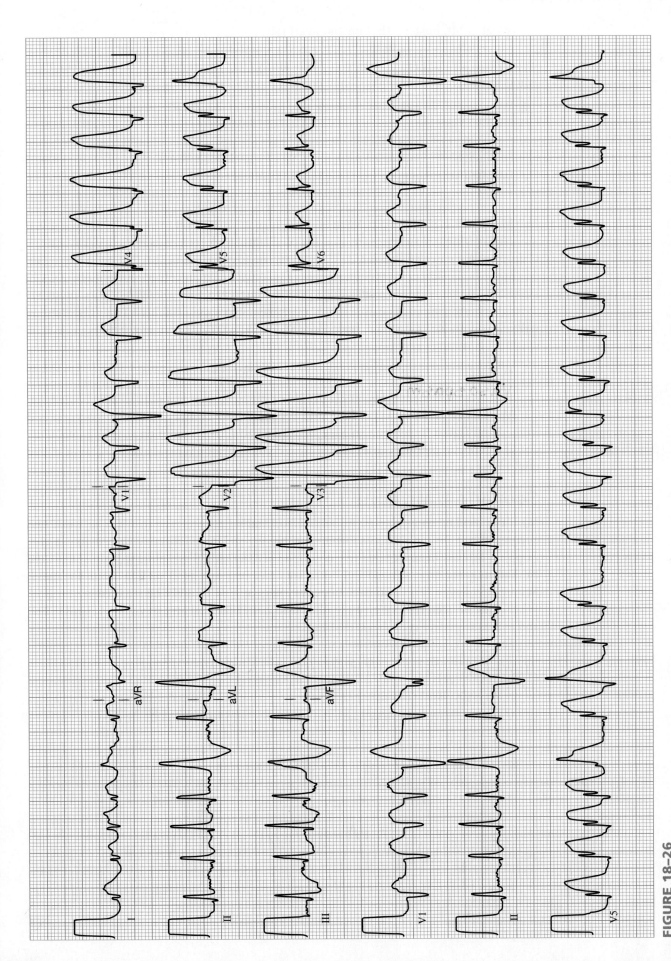

FIGURE 18–26

Mr. Foster's 12-lead EKG.

1. What is Mr. Foster's rhythm and heart rate? _____

Mr. Foster is initially unable to answer questions about his medical condition or history and the staff are unable to contact family. The ER nurse asks the physician if she wants to do elective cardioversion to convert the rhythm to sinus. The physician says no.

2. Why would she not want to shock this rhythm at this time? _____
_____

3. There is evidence of an MI on the EKG. Is it a STEMI or a non-STEMI? _____

4. Which wall or walls of the heart is/are infarcted? _____
_____

Mr. Foster is started on oxygen and given an aspirin tablet to chew. He is then given a nitroglycerine pill sublingually and the pain starts to decrease, as does his heart rate—it drops to a mean rate in the 80s. The physician advises Mr. Foster that he is having an MI and Mr. Foster is incredulous. "But I'm only 28, man! Heart attacks are for old people!" The physician explains that cocaine use greatly increases the chance of an MI even in young people who would not otherwise be considered high risk. The cardiac cath lab team is called out and Mr. Foster is taken for an angiogram, which is completely normal.

5. What effect of cocaine can cause an MI in patients with no coronary artery disease?
Vasospasm _____

Mr. Foster is sent to the ICU and recovers uneventfully. He is discharged and immediately goes into rehab to kick his drug habit. The cardiologist tells him, "This cocaine-induced coronary artery spasm gave you a heart attack at age 28. The next one could kill you."

Scenario I: Mr. Frye

Mr. Frye worked in a busy metropolitan hospital's ER as a tech. He was at work one evening when he developed shortness of breath and palpitations—"it felt like a fish flopping around in my chest," he described it later. Mr. Frye attached himself to the cardiac monitor and climbed into an empty ER bed, his head reeling from dizziness. Seeing Mr. Frye climb into bed, his coworkers at first thought he was joking around. When they noticed his pallor, they rushed to help him, starting oxygen and an IV line and evaluating Mr. Frye's heart rhythm.

See Figure 18–27.

1. What is this rhythm? _PAT (run of PACs)_____

2. What's the heart rate? _____

Vagal maneuvers were suggested as a method of terminating the rhythm.

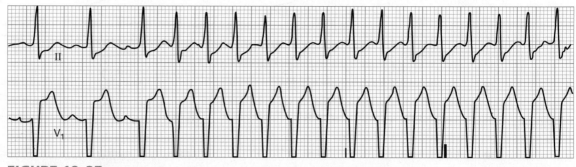

FIGURE 18–27

Mr. Frye's rhythm.

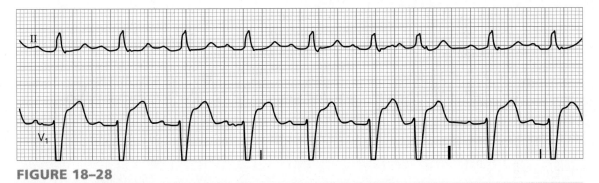

FIGURE 18–28

Mr. Frye's rhythm following the second dose of adenosine.

3. What effect does stimulation of the vagus nerve have on the heart rate? _____
_____

Mr. Frye tried the vagal maneuvers—no luck. His heart rate was still tachycardic and he was looking more and more pale. His blood pressure was 100/50—a bit below his normal of 110/70. The ER physician ordered adenosine to be given IV. Everyone watched the heart monitor as the adenosine was injected into the IV line. No change. A second dose of adenosine—double the first dose—was given.

See Figure 18–28 for Mr. Frye's rhythm following the second dose of adenosine.

4. What do you see on this strip? _____

5. What unnerving side effect can adenosine have on the rhythm and heart rate? _____
_____

6. Was that effect evident in Figure 18–28? _____

After the second dose of the medication, Mr. Frye's skin dried up, his color returned, and his shortness of breath was gone.

7. What other treatments would have been appropriate for Mr. Frye's initial rhythm? _____
_____

Scenario J: Mrs. Terry

Mr. and Mrs. Terry, age 38, had been married for 6 years. They were settled in a new house and were finally ready to have a baby. Next month, they decided, would be their last month of using birth control pills—and Mrs. Terry's last month as a smoker. The pair were browsing in the baby department at the mall when Mrs. Terry felt a crushing fatigue. "Let's just go home—I want to lie down," she told her husband. Later Mrs. Terry became woozy and very pale. Her husband, concerned his wife might have the flu, took her to the hospital. The ER physician examined her and agreed with Mr. Terry. "I think you probably just picked up the flu bug," he told her, "There's not much to do but ride it out. Just stay in bed a few days and you should feel better." So they went home and Mrs. Terry climbed into bed. The next morning she felt worse—short of breath now—so she called her family doctor and went to his office. He examined her and told her he also thought she had the flu. "You'll probably feel worse before you feel better," he told her, "Just go to bed and wait it out." So off they went back home. Mrs. Terry went straight to bed while her hubby watched TV. Mr. Terry checked in on his wife a few hours later and found her barely conscious. She was as limp as a rag doll. Mr. Terry called 911 and the paramedics arrived and attached Mrs. Terry to the cardiac monitor, which revealed the following rhythm. See Figure 18–29.

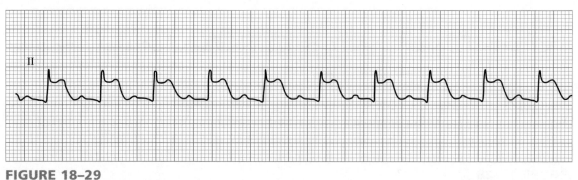

FIGURE 18–29

Mrs. Terry's rhythm strip.

1. What are the rhythm and heart rate?

   _____

2. Are there any other abnormalities on this strip? If so, what? _____

   _____

The paramedics rushed Mrs. Terry to the closest ER. En route, they did a 12-lead EKG and transmitted it to the hospital. See Figure 18–30.

3. What abnormalities does this EKG show? _____

   _____

4. Assuming the hospital is suitably equipped to handle this, what is the preferred treatment for this condition, according to the American College of Cardiology and the American Heart Association? _____

5. Mrs. Terry was found to have a large occlusion in a coronary artery. Based on the EKG, which coronary artery do you suspect was involved? _____

She was successfully treated. After assessing her risk factors for heart disease, the cardiologist concluded that Mrs. Terry's birth control pills, combined with her 2-pack-a-day smoking habit and her age, caused her MI. The cardiologist told her that her brand of birth control pills contains estrogen, known to increase the risk for blood clots, heart attacks, and strokes, especially in women who smoke. And the vague symptoms were typical of females with MIs. The cardiologist told her that because of these vague symptoms and her age, there was no red flag to raise the doctors' suspicion of an MI—until she collapsed and was picked up by paramedics. That's why she'd been misdiagnosed twice with the flu.

When she was sent home a week later, Mrs. Terry was advised to use an alternate form of birth control—no more birth control pills—and to avoid getting pregnant for at least a year in order to let her heart heal. Two years later, the Terrys became the proud parents of twin boys.

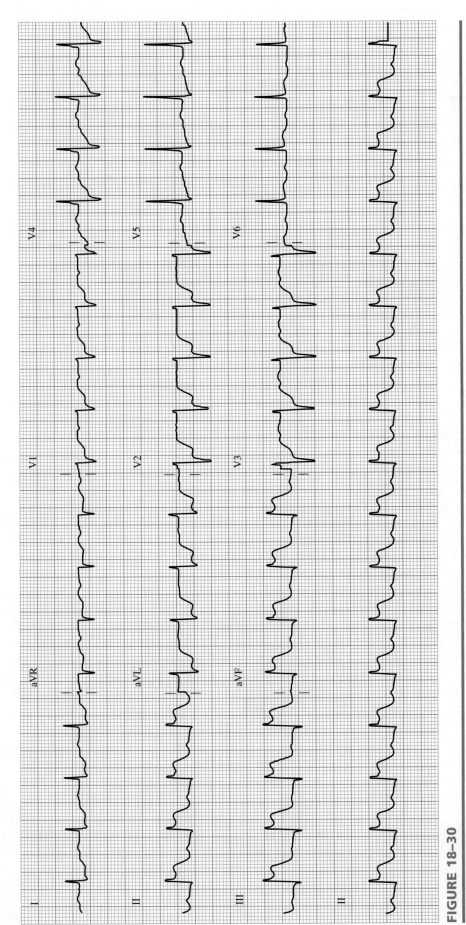

FIGURE 18–30

Mrs. Terry's EKG.

PEARSON
myhealthprofessionskit™

Use this address to access the Companion Website created for this textbook. Simply select "Basic Health Science" from the choice of disciplines. Find this book and log in using your username and password to access video clips, animations, assessment questions, and more.

Appendix

Answers to Chapter Skills Practice Questions, End-of-Chapter Practice Quizzes, and Critical Thinking Exercise Questions

CHAPTER ONE
Practice Quiz

1. The function of the heart is to **pump enough blood to meet the body's metabolic needs.**
2. The three layers of the heart are the **endocardium, myocardium,** and **epicardium.**
3. The four chambers of the heart are the **right atrium, left atrium, right ventricle,** and **left ventricle.**
4. The four heart valves are the **tricuspid, mitral, pulmonic,** and **aortic valves.**
5. The purpose of the heart valves is to **prevent backflow of blood.**
6. The five great vessels are the **aorta, pulmonary artery, pulmonary veins, superior vena cava,** and **inferior vena cava.**
7. The phases of diastole are **rapid filling, diastasis,** and **atrial kick.**
8. The phases of systole are **isovolumetric contraction, ventricular ejection, protodiastole,** and **iovolumetric relaxation.**
9. The two divisions of the autonomic nervous system are the **sympathetic** and **parasympathetic nervous systems.**
10. The three main coronary arteries are the **left anterior descending, the right coronary artery,** and **the circumflex.**

2. Here are the following structures numbered 1 to 14 in order of blood flow through the heart:
   1 superior and inferior vena cava
   3 tricuspid valve
   10 mitral valve
   12 aortic valve
   5 pulmonic valve
   14 body
   13 aorta
   6 pulmonary artery
   7 lungs
   8 pulmonary veins
   2 right atrium
   9 left atrium
   4 right ventricle
   11 left ventricle

3. If the chordae tendineae of the tricuspid and mitral valves "snapped" loose, the valves would lose their ability to remain closed during systole, allowing blood to flow backward into the atria.

Critical Thinking Exercises

1.
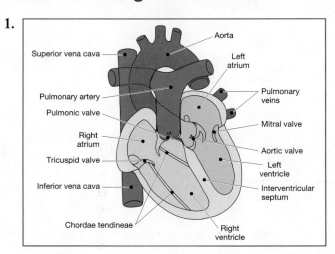

CHAPTER TWO
Waves and Complexes Practice

1.
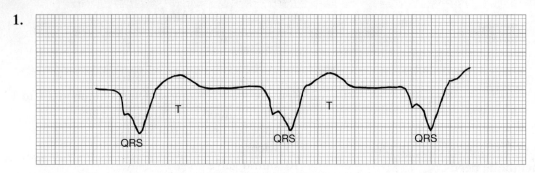

2.
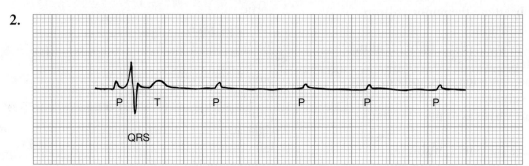

3.
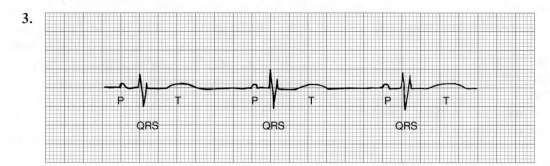

4.
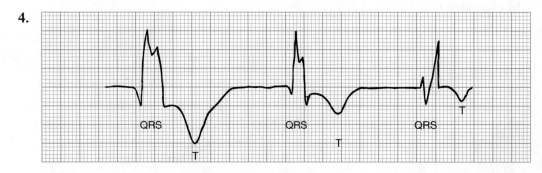

5.
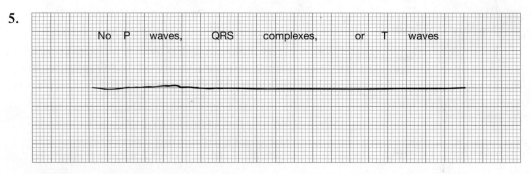

QRS Nomenclature Practice
"Name the Waves"

1. R.
2. QS. This cannot be called a Q or an S because there is no R wave to precede or follow, so the QRS complex that is completely negative is called QS.
3. QR.
4. RS.
5. QRS.
6. RSR′.

"Draw the QRS Complexes"

1.
2.
3.
4.
5.
6.

Intervals Practice

1. PR 0.12, QRS 0.08, QT 0.24.
2. PR 0.12, QRS 0.14, QT 0.32.
3. PR 0.24, QRS 0.08, QT 0.28.

Intervals Practice on Normal-Size EKG Paper

Note: For the intervals, it is acceptable if your answer is within 0.02 secs of displayed answer.

1. PR 0.20, QRS 0.08, QT 0.36.
2. PR 0.22, QRS 0.08, QT 0.32.
3. PR 0.08, QRS 0.12, QT 0.36.
4. PR 0.10, QRS 0.08, QT 0.32.
5. PR 0.16, QRS 0.06, QT 0.36.
6. PR 0.16, QRS 0.08, QT 0.30.
7. PR 0.16, QRS 0.08, QT 0.30.
8. PR 0.14, QRS 0.09, QT 0.38.
9. PR 0.16, QRS 0.10, QT 0.37.
10. PR 0.14, QRS 0.08, QT 0.30.

Practice Quiz

1. Cardiac cells at rest are electrically **negative.**
2. Depolarization and repolarization are **electrical events.**
3. Phase 4. **The cardiac cell is at rest.**

Phase 0. **Depolarization occurs when sodium rushes into the cell.**
Phase 1. **Early repolarization. Calcium is released.**
Phase 2. **The plateau phase of early repolarization. Calcium is released.**
Phase 3. **Rapid repolarization. Sodium rushes out of the cell.**

4. The P wave represents **atrial depolarization.** The QRS complex represents **ventricular depolarization.** The T wave represents **ventricular repolarization.**
5. **No impulse can result in depolarization during the absolute refractory period.**
6. The four characteristics of heart cells are **automaticity, conductivity, excitability,** and **contractility.**
7. The inherent rates of the pacemaker cells are **sinus node—60 to 100, AV junction—40 to 60, ventricle—20 to 40.**
8. The structures of the cardiac conduction pathway are **sinus node, interatrial tracts, atrium, internodal tracts, AV node, bundle of His, bundle branches, Purkinje fibers,** and **ventricle.**
9. **Escape occurs when the prevailing pacemaker slows or fails and a lower pacemaker takes over as the pacemaker at a slower rate than before.**
10. **Usurpation occurs when a lower pacemaker becomes "hyper" and fires at an accelerated rate, stealing control away from the predominant pacemaker and providing a faster heart rate than before.**

Critical Thinking Exercises

1. If the sinus node is firing at a rate of 65 and the AV junction kicks in at a rate of 70, **the AV junction will usurp the sinus node and become the heart's pacemaker.** The sinus node would be inhibited and would stop firing out impulses as long as the AV junction is faster. Remember, the fastest pacemaker at any given time is the one in control.
2. If your patient's PR interval last night was 0.16 seconds and this morning it is 0.22, **the AV node is becoming incapable of transmitting impulses at its normal rate, causing the PR interval to prolong.**
3. The heart's pumping ability can fail, but its electrical conduction ability remains **intact if there is a heart attack or other condition that damages the myocardium but leaves the conduction system unaffected.** The conduction system would send out

its impulses as usual, but the damaged myocardium would be unable to respond by pumping.

4.

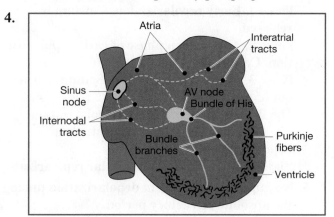

CHAPTER THREE
Lead Morphology Practice

1. **Normal morphology.**
2. **Abnormal morphology.**   Let's go lead by lead. Lead I is normal. Leads II and III are negative deflections, and they should be positive; aVR is OK, as is aVL; aVF is negative and it should be positive. The precordial leads are OK.
3. **Abnormal morphology.**   Lead I is negative and it should be positive. Leads II and III are OK; aVR is positive and it should *always* be negative; aVL is negative and should be positive; aVF is OK. V_1 is positive but should be negative. V_2 is OK, more negative than positive. V_3 is positive but should be isoelectric. V_4 is isoelectric when it should be getting more positive. V_5 and V_6 are negative when they should be positive.
4. **Abnormal morphology.**   Lead I is positive, as it should be. Leads II and III are negative but should be positive; aVR and aVL are OK; aVF is negative but should be positive. The precordial leads are all positive—this is completely abnormal.

Practice Quiz

1. **Willem Einthoven won the Nobel Prize for inventing the EKG machine.**
2. The three bipolar leads are **Leads I, II,** and **III. Lead I connects the right and left arms. Lead II connects the right arm and left leg. Lead III connects the left arm and left leg.**
3. The three augmented leads are as follows:

aVR	**Positive pole is on the right arm.**
aVL	**Positive pole is on the left arm.**
aVF	**Positive pole is on the left leg.**

4. The six leads comprising the hexiaxial diagram are **Leads I, II, III, aVR, aVL,** and **aVF.**
5. The precordial leads see the heart from the **horizontal plane.**
6. The precordial leads and their locations are as follows:

V_1	**4th ICS, RSB**
V_2	**4th ICS, LSB**
V_3	**Between V_2 and V_4**
V_4	**5th ICS, MCL**
V_5	**5th ICS, AAL**
V_6	**5th ICS, MAL**

7. The two leads most commonly used for continuous monitoring are **Leads II** and **V_1/MCL1.**
8. An impulse traveling toward a positive electrode writes a **positive** complex on the EKG.
9. aVR should have a **negative** QRS complex.
10. The QRS complexes in the precordial leads start out primarily **negative.**

Critical Thinking Exercises

1. If Lead I + Lead III do not equal Lead II, it could imply that **the electrodes were placed on the incorrect limbs.**
2. If the QRS complex in Lead III is isoelectric, **the heart's current is traveling perpendicular to that lead.**
3. If your patient has a heart rhythm in which the current starts in the left ventricle and travels upward toward the sinus node, the frontal leads would look like the following: **Lead I's QRS would be negative, Lead II would be negative, Lead III would be negative, aVR would be positive, aVL would be negative,** and **aVF would be negative.** You'll note this is the exact opposite of how the frontal leads normally look. This is because the current would be traveling away from all the positive electrodes except aVR's. Recall that aVR's positive electrode sits on the right arm and would be watching this current come straight toward it, resulting in a positive QRS in aVR.

CHAPTER FOUR
Artifact Troubleshooting Practice

1. The artifact is in Leads **I, III,** and **aVL.** Corrective action is to check for and reattach or reconnect loose or disconnected electrodes or lead wires on the **left arm.** If an electrode patch is loose or missing, put on a new patch. *Never put a used patch back on. It will*

not stick well enough to ensure good impulse transmission. How do we know the problem is on the left arm? Refer to Figure 4-6. What is the common limb shared by all these leads? Lead I connects right arm and left arm; III connects left arm and left leg; aVL involves left arm only. The common limb is the left arm. Direct corrective efforts there.

2. The artifact is in Leads **II, III,** and **aVF.** Corrective action is to check the **left leg** for loose or disconnected electrodes or lead wires and to reattach/reconnect them as necessary. What is the common limb? Lead II connects right arm and left leg; III connects left arm and left leg; aVF involves left leg only. The common limb is the left leg.

3. The artifact is in Leads **I, II,** and **aVR.** Corrective action is to check the **right arm** for loose or disconnected electrodes or lead wires and to reattach/reconnect them as necessary. What is the common limb? Lead I connects right arm and left arm; II connects right arm and left leg; III involves right arm only. The common limb is the right arm.

Practice Quiz

1. The function of the EKG machine is **to print out a representation of the electrical signals generated by the heart.**
2. Normal chart speed for running a 12-lead EKG is **25** millimeters per second.
3. The gain **adjusts the height of the waves and complexes.**
4. If the technician changes any of the settings (the chart speed or the gain) when doing an EKG, **he or she should document this on the EKG.**
5. Macroshock **is a high-voltage electrical shock that results from inadequate grounding of electrical equipment.**
6. Microshock is **a lower voltage shock that involves a conduit directly into the patient, such as a pacemaker.**
7. Artifact is **unwanted interference or jitter on the EKG tracing.**
8. The four kinds of artifact are **somatic tremors, baseline sway, 60-cycle interference,** and **broken recording.**
9. If there is artifact in I, aVR, and II, troubleshooting efforts should be directed toward the **right arm.**
10. Three ways to determine if a rhythm is real or artifact are any three of the following: **Observe the rhythm in another lead such as V_1. Check to see if the rhythm meets the normal criteria. Check the monitor wires and patches. See if the patient** has any muscle tremors that could cause artifact. Check the patient's vital signs for evidence of decreased cardiac output.

Critical Thinking Exercises

1. If your patient, who is on telemetry monitoring, is noted to have two electrodes that have fallen off—the right arm and left leg, **you would expect to see artifact in any leads that use either or both of those limbs: Lead I, Lead II, Lead III, aVR,** and **aVF.**
2. You would know that your patient is having artifact and not a life-threatening arrhythmia by **assessing the patient for signs of decreased cardiac output, checking the rhythm in another lead, checking the electrode patches and wires to see if any are loose or detached, and assessing for any muscle tremors or twitches that could mimic artifact.**

CHAPTER FIVE
Regularity Practice Strips

1. **Irregular.** The R-R intervals are all over the place, with no hint of regularity.
2. **Regular.** The R-R intervals are all about 56 little blocks.
3. **Regular but interrupted.** This is the strip shown a few pages ago as an example of regular but interrupted rhythms. Look back if you don't recognize it.
4. **Regular but interrupted.** The R-R intervals are all 28 to 29 blocks except for the long pause that interrupts this otherwise regular rhythm.
5. **Regular but interrupted.** Again, the R-R intervals are regular before and after the premature beat (and the expected short pause after it).

Calculating Heart Rate Practice

1. This is a regular rhythm, so choose any two consecutive QRS complexes and calculate the heart rate there. There are 15 little blocks between QRSs. Divide 1,500 by 15 for the little block method. The heart rate is **100.**
2. Another regular rhythm. The heart rate is **75.**
3. This is a regular rhythm interrupted by a premature beat. We therefore ignore the premature beat for the purposes of heart rate calculation. The heart rate is **107,** as there are 14 little blocks between QRS complexes.

4. Although at first glance this rhythm appears regular, closer examination reveals that the R-R intervals vary from 9 1/2 to 12 1/2 little blocks apart. Since it is an irregular rhythm, we need the heart rate range along with the mean rate. The range is **about 120 to 155, with a mean rate of 140.**

5. This is a regular rhythm interrupted by a pause, so we calculate the range and the mean rate. There are 35 little blocks during the pause, and 20 little blocks between the regular QRS complexes. The heart rate range is therefore **43 to 75, with a mean rate of 70.**

6. This is an irregular rhythm. The **mean heart rate is 80 and the range is 56 to 107.** The first two QRS complexes are the farthest apart on the strip and thus represent the slowest heart rate (56). The 6th and 7th QRS complexes are the closest together and represent the fastest heart rate on the strip (107).

7. Here the rhythm is regular. Heart rate is **50.**

8. The QRS complexes are *huge* on this strip, but the rhythm is regular. Heart rate is **75.**

9. The rhythm is irregular. Heart rate **range is 52 to 81, with a mean rate of 70.**

10. The rhythm is regular. Heart rate is **130.**

Practice Quiz

1. The three methods for calculating heart rate are the **6-second strip method,** the **little block method,** and the **memory method.**

2. The least accurate method of calculating heart rate is the **6-second strip method.**

3. When using the little block method, count the number of little blocks between QRS complexes and divide into **1,500.**

4. The memory method is **300–150–100–75–60–50–43–37–33–30.**

5. With regular rhythms interrupted by premature beats, the heart rate is calculated by **ignoring the premature beat and calculating the heart rate on an uninterrupted portion of the strip.**

6. The three types of regularity are **regular, regular but interrupted,** and **irregular.**

7. A rhythm with R-R intervals that vary throughout the strip is an **irregular** rhythm.

8. A rhythm that is regular except for premature beats or pauses is a **regular but interrupted** rhythm.

9. A rhythm in which the R-R intervals vary by only one or two little blocks is a **regular** rhythm.

10. R-R interval is defined as **the distance between two consecutive QRS complexes.**

Critical Thinking Exercises

1. A rhythm whose R-R intervals are 23, 24, 23, 23, 12, 24, 23, 24, 23, 23 would be considered **regular but interrupted (by a premature beat). The heart rate would be 65 (1500 divided by 23).** On a rhythm that's regular but interrupted by a premature beat, ignore the premature beat (the R-R interval of 12) and the short pause that normally follows it (R-R of 24) and just find an uninterrupted part of the strip. Most R-R intervals are 23, so calculate the heart rate based on this.

2. A rhythm with R-R intervals of 12, 17, 22, 45, 10, and 18 would be considered **irregular. Heart rate would be mean rate of 70 and a range of 33 to 150.** How did we come up with the mean rate? To get the first R-R of 12 requires two QRS complexes. Then each R-R is one more QRS for a total of 7 on the strip. So the mean rate is 70. Then for the heart rate range, find the two QRS complexes the farthest apart (R-R of 45) and the two closest together (R-R of 10) and divide each set into 1500. Slowest heart rate is 33; fastest is 150.

3. A rhythm with R-R intervals of 22, 23, 22, 22, 23, 22, 22, 22 would be considered **regular. Heart rate is 68 (R-R of 22 divided into 1500).**

CHAPTER SIX
Practice Quiz

1. A heart rate that is greater than 100 is said to be a **tachycardia.**

2. A heart rate less than 60 is a **bradycardia.**

3. **Is.** A sudden drop in heart rate from a tachycardia of 125 to a normal heart rate of 65 is indeed cause for concern, as it may cause the cardiac output (the amount of blood pumped out by the heart each minute) to drop. This could cause the patient to have symptoms such as low blood pressure, dizziness, cold clammy skin, or other problems.

4. Arrhythmia means **abnormal heart rhythm.**

5. The five steps to rhythm interpretation are
   - Evaluate the QRS complexes.
   - Assess rhythm regularity.
   - Calculate the heart rate.
   - Assess P waves.
   - Assess PR interval and QRS intervals.

CHAPTER SEVEN
Sinus Rhythms Practice Strips

Note: For the intervals, it is acceptable if your answer is within 0.02 secs of displayed answer.

1. **QRS complexes:** present, all shaped the same. **Regularity:** regular. **Heart rate:** 56. **P waves:** upright, matching, one per QRS; P-P interval regular. **PR:** 0.18. **QRS:** 0.12 (wider than normal). **Interpretation:** sinus bradycardia with wide QRS.

2. **QRS complexes:** present, all shaped the same. **Regularity:** regular. **Heart rate:** 125. **P waves:** upright, matching, one per QRS; P-P interval regular. **PR:** 0.14. **QRS:** 0.08. **Interpretation:** sinus tachycardia.

3. **QRS complexes:** present, all shaped the same. **Regularity:** regular. **Heart rate:** 115. **P waves:** upright, matching, one per QRS; P-P interval regular. **PR:** 0.12. **QRS:** 0.10. **Interpretation:** sinus tachycardia.

4. **QRS complexes:** present, all shaped the same. **Regularity:** regular. **Heart rate:** 45. **P waves:** upright, matching, one per QRS; P-P interval regular. **PR:** 0.16. **QRS:** 0.14 (wider than normal). **Interpretation:** sinus bradycardia.

5. **QRS complexes:** present, all shaped the same. **Regularity:** regular but interrupted (by a pause). **Heart rate:** 21 to 54, with a mean rate of 40. **P waves:** upright, matching, one per QRS; P-P interval irregular due to the pause. **PR:** 0.18. **QRS:** 0.10. **Interpretation:** sinus bradycardia with a 3.08-second sinus arrest.

6. **QRS complexes:** present, all shaped the same. **Regularity:** regular (R-R intervals vary by only two small blocks). **Heart rate:** about 68. **P waves:** upright, matching, one per QRS; P-P interval regular. **PR:** 0.16. **QRS:** 0.08. **Interpretation:** sinus rhythm.

7. **QRS complexes:** present, all shaped the same. **Regularity:** regular. **Heart rate:** about 130. **P waves:** upright and matching, one per QRS. The heart rate is so fast that the T waves and P waves merge together. Do you see the notch at the top of the T wave? That's the P wave popping out. P-P interval regular. **PR:** cannot measure. **QRS:** 0.08. **Interpretation:** sinus tachycardia.

8. **QRS complexes:** present, all shaped the same. **Regularity:** regular. **Heart rate:** 88. **P waves:** biphasic (counts as upright), matching, one per QRS; P-P interval regular. **PR:** 0.12. **QRS:** 0.10. **Interpretation:** sinus rhythm.

9. **QRS complexes:** present, all shaped the same. **Regularity:** irregular; the R-R intervals vary from 25 to 29 small blocks. **Heart rate:** 52 to 60, with a mean rate of 60. **P waves:** upright, matching, one per QRS; P-P interval irregular. **PR:** 0.16. **QRS:** 0.06. **Interpretation:** sinus arrhythmia.

10. **QRS complexes:** present, all shaped the same. **Regularity:** regular. **Heart rate:** about 47. **P waves:** upright, matching, one preceding each QRS; P-P interval regular. **PR:** 0.16. **QRS:** 0.08. **Interpretation:** sinus bradycardia.

11. **QRS complexes:** present, all shaped the same within each lead. **Regularity:** regular. **Heart rate:** 75. **P waves:** upright in Lead I and inverted in V_1 (you'll recall this is OK for this lead), matching, one per QRS; P-P interval regular. **PR:** 0.10 (unusually short). **QRS:** 0.10. **Interpretation:** sinus rhythm.

12. **QRS complexes:** present, all shaped the same within each lead. **Regularity:** irregular. **Heart rate:** 43 to 63, with a mean rate of 60. **P waves:** upright and matching, one per QRS. P-P interval irregular. **PR:** 0.16. **QRS:** 0.12. **Interpretation:** sinus arrhythmia.

13. **QRS complexes:** present, all shaped the same within each lead. **Regularity:** regular. **Heart rate:** 83. **P waves:** upright, matching, one per QRS; P-P interval regular. **PR:** 0.14. **QRS:** 0.14. **Interpretation:** sinus rhythm.

14. **QRS complexes:** present, all shaped the same within each lead. **Regularity:** regular. **Heart rate:** 71. **P waves:** upright, matching, one per QRS; P-P interval regular. **PR:** 0.16. **QRS:** 0.76. **Interpretation:** sinus rhythm.

15. **QRS complexes:** present, all shaped the same within each lead. **Regularity:** regular. **Heart rate:** 125. **P waves:** upright, matching, one preceding each QRS; P-P interval regular. **PR:** 0.12. **QRS:** 0.08. **Interpretation:** sinus tachycardia.

16. **QRS complexes:** present, all shaped the same within each lead. **Regularity:** regular. **Heart rate:** 136. **P waves:** upright, matching, one per QRS; P-P interval regular. **PR:** 0.12. **QRS:** 0.08. **Interpretation:** sinus tachycardia.

17. **QRS complexes:** present, all shaped the same within each lead. **Regularity:** regular. **Heart rate:** 42. **P waves:** upright and matching, one per QRS; P-P interval regular. **PR:** 0.16. **QRS:** 0.08. **Interpretation:** sinus bradycardia. Thank goodness this is a double-lead strip because if we had only the top strip, we'd be hard pressed to interpret it.

18. **QRS complexes:** present, all shaped the same within each lead. **Regularity:** regular. **Heart rate:** 79. **P waves:** upright, matching, one per QRS; P-P interval regular. **PR:** 0.20. **QRS:** 0.10. **Interpretation:** sinus rhythm.

19. **QRS complexes:** present, all shaped the same within each lead. **Regularity:** regular. **Heart

rate: 115. **P waves:** upright, matching, one per QRS; P-P interval regular. **PR:** 0.14. **QRS:** 0.06. **Interpretation:** sinus tachycardia.

20. **QRS complexes:** present, all shaped the same within each lead. **Regularity:** regular. **Heart rate:** 115. **P waves:** upright and matching, one per QRS; P-P interval regular. **PR:** 0.16. **QRS:** 0.12. **Interpretation:** sinus tachycardia.

21. **QRS complexes:** present, all shaped the same within each lead. **Regularity:** irregular. **Heart rate:** 48 to 71, mean rate 60. **P waves:** upright and matching, one per QRS; P-P interval irregular. **PR:** 0.16–0.18. **QRS:** 0.06. **Interpretation:** sinus arrhythmia.

22. **QRS complexes:** present, all shaped the same within each lead. **Regularity:** regular. **Heart rate:** 54. **P waves:** upright and matching, one per QRS; P-P interval regular. **PR:** 0.12. **QRS:** 0.12. **Interpretation:** sinus bradycardia.

23. **QRS complexes:** present, all shaped the same within each lead. **Regularity:** regular. **Heart rate:** 137. **P waves:** upright, matching, one per QRS; P-P regular. **PR:** 0.12. **QRS:** 0.06. **Interpretation:** sinus tachycardia.

24. **QRS complexes:** present, uniform shape within each lead. **Regularity:** regular. **Heart rate:** 88. **P waves:** matching, upright, matching, one per QRS; P-P regular. **PR:** 0.16. **QRS:** 0.08. **Interpretation:** sinus rhythm.

25. **QRS complexes:** present, uniform shape within each lead. **Regularity:** regular. **Heart rate:** 60. **P waves:** matching, upright, matching, one per QRS; P-P regular. **PR:** 0.18. **QRS:** 0.08. **Interpretation:** sinus rhythm.

Practice Quiz

1. **False.** Most rhythms from the sinus node are regular rhythms.
2. The only difference in interpretation between sinus rhythm, sinus bradycardia, and sinus tachycardia is the **heart rate.**
3. Sinus arrhythmia is typically caused by the **breathing pattern.**
4. A sinus exit block differs from a sinus arrest in that **in a sinus exit block, the pause is a multiple of the previous R-R intervals. In sinus arrest, the pause is *not* a multiple.**
5. **False.** Atropine is inappropriate for sinus tachycardia, as it would speed up the already fast heart rate even more.
6. An individual with a fever of 103°F would be expected to be in **sinus tachycardia.**

7. A regular rhythm from the sinus node with heart rate of 155 is called **sinus tachycardia.**
8. **True.** That is the most basic criterion for sinus rhythms.
9. **Atropine causes the heart rate to increase.**
10. **False.** Atropine is indicated for sinus bradycardia with symptoms. Remember, athletes very often have sinus bradycardia and tolerate it well.

Critical Thinking Exercises

1. The rhythm is **sinus rhythm.** Note the matching upright P waves and the heart rate between 60 and 100.
2. The rhythm is **sinus tachycardia,** rate 115.
3. The change in heart rate is most likely caused by **Mr. Cavernum's increasing temperature.** Recall that the heart rate speeds up about 10 beats per minute for every one degree increase in temp. Since his temp has climbed just over two degrees, his heart rate has increased by about 20 beats per minute.
4. **Acetaminophen** is the medication Mr. Cavernum needs. It will lower his body temperature and that will decrease his heart rate. Atropine is indicated for bradycardias, not tachycardias. Beta-blockers would indeed lower the heart rate, but since it is likely the heart rate is related to the fever, acetaminophen or ibuprofen is the best choice.
5. The rhythm is **sinus arrhythmia.** Note the irregularity. The first two QRS complexes are 37 little blocks apart. The last two are 41 blocks apart—enough to say this rhythm is irregular and is therefore sinus arrhythmia.
6. As long as Mr. Cavernum is tolerating the rhythm without ill effects, **he requires no emergency treatment.** If he did show signs of decreased cardiac output, however, he'd probably need atropine to speed up his heart rate. Although his heart rate is slow (between 37 and 40), it is not necessarily in need of treatment.
7. **Past history of sleep apnea** is a possible cause of sinus arrhythmia.

CHAPTER EIGHT
Atrial Rhythms Practice Strips

Note: For the intervals, it is acceptable if your answer is within 0.02 secs of displayed answer.

1. **QRS complexes:** present, all shaped the same. **Regularity:** regular. **Heart rate:** 150. **P waves:** none visible. **PR:** not applicable. **QRS:** 0.08. **Interpretation:** SVT.

2. **QRS complexes:** present, all shaped the same. **Regularity:** regular but interrupted (by a premature beat). Remember it's normal to have a short pause after a premature beat. **Heart rate:** 56. **P waves:** upright and matching, except for the fourth P wave, which is premature and shaped differently. (There is a tiny notch on the downstroke of the premature P wave.) P-P interval is irregular because of the premature beat. **PR:** 0.12. **QRS:** 0.08. **Interpretation:** sinus bradycardia with a PAC.

3. **QRS complexes:** present, all shaped the same. **Regularity:** regular. **Heart rate:** atrial rate 375; ventricular rate 79. **P waves:** none present; flutter waves present instead. **PR:** not applicable. **QRS:** 0.10. **Interpretation:** atrial flutter with 5:1 and 6:1 conduction.

4. **QRS complexes:** present, all shaped the same. **Regularity:** irregular. **Heart rate:** 88 to 137, with a mean rate of 110. **P waves:** none present; wavy baseline present instead. **PR:** not applicable. **QRS:** 0.08. **Interpretation:** atrial fibrillation.

5. **QRS complexes:** present, all shaped the same. **Regularity:** regular but interrupted (by a pause). **Heart rate:** atrial rate 300; ventricular rate 98 to 158, with a mean rate of 150. **P waves:** none present; flutter waves present instead. **PR:** not applicable. **QRS:** 0.08. **Interpretation:** atrial flutter with 2:1 and 4:1 conduction.

6. **QRS complexes:** present, all shaped the same. **Regularity:** irregular. **Heart rate:** 100 to 125, with a mean rate of 110. **P waves:** at least three different shapes; P-P interval irregular. **PR:** varies. **QRS:** 0.08. **Interpretation:** multifocal atrial tachycardia.

7. **QRS complexes:** present, all shaped the same. **Regularity:** regular but interrupted (by a pause). **Heart rate:** 43 to 83. **P waves:** upright and matching, one before each beat. See the T wave of the last beat before the pause? It's a bit taller than the other Ts. There is a P hiding inside it, distorting its normal shape. That P in the T is premature, so that makes it a PAC. **PR:** 0.16. **QRS:** 0.10. **Interpretation:** sinus rhythm with a nonconducted PAC.

8. **QRS complexes:** present, all shaped the same. **Regularity:** irregular. **Heart rate:** 52 to 75, with a mean rate of 70. **P waves:** none present; wavy baseline present instead. **PR:** not applicable. **QRS:** 0.10. **Interpretation:** atrial fibrillation.

9. **QRS complexes:** present, all shaped the same. **Regularity:** regular but interrupted (by a premature beat). **Heart rate:** 100. **P waves:** upright, all matching except for the premature P wave preceding the sixth QRS complex. There is one P wave preceding each QRS complex; P-P interval irregular. **PR:** 0.16. **QRS:** 0.08. **Interpretation:** sinus rhythm with a PAC.

10. **QRS complexes:** present, all shaped the same. **Regularity:** regular. **Heart rate:** about 150. **P waves:** Is that a tall pointy P wave distorting the T waves? Maybe. But it's also a possibility that those are flutter waves between the QRS complexes. We just can't be sure. **PR:** not applicable. **QRS:** 0.08. **Interpretation:** SVT.

11. **QRS complexes:** present, all shaped the same. **Regularity:** irregular. **Heart rate:** 22 to 75, mean rate 40. **P waves:** none noted; wavy baseline present instead. **PR:** not applicable. **QRS:** 0.08. **Interpretation:** atrial fibrillation.

12. **QRS complexes:** present, all shaped the same. **Regularity:** regular. **Heart rate:** 187. **P waves:** not seen. The wave between the QRS complexes may just be a T wave without a P wave. **PR:** not applicable. **QRS:** 0.06. **Interpretation:** SVT.

13. **QRS complexes:** present, all shaped the same. **Regularity:** regular but interrupted (by a premature beat). **Heart rate:** 75. **P waves:** biphasic, all matching except for the premature P wave preceding the fifth QRS. There is one P wave preceding each QRS; P-P interval irregular. **PR:** 0.14. **QRS:** 0.08. **Interpretation:** sinus rhythm with a PAC.

14. **QRS complexes:** present, all shaped the same. **Regularity:** irregular. **Heart rate:** 16 to 44, mean rate 30. **P waves:** none noted; wavy baseline present instead. **PR:** not applicable. **QRS:** 0.08. **Interpretation:** atrial fibrillation.

15. **QRS complexes:** present, all shaped the same. **Regularity:** regular. **Heart rate:** about 136. **P waves:** Is that a pointy P wave distorting the T waves in the top strip? Maybe—can't be sure. There are no hints of a P wave in the bottom strip. **PR:** not applicable. **QRS:** 0.10. **Interpretation:** SVT. This may indeed be a sinus tachycardia with the P wave hidden in the T wave of the preceding beat, but we can't be sure.

16. **QRS complexes:** present, all shaped the same. **Regularity:** regular. **Heart rate:** 150. **P waves:** No P waves—those are flutter waves between the QRS complexes. See the asterisks under the flutter waves toward the end of the strip on the bottom lead? **PR:** not applicable. **QRS:** 0.08. **Interpretation:** atrial flutter with 2:1 conduction. There are two flutter waves to each QRS.

17. **QRS complexes:** present, all shaped the same. **Regularity:** irregular. **Heart rate:** 136 to 231, mean rate 170. **P waves:** at least three different

shapes; P-P interval irregular. **PR:** varies. **QRS:** 0.06. **Interpretation:** multifocal atrial tachycardia.

18. **QRS complexes:** present, all shaped the same. **Regularity:** irregular. **Heart rate:** 88 to 150, mean rate 120. **P waves:** none noted; wavy baseline present instead. **PR:** not applicable. **QRS:** 0.08. **Interpretation:** atrial fibrillation.

19. **QRS complexes:** present, all shaped the same. **Regularity:** regular but interrupted by a pause. **Heart rate:** 26 to 65, mean rate 50. **P waves:** none seen. On the top strip is a very fine wavy baseline. The bottom strip has flutter waves. **PR:** not applicable. **QRS:** 0.08. **Interpretation:** This one is up for grabs. It could be either atrial fibrillation or atrial flutter (top strip looks like fib, bottom strip like flutter). It would help to have more leads to examine. Statistically, it's more likely that this is atrial flutter rather than fibrillation because atrial fib tends to be much more irregular. On this rhythm, the QRS complexes are regular except for the pause.

20. **QRS complexes:** present, all shaped the same. **Regularity:** regular but interrupted by premature beats. Remember that premature beats are followed by a short pause; that does not make the rhythm irregular. The fourth, seventh, and tenth beats are premature. **Heart rate:** 83. **P waves:** upright, matching except for the P waves on the premature beats; P-P interval irregular. **PR:** 0.14 on the sinus beats, 0.06 on the premature beats. **QRS:** 0.14. **Interpretation:** sinus rhythm with PACs.

21. **QRS complexes:** present, all shaped the same. **Regularity:** regular but interrupted by a pause. **Heart rate:** 50 to 75, mean rate 70. **P waves:** none; flutter waves present instead. **PR:** not applicable. **QRS:** 0.08. **Interpretation:** atrial flutter with 4:1 and 6:1 conduction.

22. **QRS complexes:** present, all shaped the same. **Regularity:** irregular. **Heart rate:** 40 to 115, mean rate 80. **P waves:** none; fibrillatory waves present instead. **PR:** not applicable. **QRS:** 0.08–0.10. **Interpretation:** atrial fibrillation.

23. **QRS complexes:** present, shape varies; some are smaller than others. **Regularity:** irregular. **Heart rate:** 167 to 250, mean rate 210. **P waves:** none; fibrillatory waves present instead. **PR:** not applicable. **QRS:** 0.14. **Interpretation:** atrial fibrillation.

24. **QRS complexes:** present, shape varies. **Regularity:** regular but interrupted by premature beats. **Heart rate:** 94. **P waves:** upright, shape varies. **PR:** 0.10–0.12. **QRS:** 0.12. **Interpretation:** sinus rhythm with two PACs. See the dots? Beneath them are PACs. Notice those beats pop in early and

their P wave is shaped differently from the sinus beats that surround them. The QRS shapes vary a bit also—not sure of the significance there.

25. **QRS complexes:** present, all shaped the same. **Regularity:** irregular. **Heart rate:** 45 to 94, mean rate 70. **P waves:** none; fibrillatory waves present instead. **PR:** not applicable. **QRS:** 0.10–0.12. **Interpretation:** atrial fibrillation with a wide QRS. Note the bottom half of the strip is not a rhythm—it's a printout of the patient's oxygen saturation wave as read through a sensor on the finger. So ignore this part of the strip when analyzing the rhythm.

Practice Quiz

1. The complication of atrial fibrillation that can be prevented by the use of anticoagulants is **blood clots.**
2. The rhythm that is the same as wandering atrial pacemaker except for the heart rate is **multifocal atrial tachycardia.**
3. The rhythm that produces V-shaped waves between QRS complexes is **atrial flutter.**
4. Atrial rhythms take **the normal conduction pathway to the ventricles after depolarizing the atria.**
5. All rhythms that originate in a pacemaker other than the sinus node are called **ectopic rhythms.**
6. Treatment for atrial fibrillation is dependent **on its duration—specifically whether or not the atrial fibrillation has lasted longer than 48 hours.**
7. **False.** Some PACs are nonconducted.
8. The classic cause of multifocal atrial tachycardia is **chronic lung disease.**
9. The test than can determine the presence of atrial blood clots in an emergency is **transesophageal echocardiogram.**
10. If the rhythm is regular, heart rate is 130 or greater, and P waves cannot be identified, the rhythm is called **SVT.**

Critical Thinking Exercises

1. The rhythm is **atrial fibrillation.** Heart rate varies from a **low of 71 to a high of 166. Mean rate is 110.** Note the rhythm is very irregular with a wavy baseline and no P waves between QRS complexes.
2. Mr. Baldo is relatively asymptomatic, with stable vital signs. He does feel intermittent palpitations but this is not unusual. **This is NOT an emergency.**
3. **Coumadin** (or **Heparin**), an anticoagulant, is not needed in this situation, since the duration of atrial fibrillation is less than 48 hours.

4. Appropriate treatment could include **beta-blockers, calcium channel blockers, amiodarone,** or **digitalis. Electrical cardioversion** could also be performed, but this is usually reserved for emergencies or for patients in whom medications have not been successful.

5. This rhythm strip catches Mr. Baldo converting from **atrial fibrillation to sinus rhythm.**

6. The rhythm on discharge is **sinus rhythm.**

CHAPTER NINE
Junctional Rhythms Practice Strips

Note: For the intervals, it is acceptable if your answer is within 0.02 secs of displayed answer.

1. **QRS complexes:** present, all shaped the same. **Regularity:** regular. **Heart rate:** 94. **P waves:** none visible. **PR:** not applicable. **QRS:** 0.08. **Interpretation:** accelerated junctional rhythm.

2. **QRS complexes:** present, all shaped the same. **Regularity:** regular but interrupted. **Heart rate:** 100. **P waves:** matching and upright on all except the sixth beat. That beat has no visible P wave at all. P-P interval is regular except for that sixth beat, which is premature. **PR:** 0.14. **QRS:** 0.08. **Interpretation:** sinus rhythm with a PJC.

3. **QRS complexes:** present, all shaped the same. **Regularity:** regular. **Heart rate:** 48. **P waves:** none visible. **PR:** not applicable. **QRS:** 0.08. **Interpretation:** junctional rhythm.

4. **QRS complexes:** present, all shaped the same. **Regularity:** regular but interrupted. **Heart rate:** 47. **P waves:** matching upright Ps present except on the third beat, which has an inverted P wave preceding the QRS. **PR:** 0.16 on the beats with upright Ps; 0.06 on the third beat. **QRS:** 0.08. **Interpretation:** sinus bradycardia with a PJC. Remember it is normal for the R-R cycle immediately following a premature beat to be a little longer than usual. Consider this when determining the regularity.

5. **QRS complexes:** present, all shaped the same. **Regularity:** regular. **Heart rate:** 28. **P waves:** inverted following the QRS complexes. **PR:** not applicable. **QRS:** 0.08. **Interpretation:** junctional bradycardia.

6. **QRS complexes:** present, all shaped the same. **Regularity:** regular. **Heart rate:** 75. **P waves:** none visible. **PR:** not applicable. **QRS:** 0.08. **Interpretation:** accelerated junctional rhythm.

7. **QRS complexes:** present, all shaped the same. **Regularity:** regular. **Heart rate:** 72. **P waves:** none visible. **PR:** not applicable. **QRS:** 0.10. **Interpretation:** accelerated junctional rhythm.

8. **QRS complexes:** present, all shaped the same. **Regularity:** regular. **Heart rate:** 38. **P waves:** none visible. **PR:** not applicable. **QRS:** 0.10. **Interpretation:** junctional bradycardia.

9. **QRS complexes:** present, all shaped the same. **Regularity:** regular. **Heart rate:** 100. **P waves:** inverted preceding each QRS. **PR:** 0.10–0.12. **QRS:** 0.08. **Interpretation:** accelerated junctional rhythm.

10. **QRS complexes:** present, all shaped the same. **Regularity:** regular. **Heart rate:** 150. **P waves:** none visible. **PR:** not applicable. **QRS:** 0.08. **Interpretation:** SVT. Although this could indeed be a junctional tachycardia, it is best to call it SVT since P waves cannot be seen. Had there been an inverted P wave present, we'd have known for sure the rhythm was junctional in origin. Without those P waves, we can't be sure the rhythm is junctional. It could be atrial or even sinus in origin (with the P waves hidden inside the T waves).

11. **QRS complexes:** present, all shaped the same. **Regularity:** regular. **Heart rate:** 60. **P waves:** none visible. **PR:** not applicable. **QRS:** 0.080. **Interpretation:** junctional rhythm.

12. **QRS complexes:** present, all shaped the same. **Regularity:** regular. **Heart rate:** 26. **P waves:** none visible. **PR:** not applicable. **QRS:** 0.06–0.08. **Interpretation:** junctional bradycardia. This is an extremely slow junctional bradycardia. This patient is probably either in cardiac arrest or soon will be.

13. **QRS complexes:** present, all shaped the same. **Regularity:** regular. **Heart rate:** 115 to 125. **P waves:** none visible. **PR:** not applicable. **QRS:** 0.08. **Interpretation:** junctional tachycardia.

14. **QRS complexes:** present, all shaped the same. **Regularity:** regular but interrupted by a premature beat. The third beat is early. **Heart rate:** 48. **P waves:** upright and matching on all but the premature beat. That beat has no P wave. **PR:** 0.16. **QRS:** 0.10. **Interpretation:** sinus bradycardia with one PJC.

15. **QRS complexes:** present, all shaped the same. **Regularity:** regular. **Heart rate:** 88. **P waves:** none visible. **PR:** not applicable. **QRS:** 0.08. **Interpretation:** accelerated junctional rhythm.

Practice Quiz

1. The three possible locations for the P waves in junctional rhythms are **before the QRS complex, after the QRS complex,** and **hidden inside the QRS complex.**

2. The P wave is inverted in junctional rhythms because **the impulse travels in a backward direction to reach the atria.**

3. A junctional rhythm with a heart rate greater than 100 is **junctional tachycardia.**

4. **False.** PJCs do not imply that a lethal arrhythmia is imminent.

5. A junctional rhythm with a heart rate less than 40 is **junctional bradycardia.**

6. Treatment for junctional bradycardia could consist of the following: **atropine, epinephrine or dopamine infusion if the patient is symptomatic, oxygen, discontinuing or decreasing the dosage of any medications that could slow the heart rate down, and a pacemaker.**

7. PJCs cause the regularity to be **regular but interrupted.**

8. Junctional bradycardia is usually the result of **escape.**

9. Junctional tachycardia is best called SVT if the P waves are **hidden inside the QRS.**

10. Junctional tachycardia is the result of **usurpation.**

Critical Thinking Exercises

1. The medication used to speed up the heart rate is **atropine.** That's what Mrs. Dubos would have been given.

2. The rhythm is **junctional bradycardia with a heart rate of 37.**

3. **The ER nurse was incorrect** in her assertion that the rhythm was sinus bradycardia. Recall all rhythms from the sinus node have matching upright P waves. Since this rhythm has no P waves at all, it cannot be sinus. Additionally, the heart rate is slower than the ER nurse reported.

4. The treatment in the ER would have been **atropine** and/or a **pacemaker,** which would have been appropriate for any slow rhythm that produced symptoms. So even though the nurse identified the rhythm incorrectly, the treatment was still correct.

5. Mrs. Dubos **complained of chest pain and shortness of breath, both of which imply decreased cardiac output.** If the heart rate is too slow, the myocardium is deprived of oxygen and chest pain can result. Shortness of breath is a result of the slow heart rate's inability to transport adequate oxygen throughout the body. The low blood pressure, rapid respiratory rate, and the dazed and confused demeanor are also signs of decreased cardiac output.

CHAPTER TEN
Ventricular Rhythms Practice Strips

Note: For the intervals, it is acceptable if your answer is within 0.02 secs of displayed answer.

1. **QRS complexes:** present, both shaped the same—very wide and bizarre. **Regularity:** cannot tell as only two QRS complexes are shown. **Heart rate:** 14. **P waves:** not present. **PR:** not applicable. **QRS:** 0.38. **Interpretation:** agonal rhythm.

2. **QRS complexes:** present, varying in shapes and sizes. **Regularity:** irregular. **Heart rate:** 375 to 500. **P waves:** absent. **PR:** not applicable. **QRS:** varies—some QRS intervals are not measurable; others are 0.12. **Interpretation:** torsades de pointes.

3. **QRS complexes:** present, all but the third QRS shaped the same. The third QRS is wider. **Regularity:** regular but interrupted (by a premature beat). **Heart rate:** 115. **P waves:** matching and upright on all beats except the third, which has no P wave. **PR:** 0.12 on the sinus beats. **QRS:** 0.10 on the sinus beats; 0.16 on the premature beat. **Interpretation:** sinus tachycardia with one PVC.

4. **QRS complexes:** present, wide, all shaped the same; spike noted preceding each QRS complex. **Regularity:** regular. **Heart rate:** 40. **P waves:** none noted. **PR:** not applicable. **QRS:** 0.16. **Interpretation:** ventricular pacing.

5. **QRS complexes:** absent. **Regularity:** not applicable. **Heart rate:** zero. **P waves:** upright, matching, atrial rate 26. **PR:** not applicable. **QRS:** not applicable. **Interpretation:** P wave asystole.

6. **QRS complexes:** absent; wavy baseline present instead. **Regularity:** not applicable. **Heart rate:** not measurable. **P waves:** absent. **PR:** not applicable. **QRS:** not applicable. **Interpretation:** ventricular fibrillation.

7. **QRS complexes:** present, two different shapes—some narrow, others wide and bizarre. **Regularity:** regular but interrupted (by a run of premature beats). **Heart rate:** 107 while in the narrow-QRS rhythm; 187 when in the wide-QRS rhythm. **P waves:** upright and matching on the narrow beats; none noted on the wide beats. **PR:** 0.12 on the narrow beats; not applicable on the wide beats. **QRS:** 0.06 on the narrow beats; 0.12 on the wide beats. **Interpretation:** sinus tachycardia with an 11-beat run of ventricular tachycardia.

8. **QRS complexes:** present, all shaped the same—extremely wide and bizarre. **Regularity:** regular. **Heart rate:** 28. **P waves:** absent. **PR:** not applicable. **QRS:** 0.28. **Interpretation:** idioventricular rhythm.

9. **QRS complexes:** present, every third beat wider than the rest. **Regularity:** regular but interrupted (by premature beats). **Heart rate:** 94. **P waves:** matching and upright on all narrow beats. P waves are noted in the T waves of the wide beats. **PR:** 0.16. **QRS:** 0.06 on the narrow beats; 0.14 on the wide beats. **Interpretation:** sinus rhythm with PVCs in trigeminy.

10. **QRS complexes:** present, all shaped the same—wide QRS complexes. **Regularity:** irregular. **Heart rate:** 16 to 47, with a mean rate of 30. **P waves:** none noted. **PR:** not applicable. **QRS:** 0.28. **Interpretation:** agonal rhythm. Although in places this rate exceeds 20, the very irregular nature of it points to agonal rhythm rather than idioventricular rhythm.

11. **QRS complexes:** none seen—just a coarse zigzag baseline. **Regularity:** not applicable. **Heart rate:** not measurable. **P waves:** absent. **PR:** not applicable. **QRS:** not applicable. **Interpretation:** ventricular fibrillation. (But there could be an argument for torsades de pointes. The rhythm does appear to oscillate toward the middle. It would be helpful to have a longer strip for a better look at the rhythm.)

12. **QRS complexes:** present, all but two shaped the same. Two are wider than the others. **Regularity:** regular but interrupted by premature beats. **Heart rate:** 88. **P waves:** upright and matching on the narrow-QRS beats; no P wave preceding the wide-QRS beats. **PR:** 0.20. **QRS:** 0.06 on the narrow-QRS beats; 0.16 on the wide-QRS beats. **Interpretation:** sinus rhythm with two PVCs.

13. **QRS complexes:** present, all shaped the same—very wide with a preceding spike. **Regularity:** regular. **Heart rate:** 115. **P waves:** one present—noted on the downstroke of the second T wave on the strip. **PR:** not applicable. **QRS:** 0.16. **Interpretation:** ventricular pacing.

14. **QRS complexes:** present, all shaped the same—very wide and bizarre. **Regularity:** regular. **Heart rate:** 136. **P waves:** not present. **PR:** not applicable. **QRS:** 0.28. **Interpretation:** ventricular tachycardia. Note the unusually wide QRS complexes—this is often a sign that the patient's blood potassium level is extremely high, a condition seen most often in renal failure.

15. **QRS complexes:** only one present—very wide and bizarre. **Regularity:** not applicable as only one QRS complex is shown. **Heart rate:** zero after that one beat. **P waves:** not present. **PR:** not applicable. **QRS:** 0.20. **Interpretation:** agonal rhythm, then asystole.

16. **QRS complexes:** only one present. **Regularity:** not applicable as only one QRS complex is shown. **Heart rate:** zero after that one beat. **P waves:** upright, matching, one preceding the QRS complex and then continuing on; P-P interval irregular. **PR:** 0.24 on the one beat with a QRS. **QRS:** 0.08. **Interpretation:** one beat, then P wave asystole.

17. **QRS complexes:** present, all shaped the same—very wide and bizarre. **Regularity:** regular. **Heart rate:** 150. **P waves:** not present. **PR:** not applicable. **QRS:** 0.20. If you measured a bit wider than that, rest assured it is often difficult to measure QRS complexes when they merge into the T wave so well—hard to tell where the QRS ends and the T wave begins. **Interpretation:** ventricular tachycardia.

18. **QRS complexes:** present, all shaped the same—wide and preceded by a spike. **Regularity:** regular. **Heart rate:** 68. **P waves:** upright, matching; one preceding each QRS spike; P-P interval regular. **PR:** 0.20. **QRS:** 0.12. **Interpretation:** ventricular pacing.

19. **QRS complexes:** present, all but two shaped the same—two are wide and bizarre. **Regularity:** regular but interrupted by premature beats. **Heart rate:** 94. **P waves:** upright and matching preceding the narrow-QRS beats; none preceding the wide-QRS beats. **PR:** 0.16. **QRS:** 0.06 on the narrow beats; 0.12 on the wide beats. **Interpretation:** sinus rhythm with two PVCs.

20. **QRS complexes:** very wide and bizarre. **Regularity:** not applicable as only one QRS complex is shown. **Heart rate:** zero after that one beat. **P waves:** not present. **PR:** not applicable. **QRS:** 0.16. **Interpretation:** agonal rhythm.

21. **QRS complexes:** very wide and bizarre. **Regularity:** regular. **Heart rate:** 20. **P waves:** not present. **PR:** not applicable. **QRS:** 0.20. **Interpretation:** idioventricular rhythm.

22. **QRS complexes:** none present; baseline looks like static. **Regularity:** not applicable. **Heart rate:** not measureable. **P waves:** not present. **PR:** not applicable. **QRS:** not applicable. **Interpretation:** coarse ventricular fibrillation.

23. **QRS complexes:** present, uniform shape. **Regularity:** regular. **Heart rate:** 75. **P waves:** present; pacemaker spike preceding P waves. **PR:** 0.28 (called the *AV interval* here—measure from the pacer spike to the QRS). **QRS:** 0.08. **Interpretation:** atrial pacing.

24. **QRS complexes:** present—very wide and bizarre. **Regularity:** regular. **Heart rate:** 107. **P waves:** not

present. **PR:** not applicable. **QRS:** 0.20. **Interpretation:** ventricular tachycardia.

25. **QRS complexes:** present—very wide and bizarre, uniform shape. **Regularity:** regular. **Heart rate:** 88. **P waves:** not present. **PR:** not applicable. **QRS:** 0.16. **Interpretation:** accelerated idioventricular rhythm.

Practice Quiz

1. The three main causes of PVCs are **heart disease, hypokalemia,** and **hypoxia.**
2. The rhythm that has no QRS complexes, but instead has a wavy, static-looking baseline is **ventricular fibrillation.**
3. Appropriate treatment for PVCs interrupting a sinus bradycardia with a heart rate of 32 would be **atropine** or **epinephrine** to increase the heart rate. Do not give amiodarone or lidocaine!
4. *Torsades de pointes* is a French term meaning **twisting of the points.**
5. Asystole differs from P wave asystole in that **asystole is flat line** and **P wave asystole still has P waves.**
6. For a patient with a ventricular rhythm with a heart rate of 39 and no pulse, the treatment would be **CPR, epinephrine, atropine, and oxygen.**
7. **False.** Asystole is *not* treated with electric shock to the heart. Electric shock's goal is to recoordinate the heart's electrical activity. In asystole, there is no electrical activity to coordinate.
8. The treatment of choice for ventricular fibrillation is **defibrillation.**
9. **True.** Pacemakers can pace the atrium, the ventricle, or both.
10. **False.** Antiarrhythmics should *not* be used to treat agonal rhythm. Those medications would suppress the only pacemaker this person has left—the ventricle—and would likely be fatal. Try atropine or epinephrine instead to speed up the heart rate. A pacemaker is usually not indicated for agonal rhythm, since it is likely this is a terminal event, but it can be used at the physician's discretion.

Critical Thinking Exercises

1. The rhythm is **sinus rhythm with PVCs in trigeminy and quadrigeminy.**
2. **No, this rhythm does not require emergency treatment.** The patient is stable.
3. Three causes of PVCs **are hypoxia, hypokalemia,** and **MI.**
4. **This is ventricular fibrillation.**

5. **Yes, this is an emergency.** Patients in V-fib have no pulse and no breathing.
6. Mr. Winston needs immediate defibrillation. Medications such as amiodarone or lidocaine can also be given to make defibrillation more successful, but they will not convert this lethal rhythm back to normal on their own. The treatment for V-fib is to defib!

CHAPTER ELEVEN
AV Blocks Practice Strips

Note: For the intervals, it is acceptable if your answer is within 0.02 secs of displayed answer.

1. **QRS complexes:** present, all shaped the same. **Regularity:** regular but interrupted (by a pause). **Heart rate:** 31 to 68, with a mean rate of 50. **P waves:** biphasic, matching; more than one per QRS at times; P-P interval is regular; atrial rate is 62. **PR:** varies. **QRS:** 0.08. **Interpretation:** Wenckebach. Look at the P directly preceding the second QRS complex. The PR interval there is 0.24. The PR preceding the last QRS on the strip is 0.28. The PR interval prolongs and there are blocked P waves. The rhythm starts out as 2:1 AV block and then becomes an obvious Wenckebach. The 2:1 AV block here is therefore also Wenckebach.
2. **QRS complexes:** present, all shaped the same. **Regularity:** regular. **Heart rate:** 88. **P waves:** upright, matching; one to each QRS complex; atrial rate is 88; P-P interval is regular. **PR:** 0.24. **QRS:** 0.10. **Interpretation:** sinus rhythm with first-degree AV block.
3. **QRS complexes:** present, all shaped the same. **Regularity:** regular. **Heart rate:** 83. **P waves:** upright, matching; one to each QRS; P-P interval is regular; atrial rate is 83. **PR:** 0.24. **QRS:** 0.10. **Interpretation:** sinus rhythm with first-degree AV block.
4. **QRS complexes:** present, all shaped the same. **Regularity:** regular. **Heart rate:** 33. **P waves:** upright, matching; three to each QRS; P-P interval is regular; atrial rate is 100. **PR:** 0.16. **QRS:** 0.08. **Interpretation:** Mobitz II second-degree AV block. The block here is probably at the AV node, as evidenced by the narrow QRS. This is a kind of **high-grade AV block,** a block in which more than half the P waves are not conducted.
5. **QRS complexes:** present, all shaped the same. **Regularity:** regular. **Heart rate:** 30. **P waves:** upright, matching; more than one per QRS; P-P interval is regular; atrial rate is 75. **PR:** varies.

QRS: 0.08. **Interpretation:** third-degree AV block and a junctional escape rhythm. We know the junction is the pacemaker controlling the ventricles since the QRS interval is <0.12.

6. **QRS complexes:** present, all shaped the same. **Regularity:** regular. **Heart rate:** 37. **P waves:** upright, matching; two per QRS; P-P interval is regular; atrial rate is 75. **PR:** 0.36. **QRS:** 0.08. **Interpretation:** 2:1 AV block (probably Wenckebach, since the QRS is narrow and there is a prolonged PR interval).

7. **QRS complexes:** present, all shaped the same. **Regularity:** irregular. **Heart rate:** 37 to 68. **P waves:** upright, matching; one to each QRS except for the fifth QRS, which has two P waves preceding it; P-P interval is regular; atrial rate is 60. **PR:** varies—prolongs progressively. **QRS:** 0.08. **Interpretation:** Wenckebach.

8. **QRS complexes:** present, all the same shape. **Regularity:** irregular. **Heart rate:** 25 to 75, with a mean rate of 40. **P waves:** matching, upright; one for the first two QRS complexes, then three per QRS; P-P interval is regular; atrial rate is 75. **PR:** 0.16. **QRS:** 0.16. **Interpretation:** Mobitz II second-degree AV block.

9. **QRS complexes:** present, all shaped the same. **Regularity:** regular but interrupted (by a pause). **Heart rate:** 42 to 60, with a mean rate of 50. **P waves:** matching, upright; one preceding each QRS except the fourth QRS, which has two P waves preceding it (there's a P in the T wave of the third beat); P-P interval is *irregular;* atrial rate is 60 to 125. **PR:** 0.16. **QRS:** 0.10. **Interpretation:** sinus rhythm with a nonconducted PAC. Did you think this was an AV block? It's easy to mistake a nonconducted PAC for an AV block. How do you tell the difference? AV blocks have regular P-P intervals. Here the P-P is *not regular,* is it? One P is premature. That makes it a PAC. And since there's no QRS following it, that makes it a nonconducted PAC.

10. **QRS complexes:** present, all shaped the same. **Regularity:** regular but interrupted (by pauses). **Heart rate:** 42 to 68, with a mean rate of 50. **P waves:** upright, matching; more than one per QRS at times; P-P interval is regular; atrial rate is 75. **PR:** varies. **QRS:** 0.08. **Interpretation:** Wenckebach.

11. **QRS complexes:** present, all shaped the same within each lead. **Regularity:** regular but interrupted (by a pause). **Heart rate:** 48 to 79, with a mean rate of 70. **P waves:** upright, matching; more than one per QRS at times; P-P interval is regular; atrial rate is 88. **PR:** varies. **QRS:** 0.12. **Interpretation:** Wenckebach. Look at the P wave directly preceding the first QRS complex. The PR interval there is 0.22. The PR preceding the sixth QRS (the last QRS before the pause) is 0.32. The PR interval prolongs until a P wave is blocked. This is typical of Wenckebach.

12. **QRS complexes:** present, all shaped the same within each lead. **Regularity:** regular. **Heart rate:** 68. **P waves:** upright, matching; one per QRS; P-P interval is regular. **PR:** 0.24. **QRS:** 0.08. **Interpretation:** sinus rhythm with first-degree AV block.

13. **QRS complexes:** present, all shaped the same within each lead. **Regularity:** regular but interrupted (by a pause). **Heart rate:** 38 to 68, with a mean rate of 60. **P waves:** upright, matching; more than one per QRS at times; P-P interval is regular; atrial rate is 75. **PR:** varies. **QRS:** 0.08. **Interpretation:** Wenckebach. Look at the first PR interval on the strip—it's 0.24. The PR preceding the fourth QRS is 0.36. The PR interval prolongs and there is a blocked P wave—classic Wenckebach.

14. **QRS complexes:** present, all shaped the same within each lead. **Regularity:** regular. **Heart rate:** 38. **P waves:** upright in top strip, biphasic in bottom, matching; two P waves per QRS (except first QRS has only one because the start of the strip cut off the other P wave); P-P interval is regular; atrial rate is 79. **PR:** 0.28. **QRS:** 0.12. **Interpretation:** 2:1 AV block.

15. **QRS complexes:** present, all shaped the same within each lead. **Regularity:** irregular. **Heart rate:** 30 to 37, with a mean rate of 40. **P waves:** biphasic, matching; one per QRS; P-P interval is irregular. **PR:** 0.28. **QRS:** 0.13. **Interpretation:** sinus arrhythmia with first degree AV block.

16. **QRS complexes:** present, all shaped the same within each lead. **Regularity:** regular. **Heart rate:** 37. **P waves:** upright, matching; two per QRS; P-P interval is regular; atrial rate is 75. **PR:** varies. **QRS:** 0.09. **Interpretation:** third-degree AV block. This is not 2:1 AV block because the PR intervals are not constant here, as they should be for 2:1 AV block. Notice the first PR interval on the strip is 0.20 and the last one is 0.06, with the P wave "crawling up onto" the QRS complex.

17. **QRS complexes:** present, all shaped the same within each lead. **Regularity:** regular. **Heart rate:** 41. **P waves:** upright in top strip, biphasic in bottom; matching; more than one per QRS; P-P interval is regular; atrial rate is 79. **PR:** varies.

QRS: 0.08. **Interpretation:** third-degree AV block with junctional escape rhythm.

18. **QRS complexes:** present, all shaped the same within each lead. **Regularity:** regular but interrupted (by a pause). **Heart rate:** 37 to 75, with a mean rate of 60. **P waves:** upright, matching; more than one per QRS at times; P-P interval is regular; atrial rate is 75. **PR:** varies. **QRS:** 0.10. **Interpretation:** Wenckebach. Note the first PR interval on the strip is shorter than the second and third; then there is a blocked P wave. After the pause, the PR is short again, but lengthens by the next beat.

19. **QRS complexes:** present, all shaped the same within each lead. **Regularity:** regular but interrupted (by a premature beat). **Heart rate:** 81. **P waves:** upright, all but the fifth matching (the fifth is a premature P wave of a different shape); P-P interval is irregular. **PR:** 0.28. **QRS:** 0.08. **Interpretation:** sinus rhythm with a PAC (the fifth QRS is premature) and first-degree AV block.

20. **QRS complexes:** present, all shaped the same within each lead. **Regularity:** regular but interrupted (by a pause). **Heart rate:** 36 to 75, with a mean rate of 60. **P waves:** upright, matching; more than one per QRS at times; P-P interval is regular; atrial rate is 75. **PR:** varies. **QRS:** 0.10. **Interpretation:** Wenckebach. The PR intervals prolong until a P wave is blocked.

21. **QRS complexes:** present, all shaped the same within each lead. **Regularity:** regular. **Heart rate:** 42. **P waves:** upright, matching; two per QRS; P-P interval is regular; atrial rate is 83. **PR:** 0.24. **QRS:** 0.08. **Interpretation:** 2:1 AV block. Note there are two P waves to each QRS—right after the T wave and right before the QRS.

22. **QRS complexes:** present, all shaped the same within each lead. **Regularity:** regular. **Heart rate:** 60. **P waves:** upright, matching; one per QRS; P-P interval is regular; atrial rate is 60. **PR:** 0.32. **QRS:** 0.08–0.10. **Interpretation:** sinus rhythm with first-degree AV block.

23. **QRS complexes:** present, all shaped the same within each lead. **Regularity:** regular. **Heart rate:** 25. **P waves:** upright, matching; more than one per QRS; P-P interval is regular; atrial rate is 60. **PR:** varies. **QRS:** 0.16. **Interpretation:** third-degree AV block with a ventricular escape rhythm.

24. **QRS complexes:** present, all shaped the same within each lead. **Regularity:** regular. **Heart rate:** 68. **P waves:** upright, matching; one per QRS; P-P interval is regular; atrial rate is 68. **PR:** 0.26. **QRS:** 0.16. **Interpretation:** sinus rhythm with first-degree AV block.

25. **QRS complexes:** present, all shaped the same within each lead. **Regularity:** regular. **Heart rate:** 45. **P waves:** upright, matching; more than one per QRS; P-P interval is regular; atrial rate is about 68. **PR:** varies. **QRS:** 0.12. **Interpretation:** third-degree AV block. The QRS interval is right at 0.12 seconds, so it could be either a junctional or a ventricular escape pacemaker providing the QRS. With a heart rate of 45, it's probably the junction.

Practice Quiz

1. The two typical locations for the block in AV blocks are the **AV node** and the **bundle branches.**
2. **False.** First-degree AV block causes no symptoms and does not require pacemaker insertion.
3. Wenckebach is another name for **Mobitz I second-degree AV block.**
4. AV dissociation is a hallmark of **third-degree AV block.**
5. **False.** Atropine has no effect on blocks at the bundle branches.
6. The AV block that merely results in a prolonged PR interval is **first-degree AV block.**
7. Atropine's mode of action is **to speed up the sinus node's rate of firing and to accelerate conduction through the AV node.**
8. The most dangerous type of AV block is **third-degree AV block.**
9. The least dangerous type of AV block is **first-degree AV block.**
10. **False.** First-degree AV blocks do not require atropine or epinephrine.

Critical Thinking Exercises

1. The rhythm is **sinus rhythm with first-degree AV block** (PR interval 0.24), heart rate 68.
2. **No, this is not an emergency.** First-degree AV block does not cause symptoms, and the underlying rhythm is sinus, which is normal.
3. The rhythm has changed to **Wenckebach.**
4. Both **digoxin** and **beta-blockers** can cause decreased conduction through the AV node, resulting in AV blocks. Insulin is not a likely cause of this rhythm.
5. Treatment should include **withholding digoxin until her level returns to normal, teaching her not to take extra medication without approval from her physician, and perhaps giving atropine if her heart rate slows enough to cause her symptoms.** The "funny" spell in the physician's office could have reflected a slower heart rate,

which might have been missed by the time the second rhythm strip was obtained. Atropine should be close by in case Ms. Watson needs it.

CHAPTER TWELVE
Rhythm Practice Strips

Note: For the intervals, it is acceptable if your answer is within 0.02 secs of displayed answer.

1. **QRS complexes:** present, all shaped the same. **Regularity:** regular. **Heart rate:** 68. **P waves:** matching, upright; one preceding each QRS; P-P interval regular. **PR interval:** 0.42. **QRS interval:** 0.16. **Interpretation:** sinus rhythm with first-degree AV block and a wide QRS.

2. **QRS complexes:** present, all shaped the same. **Regularity:** regular. **Heart rate:** 37. **P waves:** none seen. **PR interval:** not applicable. **QRS interval:** 0.12. **Interpretation:** junctional brady-cardia with wide QRS.

3. **QRS complexes:** present, all shaped the same. **Regularity:** regular. **Heart rate:** 71. **P waves:** matching, upright; one preceding each QRS; P-P interval regular. **PR interval:** 0.24. **QRS interval:** 0.12. **Interpretation:** sinus rhythm with first-degree AV block and wide QRS.

4. **QRS complexes:** present, all shaped the same. **Regularity:** regular. **Heart rate:** 125. **P waves:** an occasional dissociated P can be seen. **PR interval:** cannot measure. **QRS interval:** 0.22. **Interpretation:** ventricular tachycardia.

5. **QRS complexes:** present, all shaped the same. **Regularity:** irregular. **Heart rate:** 65 to 94, with a mean rate of 80. **P waves:** none present; wavy, undulating baseline is present. **PR interval:** not applicable. **QRS interval:** 0.06. **Interpretation:** atrial fibrillation.

6. **QRS complexes:** Present, all shaped the same, low voltage. **Regularity:** regular. **Heart rate:** 125. **P waves:** matching, upright; one preceding each QRS, low voltage; P-P interval regular. **PR interval:** 0.16. **QRS interval:** 0.06. **Interpretation:** sinus tachycardia.

7. **QRS complexes:** present, all shaped the same. **Regularity:** regular. **Heart rate:** 32. **P waves:** upright, matching, some nonconducted; P-P interval regular; atrial rate 125. **PR interval:** varies. **QRS interval:** 0.13. **Interpretation:** third-degree AV block and a ventricular escape rhythm.

8. **QRS complexes:** present, all shaped the same. **Regularity:** regular. **Heart rate:** 150. **P waves:** none present; regular sawtooth-shaped waves between QRS complexes present instead, two to each QRS; atrial rate about 300. **PR interval:** not applicable. **QRS interval:** 0.06. **Interpretation:** atrial flutter with 2:1 conduction. Did you think it was something else? Look at the tail end of the QRS complex. See how it looks rounded at the bottom? That rounded part looks a lot like the other rounded wave that follows it, doesn't it? Those are both flutter waves. You'll notice these flutter waves march out—they're all the same distance from one another. Always be very suspicious when the heart rate is 150—it may be atrial flutter with 2:1 conduction.

9. **QRS complexes:** present, all shaped the same. **Regularity:** regular but interrupted (by two pauses). **Heart rate:** 44 to 75, with a mean rate of 60. **P waves:** upright; one preceding each QRS; shape varies slightly, but not enough to be significant. Don't get too hyper about the P wave shapes. Slight variability can be caused by fine baseline artifact. Different P wave shapes will be much more obvious. If you have to agonize over whether the P waves are shaped the same or are different, they're probably not different enough to be significant in terms of rhythm interpretation. **PR interval:** 0.20–0.22. **QRS interval:** 0.08. **Interpretation:** sinus rhythm with two sinus pauses. Why is this not a sinus arrhythmia? Sinus arrhythmia is cyclic, with slow periods, then faster periods. And it's irregular. Here the rhythm is regular, with an R-R interval of about 20 small blocks, except during the pauses. Sinus arrhythmia would be more irregular across the strip. Pay close attention to the regularity and it should lead the way.

10. **QRS complexes:** present, all shaped the same. They look different, you say? Hold on—the explanation is coming soon. **Regularity:** irregular. **Heart rate:** 100 to 150, with a mean rate of 120. **P waves:** upright and matching on the first four beats, then changes to flutter waves after that. **PR interval:** 0.16 on the first four beats, not applicable after that. **QRS interval:** 0.08. **Interpretation:** sinus tachycardia converting after four beats to atrial flutter with variable conduction. The QRS complexes in atrial flutter here are distorted by the flutter waves. That's why they look different.

11. **QRS complexes:** present, all shaped the same. **Regularity:** regular. **Heart rate:** 44. **P waves:** upright, matching, some nonconducted; P-P interval regular; atrial rate 150. **PR interval:** varies. **QRS interval:** 0.14. **Interpretation:** third-degree AV block and a ventricular escape rhythm.

12. **QRS complexes:** present, all shaped the same. **Regularity:** regular. **Heart rate:** 125.

P waves: upright, matching; one preceding each QRS; P-P interval regular. **PR interval:** 0.16. **QRS interval:** 0.06. **Interpretation:** sinus tachycardia.

13. **QRS complexes:** present, all but three shaped the same. Three beats are wide and bizarre in shape. **Regularity:** regular but interrupted (by premature beats). **Heart rate:** 125. **P waves:** upright and matching on the narrow beats, absent on the wide beats. **PR interval:** 0.12. **QRS interval:** 0.08 on the narrow beats, 0.16 on the wide beats. **Interpretation:** sinus tachycardia with unifocal PVCs in quadrigeminy (every fourth beat is a PVC).

14. **QRS complexes:** present, all shaped the same. **Regularity:** regular. **Heart rate:** 137. **P waves:** none seen. **PR interval:** not applicable. **QRS interval:** 0.10. **Interpretation:** SVT.

15. **QRS complex:** present, all shaped the same, very low voltage. **Regularity:** regular. **Heart rate:** about 135. **P waves:** not discernible. **PR interval:** cannot measure. **QRS interval:** 0.08. **Interpretation:** SVT.

16. **QRS complex:** present, all shaped the same. **Regularity:** irregular. **Heart rate:** 56 to 71, with a mean rate of 70. **P waves:** upright, matching; one preceding each QRS; P-P interval irregular. **PR interval:** 0.12. **QRS interval:** 0.10. **Interpretation:** sinus arrhythmia. Note the longest R-R interval is between the last two QRS complexes on the strip, ending with the barely there QRS at the very end. That R-R interval is 27 small blocks. The shortest R-R is between the third and fourth QRS complexes. That R-R is 21 small blocks. Since the rhythm is irregular, the longest R-R exceeds the shortest by four or more small blocks, and this is definitely sinus in origin; it's a sinus arrhythmia. If you thought there was a sinus pause here, remember that sinus pause usually interrupts an otherwise regular rhythm. This rhythm is irregular.

17. **QRS complexes:** present, all shaped the same. **Regularity:** slightly irregular. R-R intervals vary from 22 to 25 small blocks. **Heart rate:** 60 to 68, with a mean rate of 60. **P waves:** upright, matching; one preceding each QRS. **PR interval:** 0.12. **QRS interval:** 0.10. **Interpretation:** sinus rhythm versus sinus arrhythmia. This one is a bit odd. It's really not irregular enough to call it a sinus arrhythmia, since the longest R-R interval does not exceed the shortest by four or more small blocks. On the other hand, it's a bit irregular for the typical sinus rhythm. Since we're in a gray area here, it's OK to call it one versus the other. It would be nice to have a longer rhythm strip to evaluate. If, on the longer

strip, the rhythm is an obvious sinus rhythm or an obvious sinus arrhythmia, then this little stretch of the total rhythm is probably also that same rhythm.

18. **QRS complexes:** present, all shaped the same. **Regularity:** regular. **Heart rate:** 75. **P waves:** none seen. **PR interval:** not applicable. **QRS interval:** around 0.20 to 0.28. This is a guesstimate, since it's hard to tell where the QRS ends and the ST segment begins. **Interpretation:** accelerated idioventricular rhythm.

19. **QRS complexes:** present, all shaped the same. **Regularity:** regular. **Heart rate:** 167. **P waves:** occasionally seen hidden in the T waves. Note the T waves between the first and second and eleventh and twelfth QRS complexes. Those T waves reveal the hidden P waves. **PR interval:** cannot measure, as cannot see the beginning of the P wave. **QRS interval:** 0.08. **Interpretation:** atrial tachycardia or SVT. It's probably more correct to call it atrial tachycardia, because the P waves are evident in places, but it's acceptable to say SVT.

20. **QRS complexes:** present, all shaped the same. **Regularity:** regular but interrupted (by premature beats). Remember it's normal to have a short pause following each premature beat. That's why this is not an irregular rhythm. **Heart rate:** about 85. Where did that heart rate come from? The first two beats on the strip are sinus beats with a rate of 85. From then on, every other beat is a PAC, so the heart rate cannot be determined accurately there. **P waves:** upright, two different shapes; almost every other P wave is premature and of a different shape. **PR interval:** 0.12 on the sinus beats, 0.16 on the premature beats. **QRS interval:** 0.08. **Interpretation:** sinus rhythm with frequent PACs, most of it in bigeminy.

21. **QRS complexes:** none present; wavy, static-looking baseline present instead. **Regularity:** not applicable. **Heart rate:** cannot measure, has no QRS complexes. **P waves:** none. **PR interval:** not applicable. **QRS interval:** not applicable. **Interpretation:** ventricular fibrillation.

22. **QRS complexes:** present, two different shapes. Some QRS complexes are narrow; others are wide. **Regularity:** regular but interrupted (by premature beats). **Heart rate:** 94. **P waves:** upright and matching preceding the narrow QRS complexes and seen in the T wave following the premature beats. **PR interval:** 0.18 on the narrow beats; not calculated on the premature beats, as the P is retrograde. **QRS interval:** 0.08 on the narrow beats, 0.14 on the wide beats. **Interpretation:** sinus rhythm with unifocal PVCs in trigeminy.

23. **QRS complexes:** present, all shaped the same. **Regularity:** irregular. **Heart rate:** 48 to 81, with a mean rate of 60. **P waves:** upright, matching, some nonconducted; P-P interval regular. **PR interval:** varies. **QRS interval:** 0.11. **Interpretation:** Wenckebach. Note how the PR interval gradually prolongs, and then a beat is dropped.

24. **QRS complexes:** present, all shaped the same. **Regularity:** regular. **Heart rate:** 79. **P waves:** none present; regular sawtooth-shaped waves present instead. **PR interval:** not applicable. **QRS interval:** 0.08. **Interpretation:** atrial flutter with 4:1 conduction.

25. **QRS complexes:** present, all but one having the same shape. One is very wide compared to the others. **Regularity:** regular but interrupted (by a premature beat). **Heart rate:** 107. **P waves:** upright and matching on the narrow beats, absent on the wide beat. **PR interval:** 0.12–0.14. **QRS interval:** 0.08 on the narrow beats, 0.16 on the wide beat. **Interpretation:** sinus tachycardia with one PVC.

26. **QRS complexes:** none. **Regularity:** not applicable, as there are no QRS complexes. **Heart rate:** zero. **P waves:** none. **PR interval:** not applicable. **QRS interval:** not applicable. **Interpretation:** asystole.

27. **QRS complexes:** present, all shaped the same. **Regularity:** regular. **Heart rate:** 50. **P waves:** upright, matching; P-P interval regular; one P wave is hidden inside the last QRS; atrial rate 88. **PR interval:** varies. **QRS interval:** 0.14. **Interpretation:** third-degree AV block and a ventricular escape rhythm.

28. **QRS complexes:** present, all shaped the same. **Regularity:** regular. **Heart rate:** 79. **P waves:** matching, upright; one preceding each QRS; P-P interval regular. **PR interval:** 0.28. **QRS interval:** 0.08. **Interpretation:** sinus rhythm with first-degree AV block.

29. **QRS complexes:** present, all shaped the same. **Regularity:** regular. **Heart rate:** 68. **P waves:** none present; regular sawtooth-shaped waves present instead. **PR interval:** not applicable. **QRS interval:** about 0.10. The end of the QRS is distorted by a flutter wave, making the QRS look artificially wide. **Interpretation:** atrial flutter with 4:1 conduction. Two of the flutter waves are hidden inside the QRS and T waves. So how can we tell the flutter waves are even there if we can't see them? We can definitely see two obvious flutter waves between the QRS complexes. Since we know that flutter waves are regular, we simply note the distance between the two flutter waves

we see together, and then march out where the rest of them should be.

30. **QRS complexes:** present, most shaped the same. An occasional QRS is missing the notch on the downstroke. **Regularity:** regular. **Heart rate:** 187. **P waves:** an occasional dissociated P wave is seen. **PR interval:** not applicable. **QRS interval:** 0.14. **Interpretation:** ventricular tachycardia.

31. **QRS complexes:** present, all shaped the same. **Regularity:** irregular. **Heart rate:** 48 to 60, with a mean rate of 60. **P waves:** all upright, but there are at least three different shapes; P-P interval irregular. **PR interval:** 0.24–0.28. **QRS interval:** 0.10. **Interpretation:** wandering atrial pacemaker.

32. **QRS complexes:** present, all shaped the same. **Regularity:** regular but interrupted (by a prematurely arriving beat). **Heart rate:** 71. **P waves:** none present; regular sawtooth-shaped waves present instead. **PR interval:** not applicable. **QRS interval:** 0.10. **Interpretation:** atrial flutter with 2:1 and 4:1 conduction. The one episode of the 2:1 conduction is responsible for the interruption of this otherwise regular 4:1 conduction. This beat that comes in early because of the conduction ratio change is not per se a premature beat in the way that PVCs are, but nevertheless it does arrive earlier than expected, given the surrounding R-R intervals. For this reason the regularity is called *regular but interrupted* rather than irregular. All R-R intervals except this short one are about the same.

33. **QRS complexes:** present, all shaped the same. **Regularity:** regular but interrupted (by pauses). **Heart rate:** 62 to 107, with a mean rate of 90. **P waves:** upright, matching; some nonconducted, others hidden inside T waves; P-P interval regular; atrial rate about 115. **PR interval:** varies. **QRS interval:** 0.08. **Interpretation:** Wenckebach.

34. **QRS complexes:** present, all shaped the same. **Regularity:** regular but interrupted (by premature beats). **Heart rate:** 79. **P waves:** biphasic except for the two that are inside the T wave. There are two different shapes of P waves; P-P interval varies. **PR interval:** 0.18 on the normal beats, approximately 0.22 on the premature beats. **QRS interval:** 0.08. **Interpretation:** sinus rhythm with two PACs.

35. **QRS complexes:** present, all shaped the same, one shorter than the rest. **Regularity:** regular but interrupted (by a pause). **Heart rate:** 19 to 54, with a mean rate of 50. **P waves:** upright, matching; none present on the beat ending the pause; P-P interval irregular. **PR interval:** 0.16–0.18. **QRS interval:** 0.09. **Interpretation:** sinus bradycardia with a

3.28-second sinus arrest ending with a junctional escape beat. Whenever there is a pause, the length of it must be recorded. If there is a sinus arrest, the beat ending the pause may be an escape beat from a lower pacemaker. Whichever pacemaker takes over should also be recorded.

36. **QRS complexes:** present, all shaped the same. **Regularity:** regular; the R-R intervals vary only by two small blocks. **Heart rate:** about 50. **P waves:** upright and matching; one preceding each QRS; P-P interval regular. **PR interval:** 0.20. **QRS interval:** 0.08. **Interpretation:** sinus bradycardia. A PR interval of 0.20 is still normal. There's no first-degree AV block.

37. **QRS complexes:** present, all shaped the same. **Regularity:** regular. **Heart rate:** 61. **P waves:** inverted inside ST segment following the QRS complexes. **PR interval:** not applicable. **QRS interval:** 0.12. **Interpretation:** accelerated junctional rhythm with a wide QRS.

38. **QRS complexes:** present, all shaped the same. **Regularity:** regular. **Heart rate:** 88. **P waves:** upright and matching; one preceding each QRS; P-P interval regular. **PR interval:** 0.24. **QRS interval:** 0.10. **Interpretation:** sinus rhythm with first-degree AV block.

39. **QRS complexes:** present, all shaped the same. **Regularity:** regular. The R-R intervals vary by only two small blocks. **Heart rate:** about 36. **P waves:** upright and matching; one preceding each QRS; P-P interval regular. **PR interval:** 0.16. **QRS interval:** 0.12. **Interpretation:** sinus bradycardia with a wide QRS; there's a prominent U wave following the T waves.

40. **QRS complexes:** present, all shaped the same. **Regularity:** regular. **Heart rate:** 60. **P waves:** upright, notched, and matching; one preceding each QRS; P-P interval regular. **PR interval:** 0.16. **QRS interval:** 0.08. **Interpretation:** sinus rhythm.

41. **QRS complexes:** present, all shaped the same. **Regularity:** irregular. The R-R intervals vary from 11 to 15 small blocks. **Heart rate:** 100 to 137, with a mean rate of 120. **P waves:** none seen. **PR interval:** not applicable. **QRS interval:** 0.20. **Interpretation:** ventricular tachycardia. Remember V-tach is usually regular but can be irregular at times.

42. **QRS complexes:** present, all shaped the same. **Regularity:** irregular. **Heart rate:** 39 to 88, with a mean rate of 60. **P waves:** none present; wavy, undulating baseline present instead. **PR interval:** not applicable. **QRS interval:** 0.06. **Interpretation:** atrial fibrillation.

43. **QRS complexes:** present, all shaped the same. **Regularity:** regular. **Heart rate:** 115. **P waves:** upright and matching; one preceding each QRS; P-P interval regular. **PR interval:** 0.12. **QRS interval:** 0.10. **Interpretation:** sinus tachycardia.

44. **QRS complexes:** present, all shaped the same. **Regularity:** irregular. **Heart rate:** 83 to 167, with a mean rate of 140. **P waves:** none present; wavy, undulating baseline present instead. **PR interval:** not applicable. **QRS interval:** 0.04. **Interpretation:** atrial fibrillation.

45. **QRS complexes:** present, all shaped the same. **Regularity:** regular. **Heart rate:** about 52. **P waves:** upright, matching; one preceding each QRS. **PR interval:** 0.18. **QRS interval:** 0.13. **Interpretation:** sinus bradycardia with a wide QRS.

46. **QRS complexes:** present, all shaped the same. **Regularity:** regular. **Heart rate:** 28. **P waves:** upright, matching; some nonconducted; P-P interval regular; atrial rate 83. **PR interval:** 0.16. **QRS interval:** 0.06. **Interpretation:** Mobitz II second-degree AV block.

47. **QRS complexes:** present, all but one shaped the same. **Regularity:** regular. **Heart rate:** 26. **P waves:** matching, upright, some nonconducted; P-P interval regular; atrial rate 75. **PR interval:** varies. **QRS interval:** 0.04–0.08. **Interpretation:** third-degree AV block and a junctional escape rhythm. This heart rate is extremely slow for the junction. Remember, it normally escapes at a rate of 40 to 60. This patient not only has an AV block, but also a sick AV node in terms of its pacemaking ability. Also of concern is the ventricle as a pacemaker. It normally escapes at a rate of 20 to 40. Where is it? Why didn't it kick in as the pacemaker at a faster rate than we have here? This rhythm indicates a very sick heart.

48. **QRS complexes:** present, all shaped the same. **Regularity:** regular. The R-R intervals vary by only two small blocks. **Heart rate:** 88. **P waves:** biphasic, matching; one preceding each QRS; P-P interval regular. **PR interval:** 0.12. **QRS interval:** 0.10. **Interpretation:** sinus rhythm.

49. **QRS complexes:** present, all shaped the same, although one is shorter than the other. **Regularity:** cannot assess as only two QRS complexes are present (at least three QRS complexes are needed to determine regularity). **Heart rate:** about 11. **P waves:** none present; wavy, undulating baseline present instead. **PR interval:** not applicable. **QRS interval:** 0.12. **Interpretation:** atrial fibrillation with a wide QRS. This could

also be called atrial fib-flutter, as it does look quite fluttery in places. It is best not to call this an outright atrial flutter, though, as the waves dampen out in the middle of the strip, causing the waves to look different throughout the strip. This is a drastic representation of how slow the heart rate can go with atrial fibrillation. This is a 5.6-second pause, erroneously labeled on the strip as 5.52 seconds. This patient was lucky to be asleep and had no problems. A pause this long could easily have caused symptoms of decreased cardiac output.

50. **QRS complexes:** present, all shaped the same. **Regularity:** slightly irregular. The R-R intervals vary by three small blocks. **Heart rate:** 30 to 32. **P waves:** upright, three different shapes; one preceding each QRS; P-P interval slightly irregular. **PR interval:** 0.16–0.20. **QRS interval:** 0.10. **Interpretation:** wandering atrial pacemaker.

51. **QRS complexes:** present, all shaped the same. **Regularity:** regular. **Heart rate:** 94. **P waves:** matching, biphasic; two to each QRS; atrial rate 187. **PR interval:** 0.06. **QRS interval:** 0.08. **Interpretation:** atrial tachycardia with 2:1 block. One P wave is easy to see between the QRS complexes. The other is right *on* the QRS, distorting the shape of the QRS and the P a little. It wouldn't be correct to call this atrial flutter, since there is an obvious flat baseline between the P waves. You'll recall atrial flutter has no flat isoelectric line—flutter waves all zigzag one after the other.

52. **QRS complexes:** present, all shaped the same. **Regularity:** regular. **Heart rate:** 68. **P waves:** negative; one preceding each QRS; P-P interval regular. **PR interval:** 0.24. **QRS interval:** 0.20. **Interpretation:** sinus rhythm with first-degree AV block and a wide QRS. Although the lead is not recorded on this strip, it's probably V_1. Sinus rhythms can have a negative P wave in V_1 This is a very sick heart. The AV node is sick, as evidenced by the first-degree block, but also the bundle branches are sick, as evidenced by the width of the QRS complexes. Many cardiologists believe that to some extent a patient's ventricular function can be predicted by the QRS interval. This patient was predicted to have a low-functioning heart, and that was borne out by further studies.

53. **QRS complexes:** present, all shaped the same. **Regularity:** regular. **Heart rate:** about 103. **P waves:** upright, matching; one preceding each QRS. **PR interval:** 0.16. **QRS interval:** 0.08. **Interpretation:** sinus tachycardia.

54. **QRS complexes:** present, all shaped the same. **Regularity:** irregular. **Heart rate:** 29 to 83, with a mean rate of 50. **P waves:** none present; *very* low-voltage wavy, undulating baseline present instead. **PR interval:** not applicable. **QRS interval:** 0.08. **Interpretation:** atrial fibrillation. This is an example of what's sometimes called *straight-line* atrial fibrillation. There is barely a bobble of the baseline between QRS complexes. The most obvious feature that suggests atrial fibrillation is the irregularity of the rhythm. Then you notice the fine fibrillatory waves. This patient has probably been in atrial fibrillation for years.

55. **QRS complexes:** present, all shaped the same. **Regularity:** irregular. **Heart rate:** 37 to 52, with a mean rate of 30. The strip starts in the middle of a 2.6-second pause, though, so we know the heart rate actually gets much slower at times. **P waves:** none present. Regular sawtooth-shaped waves present instead. **PR interval:** not applicable. **QRS interval:** 0.08. **Interpretation:** atrial flutter with variable conduction.

56. **QRS complexes:** present, all shaped the same. **Regularity:** regular. **Heart rate:** 94. **P waves:** upright, matching; one preceding each QRS. **PR interval:** 0.16. **QRS interval:** 0.14. **Interpretation:** sinus rhythm with wide QRS.

57. **QRS complexes:** present, all shaped the same. **Regularity:** irregular. **Heart rate:** about 19 to 23, with a mean rate of 30. **P waves:** none present. **PR interval:** not applicable. **QRS interval:** 0.28. **Interpretation:** agonal rhythm. Although the heart rate is a little fast for agonal rhythm, it must be called this because it is so irregular. Idioventricular rhythm is usually more regular.

58. **QRS complexes:** present, all shaped the same. **Regularity:** regular. R-R intervals vary by only one small block. **Heart rate:** 60. **P waves:** upright, matching; one preceding each QRS; P-P interval regular. **PR interval:** 0.12. **QRS interval:** 0.10. **Interpretation:** sinus rhythm.

59. **QRS complexes:** none present; wavy, static-looking baseline present instead. **Regularity:** not applicable. **Heart rate:** cannot measure. **P waves:** none present. **PR interval:** not applicable. **QRS interval:** not applicable. **Interpretation:** ventricular fibrillation.

60. **QRS complexes:** present, all shaped the same. **Regularity:** irregular. The R-R intervals vary by four small blocks. **Heart rate:** about 37 to 40, with a mean rate of 40. **P waves:** upright, matching; one preceding each QRS; P-P interval slightly

irregular. **PR interval:** 0.13. **QRS interval:** 0.09. **Interpretation:** sinus arrhythmia.

61. **QRS complexes:** present, all but one having the same shape. One is much wider than the others. **Regularity:** regular but interrupted (by a premature beat). **Heart rate:** 115. **P waves:** upright, matching; one preceding all QRS complexes except the wide one. **PR interval:** 0.14. **QRS interval:** 0.06 on the narrow beats, 0.14 on the wide beat. **Interpretation:** sinus tachycardia with a PVC.

62. **QRS complexes:** none present. **Regularity:** cannot determine since there are no QRS complexes. **Heart rate:** zero. **P waves:** upright and matching; P-P interval irregular. **PR interval:** not applicable. **QRS interval:** not applicable. **Interpretation:** P wave asystole.

63. **QRS complexes:** present, all shaped the same. **Regularity:** regular. **Heart rate:** about 110. **P waves:** upright, matching; one preceding each QRS; P-P interval regular. **PR interval:** 0.16. **QRS interval:** 0.08. **Interpretation:** sinus tachycardia.

64. **QRS complexes:** present, all but one shaped the same. One is wider than the others. **Regularity:** regular but interrupted (by a premature beat). **Heart rate:** 62. **P waves:** upright, matching; one preceding all QRS complexes except the premature one. There is a P wave in the premature beat's ST segment. **PR interval:** 0.20. **QRS interval:** 0.10 on the narrow beats, 0.18 on the wide beat. **Interpretation:** sinus rhythm with a PVC.

65. **QRS complexes:** present, all shaped the same. **Regularity:** irregular. **Heart rate:** 68 to 125, with a mean rate of 100. **P waves:** upright, matching, some nonconducted; P-P interval regular; atrial rate 115. **PR interval:** varies. **QRS interval:** 0.10. **Interpretation:** Wenckebach.

66. **QRS complexes:** present, all shaped the same. **Regularity:** regular. **Heart rate:** 65. **P waves:** upright, matching; one preceding each QRS; P-P interval regular. **PR interval:** 0.22. **QRS interval:** 0.10. **Interpretation:** sinus rhythm with first-degree AV block.

67. **QRS complexes:** present, all shaped the same. **Regularity:** irregular. **Heart rate:** 62 to 137, with a mean rate of 110. **P waves:** none present; wavy, undulating baseline present instead. **PR interval:** not applicable. **QRS interval:** 0.08. **Interpretation:** atrial fib-flutter. Although this may indeed be a true atrial flutter, the flutter waves are not as obvious at the beginning of the strip as they are later on, so it's possible this may be a combination of fib and flutter.

68. **QRS complexes:** present, all shaped the same. **Regularity:** regular. **Heart rate:** 44. **P waves:** upright, matching, some nonconducted; P-P interval regular; atrial rate 137. **PR interval:** 0.28–0.40. **QRS interval:** 0.14. **Interpretation:** third-degree AV block and ventricular escape rhythm. There are three P waves to each QRS. If you counted only two, look again. Note the distance between two consecutive P waves. March out where the rest of them are. There's more here than first meets the eye. Always march out the P waves!

69. **QRS complexes:** present, all shaped the same. **Regularity:** regular. **Heart rate:** 71. **P waves:** upright, matching; one preceding each QRS; P-P interval regular. **PR interval:** 0.28. **QRS interval:** 0.10. **Interpretation:** sinus rhythm with first-degree AV block.

70. **QRS complexes:** present, all shaped the same. **Regularity:** irregular. **Heart rate:** 60 to 94, with a mean rate of 70. **P waves:** none present; wavy, undulating baseline present instead. **PR interval:** not applicable. **QRS interval:** 0.10. **Interpretation:** atrial fibrillation.

71. **QRS complexes:** present, all shaped the same. **Regularity:** regular. **Heart rate:** 56. **P waves:** upright, matching; one preceding each QRS; P-P interval regular. **PR interval:** 0.14. **QRS interval:** 0.10. **Interpretation:** sinus bradycardia.

72. **QRS complexes:** present, all shaped the same. **Regularity:** regular. **Heart rate:** 79. **P waves:** none present; regular, sawtooth-shaped waves present instead. Also note the pacemaker spike preceding each QRS. **PR interval:** not applicable. **QRS interval:** 0.12. **Interpretation:** ventricular pacing with underlying atrial flutter.

73. **QRS complexes:** present, all shaped the same. **Regularity:** regular. **Heart rate:** 94. **P waves:** upright, matching; one preceding each QRS; P-P interval regular. **PR interval:** 0.12. **QRS interval:** 0.08. **Interpretation:** sinus rhythm. Baseline sway artifact is present.

74. **QRS complexes:** present, all shaped the same. **Regularity:** irregular. **Heart rate:** 75 to 107, with a mean rate of 90. **P waves:** none present; regular saw-tooth-shaped waves present instead. **PR interval:** not applicable. **QRS interval:** 0.08. **Interpretation:** atrial flutter with variable conduction.

75. **QRS complexes:** present, all shaped the same. **Regularity:** irregular. **Heart rate:** 37 to 62, with a mean rate of 60. **P waves:** upright, matching; one preceding each QRS complex; P-P interval irregular. **PR interval:** 0.12. **QRS interval:** 0.10.

Interpretation: sinus arrhythmia. If you count out the R-R intervals, you'll note they grow steadily longer throughout the strip.

76. **QRS complexes:** present, all shaped the same. **Regularity:** regular. **Heart rate:** 79. **P waves:** upright, matching; one preceding each QRS complex; P-P interval regular. **PR interval:** 0.14. **QRS interval:** 0.08. **Interpretation:** sinus rhythm.

77. **QRS complexes:** present, all shaped the same. **Regularity:** regular. **Heart rate:** 27. **P waves:** none present. **PR interval:** not applicable. **QRS interval:** 0.08. **Interpretation:** junctional bradycardia.

78. **QRS complexes:** present, all shaped the same. **Regularity:** regular. **Heart rate:** 45. **P waves:** upright, matching; one preceding each QRS; P-P interval regular. **PR interval:** 0.20. **QRS interval:** 0.08. **Interpretation:** sinus bradycardia. Note also a prominent U wave.

79. **QRS complexes:** present, all shaped the same. **Regularity:** regular. **Heart rate:** 115. **P waves:** upright, matching; one preceding each QRS; P-P interval regular. **PR interval:** 0.12. **QRS interval:** 0.06. **Interpretation:** sinus tachycardia.

80. **QRS complexes:** present, all shaped the same. **Regularity:** regular. **Heart rate:** 107. **P waves:** biphasic, matching; one preceding each QRS; P-P interval regular. **PR interval:** 0.14. **QRS interval:** 0.10. **Interpretation:** sinus tachycardia.

81. **QRS complexes:** present, all shaped the same. **Regularity:** irregular. **Heart rate:** 137 to 167, with a mean rate of 150. **P waves:** none seen. **PR interval:** not applicable. **QRS interval:** 0.08. **Interpretation:** atrial fibrillation. If you thought it was ventricular tachycardia, look again. The QRS complexes are not wide enough to be ventricular. Since it's irregular, it can't be called SVT. Although there are no obvious fibrillatory waves, it's prudent to call this atrial fibrillation because of its irregularity and lack of P waves.

82. **QRS complexes:** present, all shaped the same. **Regularity:** regular. **Heart rate:** 60. **P waves:** upright, matching; one preceding each QRS; P-P interval regular. **PR interval:** 0.12. **QRS interval:** 0.10. **Interpretation:** sinus rhythm.

83. **QRS complexes:** present, all shaped the same. **Regularity:** irregular. **Heart rate:** 88 to 115, with a mean rate of 110. **P waves:** none present; regular sawtooth-shaped waves present instead. **PR interval:** not applicable. **QRS interval:** 0.08. **Interpretation:** atrial flutter with variable conduction.

84. **QRS complexes:** present, all shaped the same. **Regularity:** irregular. **Heart rate:** 79 to 137, with a mean rate of 110. **P waves:** none present; wavy, undulating baseline present instead. **PR interval:** not applicable. **QRS interval:** 0.10. **Interpretation:** atrial fibrillation.

85. **QRS complexes:** present, all shaped the same. **Regularity:** regular. **Heart rate:** 88. **P waves:** upright, matching; one preceding each QRS; P-P interval regular. **PR interval:** 0.22. **QRS interval:** 0.12. **Interpretation:** sinus rhythm with first-degree AV block and wide QRS.

86. **QRS complexes:** present, all shaped the same. **Regularity:** regular. **Heart rate:** 60. **P waves:** none present; regular sawtooth-shaped waves present instead. **PR interval:** not applicable. **QRS interval:** 0.10. **Interpretation:** atrial flutter with variable conduction. Many of the flutter waves are lost inside the big inverted T wave.

87. **QRS complexes:** present, all shaped the same. **Regularity:** regular. **Heart rate:** 59. **P waves:** upright, matching; two to each QRS. The T wave has a double hump—do you see it? The first hump is the first P wave. The second P is right in front of the QRS. P-P interval is regular; atrial rate 115. **PR interval:** 0.24. **QRS interval:** 0.08. **Interpretation:** 2:1 AV block, probably Wenckebach.

88. **QRS complexes:** present, all shaped the same. **Regularity:** irregular. **Heart rate:** 33 to 137, with a mean rate of 50. **P waves:** none present; wavy, undulating baseline present instead. **PR interval:** not applicable. **QRS interval:** 0.08. **Interpretation:** atrial fibrillation.

89. **QRS complexes:** present, all shaped the same. **Regularity:** regular. **Heart rate:** 115. **P waves:** upright, matching; one preceding each QRS; P-P interval regular. **PR interval:** 0.16. **QRS interval:** 0.12. **Interpretation:** sinus tachycardia with wide QRS.

90. **QRS complexes:** present, all shaped the same. **Regularity:** regular. **Heart rate:** 75. **P waves:** upright, matching; one preceding each QRS; P-P interval regular. **PR interval:** 0.12. **QRS interval:** 0.06. **Interpretation:** sinus rhythm.

91. **QRS complexes:** present, sawtooth-shaped. **Regularity:** irregular. **Heart rate:** 187 to 300, with a mean rate of 230. **P waves:** none seen. **PR interval:** not applicable. **QRS interval:** cannot measure, as cannot tell where QRS ends and T wave begins. **Interpretation:** ventricular tachycardia.

92. **QRS complexes:** present. **Regularity:** regular but interrupted (by premature beats). **Heart rate:** about 85. **P waves:** inverted, matching; one preceding all the narrow QRS complexes. **PR interval:** 0.16.

Interpretation: sinus rhythm with a unifocal ventricular couplet and a PVC. Wait a minute. The P wave here is negative. Why is this not a junctional rhythm? This is V$_1$—see the notation at the top of the strip? Recall the P wave can be normally inverted in V$_1$. So that doesn't necessarily imply a junctional pacemaker. Also, a junctional rhythm would have had a shorter PR interval, less than 0.12 seconds.

93. **QRS complexes:** present, all shaped the same. **Regularity:** irregular. **Heart rate:** 29, then slower. **P waves:** none present. **PR interval:** not applicable. **QRS interval:** 0.24–0.28. **Interpretation:** agonal rhythm.

94. **QRS complexes:** present, different shapes. **Regularity:** irregular. **Heart rate:** >300 in places. **P waves:** none seen. **PR interval:** not applicable. **QRS interval:** cannot measure, as cannot tell where QRS ends and T wave begins. **Interpretation:** torsades de pointes. Remember torsades is identified more by its classic shape than by any other criteria.

95. **QRS complexes:** present, all shaped the same. **Regularity:** regular. **Heart rate:** 43. **P waves:** inverted following each QRS complex in the ST segment. **PR interval:** not applicable. **QRS interval:** 0.08. **Interpretation:** junctional rhythm.

96. **QRS complexes:** only one present—at the beginning of the strip. Then a wavy, static-looking baseline is seen. **Regularity:** not applicable. **Heart rate:** zero after that first beat. **P waves:** none present. **PR interval:** not applicable. **QRS interval:** 0.28 on the only QRS complex on the strip. **Interpretation:** one ventricular beat, then ventricular fibrillation.

97. **QRS complexes:** none present; wavy, static-looking baseline present instead. **Regularity:** not applicable. **Heart rate:** cannot measure. **P waves:** none present. **PR interval:** not applicable. **QRS interval:** not applicable. **Interpretation:** ventricular fibrillation.

98. **QRS complexes:** none present. **Regularity:** not applicable, as there are no QRS complexes. **Heart rate:** zero. **P waves:** biphasic, matching; P-P interval regular. **PR interval:** not applicable. **QRS interval:** not applicable. **Interpretation:** P wave asystole.

99. **QRS complexes:** present, all shaped the same. **Regularity:** irregular. **Heart rate:** 100 to 167, with a mean rate of 130. **P waves:** none present; wavy, undulating baseline present instead. **PR interval:** not applicable. **QRS interval:** 0.12. **Interpretation:** atrial fibrillation with wide QRS.

100. **QRS complexes:** present, all shaped the same. **Regularity:** regular. **Heart rate:** 60. **P waves:** none present. **PR interval:** not applicable. **QRS interval:** 0.16–0.22. **Interpretation:** accelerated idioventricular rhythm.

101. **QRS complexes:** present, all shaped the same. **Regularity:** regular but interrupted (by a premature beat). **Heart rate:** 68. **P waves:** upright and matching except for the last beat, which has a tiny inverted P wave. One P wave precedes each QRS; P-P interval is irregular. **PR interval:** 0.14 on all but the last beat. The PR interval of the last beat is 0.12. **QRS interval:** 0.12. **Interpretation:** sinus rhythm with a PJC and wide QRS.

102. **QRS complexes:** present, all shaped the same. **Regularity:** regular but interrupted (by a premature beat and also a pause). **Heart rate:** 39 to 100, with a mean rate of 70. **P waves:** upright and matching on all but the third beat, which has a tiny upright P wave at the end of the preceding T wave. There is also a tiny upright P wave just before the downstroke of the third T wave (inside the pause). P-P interval is irregular. **PR interval:** 0.18 on the normal beats, 0.22 on the premature beat. **QRS interval:** 0.06. **Interpretation:** sinus rhythm with a PAC and a nonconducted PAC. The third beat is the PAC. The P wave at the downstroke of the third beat's T wave is the nonconducted PAC. If you called this an AV block of some kind, remember that in AV blocks, the P-P interval is regular. Here we have two premature P waves.

103. **QRS complexes:** present, all shaped the same. **Regularity:** irregular. **Heart rate:** 28 to 38, with a mean rate of 40. **P waves:** none present; wavy, undulating baseline present instead. **PR interval:** not applicable. **QRS interval:** 0.08. **Interpretation:** atrial fibrillation.

104. **QRS complexes:** present, all shaped the same. **Regularity:** regular but interrupted (by a premature beat). **Heart rate:** 100. **P waves:** biphasic and matching on all but the third beat, which is premature and has a different shape P wave. **PR interval:** 0.14 on the normal beats, 0.12 on the premature beat. **QRS interval:** 0.06. **Interpretation:** sinus rhythm with a PAC.

105. **QRS complexes:** present, all shaped the same. **Regularity:** regular but interrupted (by premature beats and pauses). **Heart rate:** 38 to 125, with a mean rate of 80. **P waves:** upright and matching on all but the P wave following the second QRS and also the P wave preceding the sixth QRS. Those P waves have a different shape. P-P interval is irregular. **PR interval:** 0.14 on the normal beats,

0.12 on the sixth beat. **QRS interval:** 0.08. **Interpretation:** sinus rhythm with a PAC (the sixth beat) and a nonconducted PAC (the premature P after the second QRS).

106. **QRS complexes:** present, all but one shaped the same. One is wider and taller than the others. **Regularity:** regular but interrupted (by a premature beat). **Heart rate:** 125. **P waves:** upright and matching on all but the wide QRS beat, which has no P wave. **PR interval:** 0.16. **QRS interval:** 0.08 on the normal beats, 0.14 on the premature beat. **Interpretation:** sinus tachycardia with a PVC.

107. **QRS complexes:** present, all shaped the same. **Regularity:** regular. **Heart rate:** about 130. **P waves:** upright, matching; one preceding each QRS; P-P interval regular. **PR interval:** 0.14. **QRS interval:** 0.08. **Interpretation:** sinus tachycardia.

108. **QRS complexes:** present, all shaped the same. **Regularity:** irregular. **Heart rate:** 68 to 125, with a mean rate of 90. **P waves:** at least three different shapes; P-P interval irregular. **PR interval:** varies. **QRS interval:** 0.10. **Interpretation:** wandering atrial pacemaker.

109. **QRS complexes:** present, all shaped the same. **Regularity:** regular. **Heart rate:** 38. **P waves:** upright and matching directly preceding the QRS. There is an extra premature P wave at the end of each T wave. That P has a different shape—it's pointy. **PR interval:** 0.20. **QRS interval:** 0.08. **Interpretation:** sinus bradycardia with bigeminal nonconducted PACs. This strip looks like sinus bradycardia, doesn't it? But do you see the premature P wave now that it's been pointed out? Always be suspicious of T waves with humps on their downslopes. That hump might just be a P wave.

110. **QRS complexes:** present, all shaped the same. **Regularity:** irregular. **Heart rate:** 29 to 60, with a mean rate of 40. **P waves:** none present; wavy, undulating baseline present instead. **PR interval:** not applicable. **QRS interval:** 0.08. **Interpretation:** atrial fibrillation.

111. **QRS complexes:** present, most but not all shaped the same. **Regularity:** irregular. **Heart rate:** 167 to 250, with a mean rate of 200. **P waves:** none present; wavy, undulating baseline present instead. **PR interval:** not applicable. **QRS interval:** 0.06–0.08. **Interpretation:** atrial fibrillation. If you were tempted to call this SVT, remember that SVT is a regular rhythm. This strip is not regular.

112. **QRS complexes:** present, all shaped the same. **Regularity:** regular. **Heart rate:** 62. **P waves:** none seen. **PR interval:** not applicable. **QRS**

interval: 0.20. **Interpretation:** accelerated idioventricular rhythm.

113. **QRS complexes:** present, all shaped the same, although some are deeper than others. **Regularity:** regular but interrupted (by a run of premature beats). **Heart rate:** 88 when in sinus tachycardia, about 187 when in atrial tachycardia. **P waves:** upright and matching on all but the very rapid beats, whose P waves are inside the preceding T wave. **PR interval:** 0.20 on the normal beats, unable to measure on the rapid beats, as the P is inside the T wave. **QRS interval:** 0.08. **Interpretation:** sinus tachycardia with a 10-beat run of PAT. We know this is PAT, as we can see the PAC (the fourth beat) that initiates it.

114. **QRS complexes:** present, all shaped the same. **Regularity:** irregular. **Heart rate:** 150 to 250, with a mean rate of 190. **P waves:** none present; wavy, undulating baseline present instead. **PR interval:** not applicable. **QRS interval:** 0.06. **Interpretation:** atrial fibrillation.

115. **QRS complexes:** present, all shaped the same. **Regularity:** irregular. **Heart rate:** 150 to 250, with a mean rate of 190. **P waves:** none present; wavy, undulating baseline present instead. **PR interval:** not applicable. **QRS interval:** 0.06. **Interpretation:** atrial fibrillation.

116. **QRS complexes:** present, all shaped the same. **Regularity:** regular but interrupted (by a pause). **Heart rate:** 37 to 72, with a mean heart rate of 70. **P waves:** upright and matching except for the premature P wave inside the fourth T wave. **PR interval:** 0.24. **QRS interval:** 0.08. **Interpretation:** sinus rhythm with a nonconducted PAC.

117. **QRS complexes:** present, all shaped the same. **Regularity:** regular. **Heart rate:** 71. **P waves:** tiny inverted P waves present preceding the QRS complexes. **PR interval:** about 0.06. **QRS interval:** 0.10. **Interpretation:** accelerated junctional rhythm.

118. **QRS complexes:** present, all shaped the same. **Regularity:** regular but interrupted (by pauses). **Heart rate:** 48 to 88, with a mean rate of 80. **P waves:** upright and matching except for the premature P waves inside the third and sixth T waves. **PR interval:** 0.18. **QRS interval:** 0.08. **Interpretation:** sinus rhythm with two nonconducted PACs.

119. **QRS complexes:** present, all shaped the same. **Regularity:** regular. **Heart rate:** 29. **P waves:** none present. **PR interval:** not applicable. **QRS interval:** 0.28. **Interpretation:** idioventricular rhythm.

120. **QRS complexes:** present, all shaped the same. **Regularity:** regular but interrupted (by a pause).

Heart rate: 32 to 58, with a mean rate of 50. **P waves:** upright, matching; sometimes more than one per QRS; atrial rate 60. **PR interval:** varies. **QRS interval:** 0.10. **Interpretation:** Wenckebach. See how the PR interval gradually prolongs until a P wave is blocked (not followed by a QRS)?

121. **QRS complexes:** present, all shaped the same. **Regularity:** regular. **Heart rate:** 45. **P waves:** upright, matching, some nonconducted; atrial rate 137. **PR interval:** varies. **QRS interval:** 0.16. **Interpretation:** third-degree AV block and a ventricular escape rhythm. Did you think this was Mobitz II second-degree AV block? The differentiating factor here is the changing PR intervals. Mobitz II has constant PR intervals. Did you think it was Wenckebach? Wenckebach does not have regular R-R intervals. So it could only be third-degree AV block.

122. **QRS complexes:** present, all shaped the same. **Regularity:** irregular. **Heart rate:** 60 to 83, with a mean rate of 80. **P waves:** upright, matching; one per QRS; P-P interval irregular. **PR interval:** 0.14. **QRS interval:** 0.08. **Interpretation:** sinus arrhythmia.

123. **QRS complexes:** present, all shaped the same. **Regularity:** regular. **Heart rate:** 83. **P waves:** none noted. **PR interval:** not applicable. **QRS interval:** 0.16. **Interpretation:** accelerated idioventricular rhythm.

124. **QRS complexes:** present, all shaped the same. **Regularity:** regular. **Heart rate:** 125. **P waves:** none seen. **PR interval:** not applicable. **QRS interval:** 0.20. **Interpretation:** ventricular tachycardia.

125. **QRS complexes:** present, all shaped the same. **Regularity:** regular. **Heart rate:** 58. **P waves:** none seen. There's a U wave immediately following the T waves—don't confuse those with P waves. **PR interval:** not applicable. **QRS interval:** 0.10. **Interpretation:** junctional rhythm.

126. **QRS complexes:** present, all shaped the same. **Regularity:** irregular. **Heart rate:** 42 to 47, with a mean rate of 50. Wait a minute, you say. How can the mean rate be greater than the heart rate range? You're correct; it shouldn't be. This is why the mean rate should never be used alone; it is so inaccurate. The heart rate range is much more correct. **P waves:** at least three different shapes; one preceding each QRS. **PR interval:** varies. **QRS interval:** 0.10. **Interpretation:** wandering atrial pacemaker.

127. **QRS complexes:** present, all shaped the same. **Regularity:** irregular. **Heart rate:** 100 to 150, with a mean rate of 130. **P waves:** none noted; wavy, undulating baseline present instead. **PR**

interval: not applicable. **QRS interval:** 0.06. **Interpretation:** atrial fibrillation.

128. **QRS complexes:** present, all shaped the same. **Regularity:** irregular. **Heart rate:** 85 to 137, with a mean rate of 100. **P waves:** none present; sawtooth-shaped waves present between QRS complexes. **PR interval:** not applicable. **QRS interval:** 0.10. **Interpretation:** atrial flutter with variable conduction.

129. **QRS complexes:** present with differing shapes, if indeed those are real QRS complexes and not just spiked fibrillatory waves. **Regularity:** irregular. **Heart rate:** around 300 to 375, but difficult to count as QRS shapes change. **P waves:** none seen. **PR interval:** not applicable. **QRS interval:** cannot measure at times. **Interpretation:** torsades de pointes versus ventricular fibrillation. This is a judgment call, as this rhythm might well be ventricular fibrillation. You will find that torsades and V-fib can be easily mistaken for each other.

130. **QRS complexes:** present, all shaped the same. **Regularity:** regular. **Heart rate:** 79. **P waves:** upright, matching; one preceding each QRS; P-P interval regular. **PR interval:** 0.14. **QRS interval:** 0.12. **Interpretation:** sinus rhythm.

131. **QRS complexes:** present, all shaped the same. **Regularity:** regular. **Heart rate:** 51. **P waves:** none seen. **PR interval:** not applicable. **QRS interval:** 0.10. **Interpretation:** junctional rhythm.

132. **QRS complexes:** present, all shaped the same. **Regularity:** regular but interrupted (by premature beats). **Heart rate:** 65. **P waves:** upright, all except the third and fourth P waves matching. The third and fourth P waves are premature and shaped a bit differently. P-P interval is irregular. **PR interval:** 0.16–0.20. **QRS interval:** 0.06. **Interpretation:** sinus rhythm with two PACs (the third and fourth beats).

133. **QRS complexes:** present, all shaped the same. **Regularity:** irregular. **Heart rate:** 71 to 110, with a mean rate of 90. **P waves:** none present; wavy, undulating baseline present instead. **PR interval:** not applicable. **QRS interval:** 0.08. **Interpretation:** atrial fibrillation. In places it looks pretty fluttery, doesn't it? You might have been tempted to call this atrial flutter. The problem is that the fluttery pattern is not consistent. Its waves could never be marched out, as they dampen out so much in places. It's safer to call this atrial fibrillation (or fib-flutter).

134. **QRS complexes:** present, all shaped the same. **Regularity:** regular. **Heart rate:** 60. **P waves:** none noted. **PR interval:** not applicable.

QRS interval: 0.20. **Interpretation:** accelerated idioventricular rhythm.

135. **QRS complexes:** present, all shaped the same, although two are distorted by artifact. **Regularity:** regular. **Heart rate:** 137. **P waves:** none seen. **PR interval:** not applicable. **QRS interval:** 0.18. **Interpretation:** ventricular tachycardia.

136. **QRS complexes:** present, all shaped the same. **Regularity:** regular. **Heart rate:** 60. **P waves:** none seen; wavy, undulating baseline present instead. **PR interval:** not applicable. **QRS interval:** 0.10. **Interpretation:** atrial fibrillation. Although normally atrial fibrillation is an irregular rhythm, you can see that it may look regular at times. This is not common, but you should be aware it does happen sometimes, typically in individuals who've been in atrial fibrillation for years.

137. **QRS complexes:** present, all shaped the same. **Regularity:** regular. **Heart rate:** 137. **P waves:** upright, matching; one preceding each QRS; P-P interval regular. **PR interval:** 0.16. **QRS interval:** 0.08. **Interpretation:** sinus tachycardia.

138. **QRS complexes:** present, all shaped the same. **Regularity:** regular. **Heart rate:** 42. **P waves:** upright, matching (some a little distorted by artifact); one preceding each QRS; P-P interval regular. **PR interval:** 0.16. **QRS interval:** 0.10. **Interpretation:** sinus bradycardia.

139. **QRS complexes:** present, all shaped the same. **Regularity:** regular. **Heart rate:** 60. **P waves:** upright, matching; one preceding each QRS; P-P interval regular. **PR interval:** 0.14. **QRS interval:** 0.08. **Interpretation:** sinus rhythm.

140. **QRS complexes:** present, all shaped the same. **Regularity:** irregular. **Heart rate:** 71 to 107, with a mean rate of 90. **P waves:** none present; sawtooth waves present instead. **PR interval:** not applicable. **QRS interval:** 0.06. **Interpretation:** atrial flutter with variable conduction.

141. **QRS complexes:** present, all shaped the same. **Regularity:** regular. **Heart rate:** about 73. **P waves:** none noted; sawtooth waves present instead. **PR interval:** not applicable. **QRS interval:** 0.12, although difficult to measure as QRS is distorted by flutter waves. **Interpretation:** atrial flutter with variable conduction and a possible wide QRS.

142. **QRS complexes:** cannot distinguish. **Regularity:** cannot tell. **Heart rate:** cannot tell. **P waves:** cannot distinguish. **PR interval:** not applicable. **QRS interval:** not applicable. **Interpretation:** unknown rhythm with artifact. Why is this strip even in here if you can't possibly tell what it is? Because it's important for you to know *not to even try to interpret a rhythm this obscured by artifact.* There is no way to tell what the underlying rhythm is here. Check the patient's monitor lead wires and electrode patches or change the lead the patient is being monitored in to get a better tracing, and try again with a clearer strip.

143. **QRS complexes:** present, all shaped the same. **Regularity:** regular. **Heart rate:** about 130. **P waves:** upright, matching; one preceding each QRS; P-P interval regular. **PR interval:** 0.16. **QRS interval:** 0.06. **Interpretation:** sinus tachycardia.

144. **QRS complexes:** present, all shaped the same. **Regularity:** regular. **Heart rate:** 83. **P waves:** upright, matching; one preceding each QRS; P-P interval regular. **PR interval:** 0.10. **QRS interval:** 0.08. **Interpretation:** sinus rhythm with short PR interval.

145. **QRS complexes:** present, all shaped the same. **Regularity:** regular. **Heart rate:** 88. **P waves:** upright, matching; one preceding each QRS; P-P interval regular. **PR interval:** 0.12. **QRS interval:** 0.12. **Interpretation:** sinus rhythm with wide QRS.

146. **QRS complexes:** present, all shaped the same. **Regularity:** regular. **Heart rate:** 60. **P waves:** upright, matching; one preceding each QRS; P-P interval regular. **PR interval:** 0.16. **QRS interval:** 0.08. **Interpretation:** sinus rhythm.

147. **QRS complexes:** present, all shaped the same. **Regularity:** regular. **Heart rate:** 68. **P waves:** upright, matching; one preceding each QRS; P-P interval regular. **PR interval:** 0.18. **QRS interval:** 0.14. **Interpretation:** sinus rhythm with wide QRS.

148. **QRS complexes:** present, all shaped the same. **Regularity:** regular. **Heart rate:** about 57. **P waves:** upright, matching; one preceding each QRS; P-P interval regular. **PR interval:** 0.16. **QRS interval:** 0.08. **Interpretation:** sinus bradycardia.

149. **QRS complexes:** present, all shaped the same. **Regularity:** irregular. **Heart rate:** 56 to 83, with a mean rate of 70. **P waves:** none noted; wavy, undulating baseline present instead. **PR interval:** not applicable. **QRS interval:** 0.10. **Interpretation:** atrial fibrillation.

150. **QRS complexes:** present, all shaped the same. **Regularity:** regular. **Heart rate:** 43. **P waves:** upright, matching; one preceding each QRS; P-P interval regular. **PR interval:** 0.16. **QRS interval:** 0.08. **Interpretation:** sinus bradycardia.

151. **QRS complexes:** present, all shaped the same. **Regularity:** regular. **Heart rate:** 83. **P waves:** upright, matching; one preceding each QRS; P-P interval regular. **PR interval:** 0.14. **QRS interval:** 0.10. **Interpretation:** sinus rhythm.

152. **QRS complexes:** present, all shaped the same. **Regularity:** regular. **Heart rate:** about 35. **P waves:** upright, matching; one preceding each QRS; P-P interval regular. **PR interval:** 0.16. **QRS interval:** 0.10. **Interpretation:** sinus bradycardia.

153. **QRS complexes:** present, most but not all shaped the same. Some have an S wave, but others do not. **Regularity:** irregular. **Heart rate:** 150 to 250, with a mean rate of 190. **P waves:** none noted; wavy, undulating baseline present instead. **PR interval:** not applicable. **QRS interval:** 0.06 to 0.08. **Interpretation:** atrial fibrillation.

154. **QRS complexes:** present, all shaped the same. **Regularity:** regular. **Heart rate:** 62. **P waves:** upright, matching; one preceding each QRS; P-P interval regular. **PR interval:** 0.20. **QRS interval:** 0.08. **Interpretation:** sinus rhythm.

155. **QRS complexes:** present, all shaped the same. **Regularity:** regular. **Heart rate:** 115. **P waves:** upright, matching; one preceding each QRS; P-P interval regular. **PR interval:** 0.12. **QRS interval:** 0.10. **Interpretation:** sinus tachycardia.

156. **QRS complexes:** present, all shaped the same. **Regularity:** irregular. **Heart rate:** 107 to 167, with a mean rate of 140. **P waves:** none seen; wavy, undulating baseline present instead. **PR interval:** not applicable. **QRS interval:** 0.08. **Interpretation:** atrial fibrillation.

157. **QRS complexes:** one present; wavy, static-looking baseline present instead. **Regularity:** not applicable. **Heart rate:** cannot determine, as there is only one QRS complex. **P waves:** none seen. **PR interval:** not applicable. **QRS interval:** not applicable. **Interpretation:** ventricular fibrillation.

158. **QRS complexes:** present, all shaped the same. **Regularity:** irregular. **Heart rate:** 36 to 42, with a mean rate of 40. **P waves:** upright, matching; one preceding each QRS; P-P interval irregular. **PR interval:** 0.16. **QRS interval:** 0.10. **Interpretation:** sinus arrhythmia.

159. **QRS complexes:** present, all shaped the same. **Regularity:** regular but interrupted (by pauses). **Heart rate:** 75 to 125, with a mean rate of 110. **P waves:** upright, many hidden in T waves. Some P waves are nonconducted. P-P interval is regular; atrial rate 137. **PR interval:** varies. **QRS interval:** 0.06. **Interpretation:** Wenckebach. This is not an obvious Wenckebach, is it? See the pause between the third and fourth QRS complexes? Note the P wave preceding the fourth QRS. Now back up to the T wave of the third beat. See how deformed the T wave's shape is? That's because there's a P wave inside it. Note the P-P interval between those two P waves and you can march out where the rest of the P waves are. You'll find the P-P intervals are all regular and the PR intervals gradually prolong until a beat is dropped.

160. **QRS complexes:** present, all shaped the same. **Regularity:** irregular. **Heart rate:** 75 to 107, with a mean rate of 100. **P waves:** none noted; wavy, undulating baseline present instead. **PR interval:** not applicable. **QRS interval:** 0.10. **Interpretation:** atrial fibrillation.

161. **QRS complexes:** present, all shaped the same. **Regularity:** regular. **Heart rate:** about 130. **P waves:** none seen. **PR interval:** not applicable. **QRS interval:** 0.08. **Interpretation:** SVT.

162. **QRS complexes:** cannot be sure if there are QRS complexes of varying shapes or if it is just a static-looking baseline without QRS complexes. **Regularity:** irregular. **Heart rate:** 250 to 300, with a mean rate of about 280. **P waves:** none seen. **PR interval:** not applicable. **QRS interval:** 0.12 or greater. **Interpretation:** either torsades de pointes or ventricular fibrillation. It oscillates like torsades but looks more uncoordinated, like V-fib. The treatment for these is similar, thankfully, so calling it either torsades or V-fib would still get appropriate treatment for the patient.

163. **QRS complexes:** present, all shaped the same. **Regularity:** irregular. **Heart rate:** 60 to 107, with a mean rate of 90. **P waves:** none seen; wavy, undulating baseline present instead. **PR interval:** not applicable. **QRS interval:** 0.06. **Interpretation:** atrial fibrillation.

164. **QRS complexes:** present, all shaped the same. **Regularity:** regular. **Heart rate:** about 80. **P waves:** none seen; wavy, undulating baseline present instead. **PR interval:** not applicable. **QRS interval:** 0.10. **Interpretation:** atrial fibrillation. This is another example of a regular spell of atrial fibrillation.

165. **QRS complexes:** present, all but one shaped the same. One is shorter than the rest. **Regularity:** irregular. **Heart rate:** 45 to 65, with a mean rate of 50. **P waves:** none noted; wavy, undulating baseline present instead. **PR interval:** not applicable. **QRS interval:** 0.08. **Interpretation:** atrial fibrillation.

166. **QRS complexes:** present, all shaped the same. **Regularity:** regular. **Heart rate:** 75. **P waves:** upright, matching; one preceding each QRS; P-P interval regular. **PR interval:** 0.16. **QRS interval:** 0.14. **Interpretation:** sinus rhythm with wide QRS.

167. **QRS complexes:** present, all shaped the same. **Regularity:** irregular. **Heart rate:** 88 to 187, with

a mean rate of 120. **P waves:** present, at least three different shapes; P-P interval irregular. **PR interval:** varies. **QRS interval:** 0.08. **Interpretation:** multifocal atrial tachycardia.

168. **QRS complexes:** present, all shaped the same. **Regularity:** regular. **Heart rate:** around 90. **P waves:** upright, matching; one preceding each QRS; P-P interval regular. **PR interval:** 0.14. **QRS interval:** 0.08. **Interpretation:** sinus rhythm.

169. **QRS complexes:** present, all shaped the same. **Regularity:** irregular. **Heart rate:** 83 to 137, with a mean rate of 110. **P waves:** none noted; sawtooth waves present instead. **PR interval:** not applicable. **QRS interval:** 0.08. **Interpretation:** atrial flutter with variable conduction.

170. **QRS complexes:** present, all shaped the same. **Regularity:** regular. **Heart rate:** 150. **P waves:** upright, matching; one preceding each QRS; P-P interval regular. **PR interval:** 0.10. **QRS interval:** 0.10. **Interpretation:** sinus tachycardia with short PR interval.

171. **QRS complexes:** present, all shaped the same. **Regularity:** regular. **Heart rate:** 45. **P waves:** upright, matching, two preceding each QRS; P-P interval regular; atrial rate 88. **PR interval:** 0.36. **QRS interval:** 0.08. **Interpretation:** 2:1 AV block.

172. **QRS complexes:** present, all shaped the same. **Regularity:** regular but interrupted (by pauses). **Heart rate:** 44 to 83, with a mean rate of 60. **P waves:** upright, matching, some nonconducted; P-P interval regular; atrial rate 88. **PR interval:** 0.36. **QRS interval:** 0.08. **Interpretation:** Mobitz II second-degree AV block.

173. **QRS complexes:** present, all shaped the same. **Regularity:** regular. **Heart rate:** 137. **P waves:** none seen. **PR interval:** not applicable. **QRS interval:** 0.06. **Interpretation:** SVT.

174. **QRS complexes:** only one mammoth QRS on the strip. Believe it or not, that huge wave at the beginning of the strip is a QRS and T wave. **Regularity:** cannot determine. **Heart rate:** cannot determine. **P waves:** none seen. **PR interval:** not applicable. **QRS interval:** about 0.60, but that's a guesstimate. **Interpretation:** agonal rhythm. It is unusual for an agonal rhythm's QRS complexes to be this wide. It's likely this patient has an *extremely elevated* potassium level in his or her bloodstream, which can cause the QRS to widen out more than usual.

175. **QRS complexes:** none seen. **Regularity:** not applicable. **Heart rate:** zero. **P waves:** none seen. **PR interval:** not applicable. **QRS interval:** not applicable. **Interpretation:** asystole.

176. **QRS complexes:** present, differing shapes. **Regularity:** irregular. **Heart rate:** about 375. **P waves:** none seen. **PR interval:** not applicable. **QRS interval:** 0.12 or greater. **Interpretation:** torsades de pointes.

177. **QRS complexes:** none; wavy, static-looking baseline present instead. **Regularity:** not applicable. **Heart rate:** cannot measure. **P waves:** none seen. **PR interval:** not applicable. **QRS interval:** not applicable. **Interpretation:** ventricular fibrillation.

178. **QRS complexes:** none; wavy, static-looking baseline present instead. **Regularity:** not applicable. **Heart rate:** cannot measure. **P waves:** none seen. **PR interval:** not applicable. **QRS interval:** not applicable. **Interpretation:** ventricular fibrillation.

179. **QRS complexes:** present, all shaped the same. **Regularity:** regular. **Heart rate:** just a hair over 100. **P waves:** upright, matching; one preceding each QRS; P-P interval regular. **PR interval:** 0.22. **QRS interval:** 0.10. **Interpretation:** sinus tachycardia with a first-degree AV block.

180. **QRS complexes:** present, all shaped the same. **Regularity:** irregular. **Heart rate:** 80 to 167, with a mean rate of 110. **P waves:** present, at least three different shapes. **PR interval:** not applicable. **QRS interval:** 0.06. **Interpretation:** multifocal atrial tachycardia. If you thought it was atrial fibrillation, remember that *atrial fibrillation has no P waves.* There are obvious P waves on this strip.

181. **QRS complexes:** present, all shaped the same. **Regularity:** regular. **Heart rate:** 68. **P waves:** none seen. **PR interval:** not applicable. **QRS interval:** 0.18. **Interpretation:** accelerated idioventricular rhythm.

182. **QRS complexes:** present, all shaped the same. **Regularity:** regular. **Heart rate:** 125. **P waves:** upright, matching; one preceding each QRS; P-P interval regular. **PR interval:** 0.16. **QRS interval:** 0.06. **Interpretation:** sinus tachycardia.

183. **QRS complexes:** present, all shaped the same. **Regularity:** regular. **Heart rate:** 56. **P waves:** upright, matching; one preceding each QRS; P-P interval regular; P waves are small. **PR interval:** 0.16. **QRS interval:** 0.16. **Interpretation:** sinus bradycardia with wide QRS. Look again at this strip if you thought this was atrial fibrillation. There are obvious, although tiny, P waves. And if you thought this was a ventricular rhythm of some kind because of the QRS width, note the matching upright P waves. Ventricular rhythms don't have that. Remember—the width of the QRS does not

determine whether a rhythm can be sinus. The P waves are the key criterion.

184. **QRS complexes:** present, all shaped the same. **Regularity:** regular. **Heart rate:** 83. **P waves:** upright, matching; one preceding each QRS; P-P interval regular. **PR interval:** 0.13. **QRS interval:** 0.10. **Interpretation:** sinus rhythm. Did you think this was a 2:1 AV block? The T wave does look like the P wave, doesn't it? Remember AV blocks have regular P-P intervals. If this T wave were hiding a P wave, the P-P intervals would not be regular. So it's not an AV block.

185. **QRS complexes:** present, all shaped the same. **Regularity:** regular. **Heart rate:** 167. **P waves:** upright, matching; one preceding each QRS; P-P interval regular. **PR interval:** 0.12. **QRS interval:** 0.06. **Interpretation:** atrial tachycardia. Remember, the sinus node does not usually fire at rates above 160 in supine resting adults. Since this rate is above 160, we must call it atrial tachycardia.

186. **QRS complexes:** present, all shaped the same. **Regularity:** irregular. **Heart rate:** 20 to 75, with a mean rate of 50. **P waves:** none seen; very fine wavy, undulating baseline present instead. **PR interval:** not applicable. **QRS interval:** 0.08. **Interpretation:** atrial fibrillation.

187. **QRS complexes:** present, all shaped the same. **Regularity:** irregular. **Heart rate:** 28 to 62, with a mean rate of 50. **P waves:** none seen; wavy, undulating baseline present instead. **PR interval:** not applicable. **QRS interval:** 0.10. **Interpretation:** atrial fibrillation.

188. **QRS complexes:** present, all shaped the same. **Regularity:** irregular. **Heart rate:** 60 to 79, with a mean rate of 70. **P waves:** upright, matching; one preceding each QRS; P-P interval regular. **PR interval:** 0.18. **QRS interval:** 0.08. **Interpretation:** sinus arrhythmia.

189. **QRS complexes:** present, all shaped the same. **Regularity:** regular. **Heart rate:** 60. **P waves:** upright, matching (the ones that can be seen); one preceding each QRS; P-P interval regular, as far as can be seen. **PR interval:** 0.18. **QRS interval:** 0.08. **Interpretation:** sinus rhythm partially obscured by artifact. Unlike some strips with artifact, this strip has measurable waves and complexes. Since we can pick out the QRS complexes throughout the strip, we can deduce that the P waves continue as well during the artifact spells. Even so, it would be better not to mount a strip like this in the patient's chart, since one cannot be entirely sure what is happening during the periods of artifact.

190. **QRS complexes:** present, all shaped the same. **Regularity:** regular but interrupted (by pauses). **Heart rate:** 75 to 125. **P waves:** upright, some hidden in T waves, some nonconducted; P-P interval regular; atrial rate 137. **PR interval:** varies. **QRS interval:** 0.06. **Interpretation:** Wenckebach.

191. **QRS complexes:** present, all but two shaped the same (two are taller and wider). **Regularity:** regular but interrupted (by premature beats). **Heart rate:** 88. **P waves:** upright and matching on the narrow beats, none on the wide beats; P-P regular. **PR interval:** 0.24. **QRS interval:** 0.08 on the narrow beats, 0.14 on the wide beats. **Interpretation:** sinus rhythm with PVCs and a first-degree AV block.

192. **QRS complexes:** present, all shaped the same. **Regularity:** regular. **Heart rate:** 88. **P waves:** notched, matching; one preceding each QRS; P-P interval regular. **PR interval:** 0.20. **QRS interval:** 0.08. **Interpretation:** sinus rhythm.

193. **QRS complexes:** present, all shaped the same. **Regularity:** regular. **Heart rate:** 71. **P waves:** upright, matching; one preceding each QRS; P-P interval regular. **PR interval:** 0.22. **QRS interval:** 0.08. **Interpretation:** sinus rhythm with a first-degree AV block.

194. **QRS complexes:** present, all shaped the same. **Regularity:** regular. **Heart rate:** 36. **P waves:** upright, matching; one preceding each QRS; P-P interval regular. **PR interval:** 0.16. **QRS interval:** 0.10. **Interpretation:** sinus bradycardia.

195. **QRS complexes:** only one seen on the strip. **Regularity:** cannot determine. **Heart rate:** cannot determine from just one QRS complex. **P waves:** cannot distinguish due to artifact. **PR interval:** not applicable. **QRS interval:** cannot measure, as it's distorted by artifact. **Interpretation:** probably agonal rhythm obscured by CPR artifact. This strip looks a lot like the example of CPR artifact in Chapter 3, doesn't it? In order to know for sure what this rhythm is, CPR would need to be stopped briefly to allow a strip without artifact to be analyzed.

196. **QRS complexes:** none present; wavy, static-looking baseline present instead. **Regularity:** not applicable. **Heart rate:** not applicable. **P waves:** none seen. **PR interval:** not applicable. **QRS interval:** not applicable. **Interpretation:** ventricular fibrillation.

197. **QRS complexes:** present, all shaped the same. **Regularity:** regular but interrupted (by a premature beat). **Heart rate:** 75 **P waves:** upright and matching except for the premature P wave on the seventh beat; P-P interval irregular because of this premature beat. **PR interval:** 0.16. **QRS interval:** 0.10. **Interpretation:** sinus rhythm with a PAC.

198. **QRS complexes:** present, all shaped the same. **Regularity:** regular but interrupted (by a premature beat). **Heart rate:** about 77. **P waves:** tiny, biphasic, and matching except for the third beat, which is premature. The P-P interval is irregular because of this premature beat. **PR interval:** 0.14–0.16. **QRS interval:** 0.06. **Interpretation:** sinus rhythm with a PAC. This premature beat is not a PJC because the PR interval of that beat is greater than 0.12.

199. **QRS complexes:** present, two different shapes. **Regularity:** regular but interrupted (by premature beats). **Heart rate:** 115. **P waves:** upright and matching on the narrow beats, none on the wide beats. **PR interval:** 0.14. **QRS interval:** 0.08 on the narrow beats, 0.16 on the wide beats. **Interpretation:** sinus tachycardia with two PVCs.

200. **QRS complexes:** present, all shaped the same. **Regularity:** irregular. **Heart rate:** 79 to 125, with an atrial rate of 100. **P waves:** none present, sawtooth waves present instead. **PR interval:** not applicable. **QRS interval:** 0.08. **Interpretation:** atrial flutter with variable conduction.

201. **QRS complexes:** present, all shaped the same within each lead. **Regularity:** regular. **Heart rate:** 38. **P waves:** upright in Lead II, biphasic in V_1, matching within each lead. **PR interval:** 0.26. **QRS interval:** 0.10. **Interpretation:** sinus bradycardia with first-degree AV block.

202. **QRS complexes:** present, all shaped the same. **Regularity:** regular. **Heart rate:** 65. **P waves:** upright, matching. **PR interval:** 0.10. **QRS interval:** 0.10. **Interpretation:** sinus rhythm.

203. **QRS complexes:** present, all shaped the same within each lead. **Regularity:** regular. **Heart rate:** 150. **P waves:** none noted. **PR interval:** not applicable. **QRS interval:** 0.06. **Interpretation:** SVT.

204. **QRS complexes:** absent. **Regularity:** not applicable. **Heart rate:** zero. **P waves:** none present. **PR interval:** not applicable. **QRS interval:** not applicable. **Interpretation:** asystole.

205. **QRS complexes:** present, all shaped the same within each lead. **Regularity:** regular. **Heart rate:** 65. **P waves:** upright in Lead II, biphasic in V_1, matching within each lead. **PR interval:** 0.20. **QRS interval:** 0.10. **Interpretation:** sinus rhythm.

206. **QRS complexes:** present, all shaped the same within each lead. **Regularity:** irregular. **Heart rate:** 41 to 68, with a mean rate of 50. **P waves:** upright in Lead II, biphasic in V_1, matching within each lead. P-P interval is regular; atrial rate 79. **PR interval:** varies. **QRS interval:** 0.14. **Interpretation:** Wenckebach with wide QRS.

207. **QRS complexes:** present, all shaped the same within each lead. **Regularity:** regular but interrupted by a pause. **Heart rate:** 36 to 79, with a mean rate of 50. **P waves:** upright, matching; P-P interval regular; atrial rate 75. **PR interval:** varies. **QRS interval:** 0.10. **Interpretation:** Wenckebach.

208. **QRS complexes:** present, all shaped the same within each lead. **Regularity:** regular but interrupted by a premature beat. The fifth QRS complex is premature. **Heart rate:** 75. **P waves:** upright in Lead II, biphasic in V_1, matching within each lead except for the fifth P wave, which is shaped differently and is premature. **PR interval:** 0.12. **QRS interval:** 08. **Interpretation:** sinus rhythm with PAC.

209. **QRS complexes:** present, all shaped the same within each lead. **Regularity:** regular. **Heart rate:** 38. **P waves:** upright in Lead II, biphasic in V_1, matching within each lead. P-P interval is regular; atrial rate 79. **PR interval:** 0.28. **QRS interval:** 0.14. **Interpretation:** 2:1 AV block with wide QRS.

210. **QRS complexes:** present, all shaped the same within each lead. **Regularity:** regular. **Heart rate:** 102. **P waves:** matching, inverted following the QRS in both leads. **PR interval:** not applicable. **QRS interval:** 0.08. **Interpretation:** junctional tachycardia. See the blips following the QRS complexes? Those are the inverted P waves.

211. **QRS complexes:** present, all shaped the same within each lead. **Regularity:** regular. **Heart rate:** 71. **P waves:** cannot see in Lead II, inverted in V_1. **PR interval:** 0.11. **QRS interval:** 0.06. **Interpretation:** accelerated junctional rhythm.

212. **QRS complexes:** present, all shaped the same. **Regularity:** irregular. **Heart rate:** 71 to 125, with a mean rate of 90. **P waves:** none noted; wavy baseline present between QRS complexes. **PR interval:** not applicable. **QRS interval:** 0.10. **Interpretation:** atrial fibrillation.

213. **QRS complexes:** present, all shaped the same. **Regularity:** regular. **Heart rate:** 65. **P waves:** matching, upright. **PR interval:** 0.20. **QRS interval:** 0.12. **Interpretation:** sinus rhythm with borderline first-degree and wide QRS.

214. **QRS complexes:** present, all shaped the same. **Regularity:** regular but interrupted by premature beats. **Heart rate:** 88. **P waves:** matching on all but the second, fourth, and sixth beats—those P waves are shaped differently. **PR interval:** 0.13. **QRS interval:** 0.14. **Interpretation:** sinus rhythm with three PACs and wide QRS.

215. **QRS complexes:** present, all shaped the same. **Regularity:** regular but interrupted by a run of rapid beats. **Heart rate:** 68, then 150. **P waves:** upright

and matching on the first four beats, then shaped differently during the tachycardia. **PR interval:** 0.16. **QRS interval:** 0.10. **Interpretation:** sinus rhythm, then atrial tachycardia (the fifth beat is a PAC, which starts off a run of PACs—this run of PACs is called atrial tachycardia).

216. **QRS complexes:** present, all shaped the same. **Regularity:** regular. **Heart rate:** 83. **P waves:** upright, matching; one preceding each QRS. **PR interval:** 0.16. **QRS interval:** 0.08. **Interpretation:** sinus rhythm.

217. **QRS complexes:** present, all shaped the same within each lead. **Regularity:** regular. **Heart rate:** 94. **P waves:** cannot see in Lead I, inverted preceding the QRS in Lead II. **PR interval:** 0.08. **QRS interval:** 0.06. **Interpretation:** accelerated junctional rhythm.

218. **QRS complexes:** present, all different shapes. **Regularity:** irregular. **Heart rate:** up to 500. **P waves:** none seen. **PR interval:** not applicable. **QRS interval:** 0.04–0.08 (hard to measure). **Interpretation:** torsades de pointes. Note the characteristic oscillating (bigger-smaller-bigger) pattern.

219. **QRS complexes:** None present—chaotic, wavy baseline noted instead. **Regularity:** not applicable as no QRS complexes. **Heart rate:** cannot measure. **P waves:** none. **PR interval:** not applicable. **QRS interval:** not applicable. **Interpretation:** ventricular fibrillation. Note the sudden wild change in baseline on the strip along with the notation of a shock delivered to the heart. This was an attempt to defibrillate the heart. Note that the V-fib continues even after the shock.

220. **QRS complexes:** present, all shaped the same within each lead. **Regularity:** regular. **Heart rate:** 187. **P waves:** an occasional dissociated P wave is noted. See the blip following the 5th, 8th, 10th, 12th, and 14th QRS complexes? Those are P waves. **PR interval:** not applicable. **QRS interval:** 0.14. **Interpretation:** ventricular tachycardia.

221. **QRS complexes:** present, all shaped the same within each lead. **Regularity:** irregular. **Heart rate:** from less than 30 to 62, with a mean rate of 40. **P waves:** none seen; wavy baseline noted between QRS complexes. **PR interval:** not applicable. **QRS interval:** 0.06. **Interpretation:** atrial fibrillation.

222. **QRS complexes:** present, all shaped the same within each lead. **Regularity:** regular. **Heart rate:** 88. **P waves:** matching and upright in both leads. **PR interval:** 0.18. **QRS interval:** 0.10. **Interpretation:** sinus rhythm.

223. **QRS complexes:** present, all shaped the same within each lead. **Regularity:** regular. **Heart rate:** 75. **P waves:** matching, upright in both leads.

PR interval: 0.16. **QRS interval:** 0.12. **Interpretation:** sinus rhythm with wide QRS.

224. **QRS complexes:** present, all shaped the same within each lead. **Regularity:** irregular. **Heart rate:** 68 to 94, with a mean rate of 80. **P waves:** none present; wavy baseline noted between QRS complexes. **PR interval:** not applicable. **QRS interval:** 0.09. **Interpretation:** atrial fibrillation.

225. **QRS complexes:** present, all shaped the same within each lead. **Regularity:** regular. **Heart rate:** 68. **P waves:** matching, upright in both leads. **PR interval:** 0.14. **QRS interval:** 0.06. **Interpretation:** sinus rhythm.

226. **QRS complexes:** present, all shaped the same within each lead. **Regularity:** regular. **Heart rate:** 62. **P waves:** matching, right in both leads. **PR interval:** 0.12. **QRS interval:** 0.10. **Interpretation:** sinus rhythm.

227. **QRS complexes:** present, all shaped the same within each lead. **Regularity:** regular but interrupted by a premature beat. **Heart rate:** 75. **P waves:** matching, upright in both leads. **PR interval:** 0.22. **QRS interval:** 0.08. **Interpretation:** sinus rhythm with first-degree AV block.

228. **QRS complexes:** present, all shaped the same within each lead. **Regularity:** regular. **Heart rate:** 83. **P waves:** matching, upright in both leads. **PR interval:** 0.12. **QRS interval:** 0.08. **Interpretation:** sinus rhythm.

229. **QRS complexes:** present, all shaped the same. **Regularity:** regular. **Heart rate:** 62. **P waves:** matching, M-shaped. **PR interval:** 0.20. **QRS interval:** 0.10. **Interpretation:** sinus rhythm.

230. **QRS complexes:** present, all shaped the same within each lead. **Regularity:** regular. **Heart rate:** 88. **P waves:** none seen. **PR interval:** not applicable. **QRS interval:** 0.08. **Interpretation:** accelerated junctional rhythm.

231. **QRS complexes:** none noted. **Regularity:** not applicable. **Heart rate:** zero. **P waves:** none. **PR interval:** not applicable. **QRS interval:** not applicable. **Interpretation:** asystole.

232. **QRS complexes:** present, all shaped the same within each lead. **Regularity:** regular. **Heart rate:** 107. **P waves:** matching, inverted following the QRS in both leads. **PR interval:** not applicable. **QRS interval:** 0.08. **Interpretation:** junctional tachycardia. See the blips following the QRS complexes? Those are the inverted P waves.

233. **QRS complexes:** present, all shaped the same within each lead. **Regularity:** regular. **Heart rate:** 100. **P waves:** matching, upright in both leads. **PR interval:** 0.20. **QRS interval:** 0.08. **Interpretation:** sinus rhythm.

234. **QRS complexes:** present, all shaped the same within each lead. **Regularity:** regular. **Heart rate:** 137. **P waves:** none seen. **PR interval:** not applicable. **QRS interval:** hard to measure, but probably about 0.20. **Interpretation:** ventricular tachycardia.

235. **QRS complexes:** present, all shaped the same. **Regularity:** regular. **Heart rate:** 150. **P waves:** matching, upright. **PR interval:** 0.12. **QRS interval:** 0.08. **Interpretation:** sinus tachycardia.

236. **QRS complexes:** present, all shaped the same within each lead. **Regularity:** regular. **Heart rate:** 43. **P waves:** upright and matching in Lead II, biphasic and matching in V_1. **PR interval:** 0.26. **QRS interval:** 0.10. **Interpretation:** sinus bradycardia with first-degree AV block.

237. **QRS complexes:** present, all shaped the same. **Regularity:** irregular. **Heart rate:** 45 to 54, with a mean rate of 50. **P waves:** matching, upright. **PR interval:** 0.18. **QRS interval:** 0.10. **Interpretation:** sinus bradycardia.

238. **QRS complexes:** present, all shaped the same within each lead. **Regularity:** irregular. **Heart rate:** 35 to 60, with mean rate of 50. **P waves:** upright and matching in both leads. The fourth QRS has a P wave at the top of its T wave. P-P interval is regular; atrial rate 60. **PR interval:** 0.24. **QRS interval:** 0.08. **Interpretation:** Mobitz II second-degree AV block.

239. **QRS complexes:** present, all shaped the same within each lead. **Regularity:** irregular. **Heart rate:** 54 to 68, with a mean rate of 60. **P waves:** matching, upright in both leads. **PR interval:** 0.16. **QRS interval:** 0.08. **Interpretation:** sinus arrhythmia.

240. **QRS complexes:** present, all shaped the same within each lead. **Regularity:** irregular. **Heart rate:** 100 to 150, with a mean rate of 140. **P waves:** none noted. **PR interval:** not applicable. **QRS interval:** 0.12. **Interpretation:** ventricular tachycardia.

241. **QRS complexes:** present, all shaped the same within each lead. **Regularity:** regular. **Heart rate:** 107. **P waves:** matching, inverted preceding the QRS. **PR interval:** 0.09. **QRS interval:** 0.08. **Interpretation:** junctional tachycardia.

242. **QRS complexes:** present, all shaped the same within each lead. **Regularity:** regular. **Heart rate:** 137. **P waves:** none noted. **PR interval:** not applicable. **QRS interval:** 0.10. **Interpretation:** SVT.

243. **QRS complexes:** present, all shaped the same within each lead. **Regularity:** irregular. **Heart rate:** 86 to 150, with a mean rate of 120. **P waves:** none seen; wavy baseline noted between QRS complexes. **PR interval:** not applicable. **QRS interval:** 0.08. **Interpretation:** atrial fibrillation.

244. **QRS complexes:** present, all shaped the same. **Regularity:** regular. **Heart rate:** 102. **P waves:** none noted; sawtooth-shaped waves noted between QRS complexes. **PR interval:** not applicable. **QRS interval:** 0.08. **Interpretation:** atrial flutter.

245. **QRS complexes:** present, all shaped the same. **Regularity:** regular. **Heart rate:** 79. **P waves:** matching, upright in Lead II, cannot see Ps in V_1. **PR interval:** 0.14. **QRS interval:** 0.12. **Interpretation:** sinus rhythm with wide QRS.

246. **QRS complexes:** present, all shaped the same within each lead except for beat number 3, which is a different shape. **Regularity:** regular but interrupted by a premature beat. **Heart rate:** 50. **P waves:** matching, upright in Lead II, biphasic in V_1. The third QRS has no P wave. **PR interval:** 0.14. **QRS interval:** 0.08. **Interpretation:** sinus bradycardia with a PJC. The PJC beat has a wide QRS.

247. **QRS complexes:** present, all shaped the same within each lead. **Regularity:** regular. **Heart rate:** 107. **P waves:** matching, upright in both leads. **PR interval:** 0.14. **QRS interval:** 0.08. **Interpretation:** sinus tachycardia.

248. **QRS complexes:** present, all but the sixth shaped the same. The sixth QRS is wider. **Regularity:** regular but interrupted by a premature beat. **Heart rate:** 71. **P waves:** upright and matching in both leads. **PR interval:** 0.14. **QRS interval:** 0.08. **Interpretation:** sinus rhythm with PVC.

249. **QRS complexes:** only one present; then chaotic, spiked, wavy baseline. **Regularity:** not applicable. **Heart rate:** unable to calculate, as only one QRS. **P waves:** none noted. **PR interval:** not applicable **QRS interval:** 0.06 on the one QRS. **Interpretation:** one sinus beat, then V-fib.

250. **QRS complexes:** present, the first two and the last one shaped the same. In between is a run of differently shaped beats. **Regularity:** irregular. **Heart rate:** 94 for the first two beats, then 187 on the run of beats. **P waves:** matching and upright on the first two and the last one beat; no Ps on the other beats. **PR interval:** 0.16. **QRS interval:** 0.10 on the narrow beats, 0.12 on the other beats. **Interpretation:** sinus rhythm with a run of V-tach.

CHAPTER THIRTEEN
Axis Practice EKGs

1. **Left axis deviation.** Lead I is positive and aVF is negative, so there is a left axis deviation.

2. **Normal axis.** Leads I and aVF are both positive, so the axis is in the normal quadrant.

3. **Indeterminate axis.** Leads I and aVF are both negative, so there is indeterminate axis.

4. **Left axis deviation.** Lead I is positive and aVF is negative, giving us a left axis deviation.

5. **Right axis deviation.** Lead I is negative and aVF is positive, so there is a right axis deviation.

6. **Normal axis.** Leads I and aVF are both positive, so the axis is in the normal quadrant.

7. **Normal axis.** Again, Leads I and aVF both are positive, so axis is normal.

BBB/HB Practice

1. **No BBB. LAHB present.** The QRS interval is normal (about 0.10 seconds), so there is no BBB. But there is a small Q in Lead I and a small R in Lead III, so there's a LAHB.

2. **RBBB and LAHB.** There is not the typical RSR′ configuration in V_1—the initial R wave is missing—but it is still a RBBB. The QRS is wide (about 0.12 seconds) and the T wave slopes off opposite the final wave of the QRS complex. There is left axis deviation, which, in the presence of a RBBB, almost always implies a coexisting LAHB.

3. **LBBB.** There is a wide QRS (about 0.14 seconds), and a QS complex in V_1. The T wave is opposite the final part of the QRS.

4. **LBBB.** Again, there is a wide QRS of about 0.13 seconds, a QS in V_1. The T wave is opposite the final wave of the QRS complex.

5. **RBBB and LPHB.** There is a wide QRS with a QR configuration in V_1. Also there's a right axis deviation, which implies LPHB here.

6. **RBBB.** Note the RSR′ configuration in V_1, along with the QRS interval of 0.12 seconds and the T wave opposite the terminal wave of the QRS. The axis here is indeterminate, which does not imply a hemiblock.

7. **LBBB.** Note the QS configuration in V_1 with the QRS interval of 0.14 seconds and the T wave opposite the terminal QRS wave.

8. **RBBB.** Note the RR′ configuration in V_1 along with a QRS interval of about 0.12 seconds and a T wave opposite the terminal QRS wave. The indeterminate axis does not imply hemiblock.

9. **RBBB.** There's an RSR′ in V_1, the QRS interval is 0.16 seconds, and the T wave is opposite the terminal QRS wave. Axis is normal, so no hemiblock.

10. **No BBB or HB.** The QRS interval is normal, about 0.08 seconds.

Hypertrophy Practice

1. **LVH.** The QRS in V_1 is about 8 mm deep, and the R wave in V_5 is 41 mm tall (it extends up beyond the QRS in V_4). Total is greater than 35 mm, so this EKG meets and exceeds the criteria for LVH.

2. **Low voltage.** The QRS complexes are short in all leads, especially aVL, which is tiny.

3. **Normal.** There is no hypertrophy or low voltage.

4. **RVH.** The R wave in V_1 is as tall as, if not slightly taller than, the S wave is deep and there is right axis deviation. The T wave is not inverted here as it often is, but that is not an absolute requirement for RVH.

5. **LVH.** The QRS in V_1 is 23 mm deep and in V_5 is 15 mm tall, for a total of 38 mm, more than enough to meet the voltage criteria for LVH.

Practice Quiz

1. If the QRS complexes in Leads I and aVF are both negative, **the axis is in the indeterminate axis quadrant.**

2. **False.** Right bundle branch block can be a normal variant, seen in normal hearts.

3. Sagging ST segments are associated with **digitalis effect.**

4. **False.** Tall pointy T waves are typical of hyperkalemia, not RBBB.

5. Three causes of axis deviations are any three of the following: **normal variant, advanced pregnancy or obesity, myocardial infarction, hypertrophy, arrhythmias, chronic lung disease,** and **pulmonary embolism.**

6. The voltage criteria for LVH is the following: **If the S wave in V_1 added to the R wave in V_5 or V_6 (whichever is taller) is greater than or equal to 35, there is LVH.**

7. **False.** RVH is not always associated with an inverted T wave.

8. Hypertrophy is **excessive growth of tissue.**

9. Hypokalemia **causes the T wave to flatten.**

10. In a BBB, the **QRS interval must be at least 0.12 seconds.**

Critical Thinking Exercises

1. If both bundle branches became blocked simultaneously and no lower pacemaker took over, the rhythm would initially be **P wave asystole, then eventually asystole.** The sinus node, unaffected by the BBB, would continue sending out its impulses as usual for awhile. This would provide the P waves. There would be no QRS complexes following these P waves because the bundle branch blocks would prevent the sinus impulses from reaching the ventricles. Thus the rhythm is initially P wave asystole.

Eventually the sinus node would slow down and stop, as it becomes more and more compromised by the lack of blood flow. Thus the P waves would stop. This would be asystole. Remember, if there are no QRS complexes, there is no pulse and no blood flow. The sinus node, like all heart tissues, requires blood flow to function. Thus the sinus node would eventually fail because of a lack of perfusion.

2.

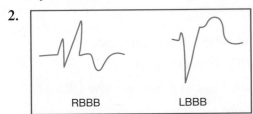

RBBB   LBBB

3. What happened is **she delivered the baby and her axis, which had been deviated to the left because of advanced pregnancy, is now back to normal.**

CHAPTER FOURTEEN
MI Practice

1. **Extensive anterior STEMI, acute.** Note the ST segment elevation in Leads I, aVL, V_1 to V_6, along with reciprocal ST depression in II, III, and aVF. The T waves are upright.

2. **Inferior STEMI, age indeterminate.** Note the significant Q waves in II, III, and aVF, along with inverted T waves. The ST segment is at baseline. Remember STEMIs develop Q waves as they evolve, and the ST segment retreats toward the baseline.

3. **Lateral wall STEMI, acute.** Note the ST elevation, significant Q waves, and inverted T waves in I, aVL, and V_5 to V_6, along with reciprocal ST depression in II, III, and aVF.

4. **Anteroseptal STEMI, acute.** Note the ST elevation and inverted T in V_1 to V_2, along with reciprocal ST depression in II, III, and aVF.

5. **No MI. Lateral wall ischemia present.** Note the T wave inversion in I, aVL, and V_5 to V_6. Remember that T wave inversion represents ischemia. There is no ST elevation or depression and no significant Q waves.

6. **Anteroseptal and inferior STEMI, both old.** Note the significant Q waves in V_1 to V_4 (anterior and septal leads), along with essentially normal ST segments. The ST does slope upward a bit in V_1 to V_4, but it is not frankly elevated. There is also an old inferior MI. There are significant Q waves in III and aVF, but not in II; aVF is tiny, but you can see a Q wave there. That Q wave in aVF is significant because it is about half the size of the R wave—more than deep enough to meet the criteria. The T waves in the inferior leads are not inverted.

7. **Inferior and anterior-lateral STEMI, acute.** There is ST elevation in II, III, and aVF (inferior leads) and ST elevation and QS complexes in V_3 to V_6 (anterior and lateral leads). Leads V_1 and V_2 both have tiny R waves—those are not QS complexes there. It appears this patient started off with an anterior-lateral MI, which then extended into the inferior wall. The Q waves in V_3 to V_6 indicate that that infarct area is older than that in the inferior leads, where there are no significant Q waves.

8. **Inferior STEMI, acute.** There is ST elevation in II, III, and aVF, along with upright T waves and no significant Q waves as yet. Also note the reciprocal ST depression in I, aVL, and V_1 to V_3.

9. **Inferior-lateral STEMI, old.** There are significant Q waves in II, III, aVF (inferior leads), and V_6 (lateral lead) with upright T waves and baseline ST segments. Lead V_5 looks like it has a tiny R wave, not a Q wave. Also note the essentially nonexistent R wave progression in the precordial leads. This could imply an additional old anterior MI, or it could be caused by other factors.

10. **Inferior STEMI, acute.** Note the ST elevation in II, III, and aVF with reciprocal ST depression in I, aVL, and V_1 to V_3. There is a significant Q in III, but not yet in II or aVF.

Practice Quiz

1. The three Is of infarction are **ischemia, injury,** and **infarction.**

2. **A STEMI causes ST elevation, T wave inversion, and significant Q waves to develop on the EKG. The NSTEMI does not cause development of significant Q waves.**

3. Occlusion of the **left anterior descending coronary artery** causes anterior MI.

4. The normal indicative changes of an MI are **ST elevation, significant Q waves,** and **T wave inversions.**

5. Reciprocal changes are seen **in the area electrically opposite the damaged area.**

6. If there is ST elevation in II, III, and aVF, **the MI is acute inferior.**

7. If there is a significant Q wave in V_1 to V_3 with baseline ST segments and upright T waves, **the MI is an old anteroseptal MI.**

8. If the transition zone is in V_1 to V_2, **there is counterclockwise rotation of the heart.**

9. The kind of MI that can be diagnosed by inverting (turning over) the EKG and looking at Leads V_1 and V_2 from behind is the **posterior MI.**

10. The **circumflex coronary artery** supplies the lateral wall of the left ventricle.

Critical Thinking Exercises

1.
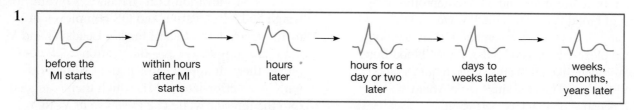

2. If Mr. Milner, a 69-year-old man with a history of chest pain, arrives in your ER with newly inverted T waves in Leads II, III, and aVF, it is likely **he has new ischemia in the inferior wall of the left ventricle.**

3. If an hour later Mr. Milner is doubled over with crushing chest pain and his EKG now shows marked ST elevation in II, III, aVF and V_{5-6}, **he is now injuring the inferior and lateral wall of the left ventricle.** This is an acute MI in progress, which is reversible if he receives PCI or thrombolytic medications. If the MI in progress is untreated, myocardial tissue will die and significant Q waves will develop in the inferior and lateral leads on his EKG.

4. Mr. Jones's EKG shows inverted T waves in II, III, and aVF—changes consistent with ischemia.

5. He is now having an MI. Leads II, III, and aVF show ST segment elevations and upright T waves. Notice that the T waves, which were inverted on the first EKG showing ischemia, now become upright. This is common once myocardial injury begins.

CHAPTER FIFTEEN
12-Lead EKG Practice

Note: For the intervals, it is acceptable if your answer is within 0.02 secs of displayed answer.

EKG 1

- **Rhythm and rate:** Sinus rhythm with first-degree AV block, rate 62.
- **PR:** 0.20–0.24 **QRS:** 0.16 **QT:** 0.44–0.48.
- **Axis:** Normal. Both Leads I's and aVF's QRS complexes are positive.
- **BBB/HB:** Left bundle branch block.
- **Hypertrophy:** None.
- **Miscellaneous effects:** None. The widened QRS here is from the LBBB, not from hyperkalemia.
- **Infarction:** No evidence of ischemia or infarction.

EKG 2

- **Rhythm and rate:** Sinus rhythm, rate 94.
- **PR:** 0.12 **QRS:** 0.06 **QT:** 0.34.
- **Axis:** Normal. I and aVF have positive QRSs.
- **BBB/HB:** None.
- **Hypertrophy:** None.
- **Miscellaneous effects:** None.
- **Infarction:** No evidence of ischemia or infarction.

EKG 3

- **Rhythm and rate:** Sinus rhythm, rate 94.
- **PR:** 0.16 **QRS:** 0.14 **QT:** 0.40.
- **Axis:** Left axis deviation. Lead I is positive; aVF is negative.
- **BBB/HB:** RBBB and LAHB. A RBBB with a left axis deviation is almost always LAHB.
- **Hypertrophy:** None.
- **Miscellaneous effects:** None.
- **Infarction:** No evidence of ischemia or infarction. There is ST depression in many leads, but this is probably bundle related rather than true ischemia.

EKG 4

- **Rhythm and rate:** Sinus rhythm, rate 68.
- **PR:** 0.16 **QRS:** 0.08 **QT:** 0.40
- **Axis:** Normal. I and aVF are both positive.
- **BBB/HB:** None.
- **Hypertrophy:** None.
- **Miscellaneous effects:** None.
- **Infarction:** No evidence of ischemia or infarction.

EKG 5

- **Rhythm and rate:** Sinus tachycardia, rate 150.
- **PR:** 0.14 **QRS:** 0.06 **QT:** 0.24.
- **Axis:** Normal.
- **BB/HB:** None.

- **Hypertrophy:** None. In fact, the voltage is pretty low throughout most leads.
- **Miscellaneous effects:** None.
- **Infarction:** No evidence of ischemia or infarction. Those are not Q waves in V_1 to V_2, in case you thought it was an anteroseptal MI. There's a teeny R wave there.

EKG 6

- **Rhythm and rate:** Sinus rhythm, rate 71.
- **PR:** 0.20 **QRS:** 0.12 **QT:** 0.40.
- **Axis:** Left axis deviation. Lead I is positive, and aVF is negative.
- **BBB/HB:** LBBB.
- **Hypertrophy:** None.
- **Miscellaneous effects:** None.
- **Infarction:** No evidence of ischemia or infarction.

EKG 7

- **Rhythm and rate:** Atrial flutter with 2:1 conduction. Atrial rate 250, ventricular rate 115.
- **PR:** 0.16 **QRS:** 0.10 **QT:** 0.28.
- **Axis:** Left axis deviation. Lead I is positive, and aVF is negative.
- **BBB/HB:** None.
- **Hypertrophy:** LVH by voltage criteria.
- **Miscellaneous effects:** No miscellaneous effects. The incredibly tall, pointy T wave in V_3 is related to the huge QRS voltage in that lead.
- **Infarction:** Anteroseptal and inferior wall MI. Note the ST segment elevation in II, III, aVF, and V_1 to V_4. There are already significant Q waves in V_1 to V_3. This is a massive MI.

EKG 8

- **Rhythm and rate:** Sinus rhythm, rate 75.
- **PR:** 0.18 **QRS:** 0.13 **QT:** 0.42.
- **Axis:** Left axis deviation. Lead I is positive, and aVF is negative.
- **BBB/HB:** RBBB.
- **Hypertrophy:** None by our voltage criteria.
- **Miscellaneous effects:** None.
- **Infarction:** Probable old anteroseptal MI, as there is a loss of the normal small R wave in V_1 to V_2.

EKG 9

- **Rhythm and rate:** Sinus rhythm, rate 65.
- **PR:** 0.18 **QRS:** 0.06 **QT:** 0.36.
- **Axis:** Normal. Leads I and aVF are both positive.
- **BBB/HB:** None.
- **Hypertrophy:** LVH. The S wave in V_2 is 11; the R wave in V_5 is 26. Total is 37.
- **Miscellaneous effects:** None.
- **Infarction:** Probable early repolarization. Note the very slight concave ST elevation in II, III, aVF, and V_3 to V_5. It would help to know the age of this patient and the symptoms (if any) to identify this with a higher probability of accuracy.

EKG 10

- **Rhythm and rate:** Atrial flutter with 2:1 conduction. No way, you say? Look at V_1. See the teeny spike in the ST segment? That's a flutter wave. There's another one before the QRS. If the gain had been turned up higher, this would have been much more obvious. Atrial rate is about 250; ventricular rate is 125.
- **PR:** Not applicable **QRS:** 0.06 **QT:** 0.24.
- **Axis:** Left axis deviation. Lead I is positive, and aVF is negative.
- **BBB/HB:** *Maybe* a LAHB, but not sure we can really say there's a Q wave in Lead I.
- **Hypertrophy:** None. In fact, the voltage is rather low in the frontal leads.
- **Miscellaneous effects:** None.
- **Infarction:** Acute anterior-septal-lateral MI. Note the ST elevation in V_1 to V_6. There are significant Q waves in V_1 to V_5. There is also *very slight* ST coving in III and aVF, so there may also be an inferior MI starting up.

EKG 11

- **Rhythm and rate:** Sinus tachycardia, rate 101.
- **PR:** 0.12 **QRS:** 0.06 **QT:** 0.32.
- **Axis:** Left axis deviation. Lead I is positive, and aVF is negative.
- **BBB/HB:** None.
- **Hypertrophy:** None.
- **Miscellaneous effects:** None.
- **Infarction:** Old inferior MI and old anterior MI. Note the significant Q waves in Leads III and aVF and also in V_2 to V_3. Also note the poor R wave progression.

The transition zone is V_5 and should be around V_3 to V_4.

EKG 12

- **Rhythm and rate:** Sinus rhythm, rate 60.
- **PR:** 0.20 **QRS:** 0.14 **QT:** 0.46.
- **Axis:** Left axis deviation. Lead I is positive, and aVF is negative.
- **BBB/HB:** RBBB and LAHB. There is a QR configuration in V_1.
- **Hypertrophy:** None.
- **Miscellaneous effects:** None.
- **Infarction:** Acute anterior-septal-lateral MI. Note the ST elevation in V_1 to V_5. There are significant Q waves in V_1 to V_3.

EKG 13

- **Rhythm and rate:** Sinus rhythm, rate 75.
- **PR:** 0.12 **QRS:** 0.14 **QT:** 0.42.
- **Axis:** Normal.
- **BBB/HB:** LBBB. Note the *huge* QS wave in V_1.
- **Hypertrophy:** None.
- **Miscellaneous effects:** None.
- **Infarction:** None.

EKG 14

- **Rhythm and rate:** Sinus rhythm, rate 83.
- **PR:** 0.14 **QRS:** 0.08 **QT:** 0.34.
- **Axis:** Normal.
- **BBB/HB:** None.
- **Hypertrophy:** None.
- **Miscellaneous effects:** None.
- **Infarction:** Acute inferior MI. Note the ST elevation in II, III, and aVF, along with reciprocal ST depression in I, aVL, and V_2 to V_6.

EKG 15

- **Rhythm and rate:** Atrial fibrillation with uncontrolled ventricular response.
- **PR:** Not applicable **QRS:** 0.04 **QT:** 0.16.
- **Axis:** Normal.
- **BBB/HB:** None.

- **Hypertrophy:** None. In fact, the voltage is rather low in the frontal leads.
- **Miscellaneous effects:** Digitalis effect? ST segments look a bit scooped in Leads II and V_6. This may be simply from the rapid heart rate, however.
- **Infarction:** None. There are widespread inverted T waves, but this isn't a surprise, given the heart rate. Some ischemia may be occurring.

EKG 16

- **Rhythm and rate:** Atrial fibrillation, rate 100 to150, mean rate 130.
- **PR:** Not applicable **QRS:** 0.06 **QT:** 0.28.
- **Axis:** Normal.
- **BBB/HB:** None.
- **Hypertrophy:** None. In fact, the voltage is rather low in the frontal leads.
- **Miscellaneous effects:** None.
- **Infarction:** None.

EKG 17

- **Rhythm and rate:** Sinus rhythm, rate 75.
- **PR:** 0.16 **QRS:** 0.14 **QT:** 0.40.
- **Axis:** Left axis deviation. Lead I is slightly more positive than negative, and aVF is slightly more negative than positive.
- **BBB/HB:** RBBB and LAHB.
- **Hypertrophy:** None.
- **Miscellaneous effects:** None.
- **Infarction:** Acute anterior MI. Note the ST elevation in V_2 to V_4.

EKG 18

- **Rhythm and rate:** Sinus rhythm, rate 94.
- **PR:** 0.16 **QRS:** 0.10 **QT:** 0.36.
- **Axis:** Normal. The aVF's QRS has a little blip downward and then is positive.
- **BBB/HB:** None.
- **Hypertrophy:** None.
- **Miscellaneous effects:** None.
- **Infarction:** Acute inferior-lateral MI. Note the ST elevation in II, III, aVF, and V_5 to V_6. V_5 to V_6 is much shallower elevation than II, III, and aVF, so you might miss it at first. But do you see it now?

EKG 19

- **Rhythm and rate:** Sinus rhythm, rate 88, with one PVC.
- **PR:** 0.12 **QRS:** 0.08 **QT:** 0.32.
- **Axis:** Left axis deviation. Lead I is positive, and aVF is negative.
- **BBB/HB:** None.
- **Hypertrophy:** None. In fact, the voltage is rather low in the frontal leads.
- **Miscellaneous effects:** None.
- **Infarction:** None.

EKG 20

- **Rhythm and rate:** Sinus rhythm, rate 65.
- **PR:** 0.16 **QRS:** 0.06 **QT:** 0.36.
- **Axis:** Normal.
- **BBB/HB:** None.
- **Hypertrophy:** None.
- **Miscellaneous effects:** None.
- **Infarction:** None.

CHAPTER SIXTEEN
DDD versus VVI Practice

1. **Cannot tell which kind of pacemaker.** Since there are no paced beats at all, it is not possible to tell if it's a DDD or a VVI pacemaker.
2. **VVI.** There are pacemaker spikes preceding the QRS complexes, and there are no P waves in sight. Had this been a DDD pacemaker, there should have been some paced P waves also.
3. **DDD.** There are pacemaker spikes preceding the P waves and the QRS complexes.
4. **VVI.** There are four intrinsic beats and two paced beats on the strip. The paced beats pace only the ventricle. With this long a pause before a paced beat kicks in, a DDD pacemaker would have provided a paced P wave as well.
5. **DDD.** This strip has a little of everything. The first beat is all intrinsic. The second beat paces atrium and ventricle, as evidenced by the pacemaker spikes preceding the P wave and the QRS. The third beat has a paced P wave and an intrinsic QRS. The fourth, sixth, and seventh beats are all intrinsic. The fifth beat has an intrinsic P wave followed by a paced QRS.

Pacemaker Malfunctions Practice

1. **Undersensing and loss of capture.** We have pacemaker spikes in inappropriate places, such as inside the first QRS complex. It is clear this pacemaker is not sensing the QRS complexes, since it does nothing in response to those intrinsic complexes. The pacemaker should have been inhibited by the patient's intrinsic QRS complexes. Also note the spikes are regular at a rate of 60. This is essentially a fixed-rate pacemaker now because it's not sensing anything. In addition, there is loss of capture, as evidenced by the pacemaker spikes not followed by Ps or QRSs at times when they should have been. The patient's underlying rhythm is idioventricular rhythm with a rate of 23.
2. **No malfunction at this time.** This strip shows a normally functioning DDD pacemaker. Note the upward atrial spikes followed by a tiny blip of a P wave, then a ventricular spike followed by a wide QRS. Although the pacemaker seems fine right now, it could be that it malfunctions intermittently, causing the symptoms, so the patient will still need close observation. It is also possible that the patient's dizziness and syncope were caused by something totally unrelated to the pacemaker.
3. **No malfunction noted.** This strip shows a normally functioning DDD pacemaker. See the small intrinsic P waves preceding each QRS? The pacemaker senses them and tracks them, providing the paced QRS to follow those Ps since the patient does not have her own QRS complexes in the programmed time.
4. **Failure to fire.** There are two intrinsic P waves on this strip. The pacemaker should have sensed them and provided a paced QRS to follow them. In addition, it should have paced the atrium and then the ventricle, as necessary, at its programmed rate of 70. It didn't. There's not a pacemaker spike in sight.
5. **No malfunction noted.** The pacemaker rate is set at 60, and it fires at 60 when the atrial fibrillation slows down. Note the pacing interval from spike to spike on the three paced beats. Now look at the interval between the second QRS and the paced beat that follows. It's exactly the same interval. The pacemaker is therefore sensing the underlying rhythm, and it's firing and capturing appropriately.

Practice Quiz

1. Digitalis is classified as a **cardiac glycoside.**
2. Class I antiarrhythmic medications **affect phase 0 of the action potential by blocking the influx of sodium into the cardiac cell.**
3. Atropine **increases the heart rate.**
4. Vasoconstriction **causes the blood pressure to increase.**
5. **True.** The AED is meant for use by the lay public.
6. Class III antiarrhythmic medications **affect phase 3 of the action potential. They interfere with the movement of potassium into the cardiac cell during repolarization.**
7. **Therapeutic hypothermia is used in post–cardiac arrest patients who regain spontaneous circulation. Their body temperature is lowered to 90 to 93 degrees in order to decrease ischemia, particularly of the brain, that can result from the cardiac arrest.**
8. The 3 letters of the pacemaker code refer to **the chamber paced, the chamber sensed,** and **the response to sensed events.**
9. Cardioversion differs from defibrillation in that **cardioversion is synchronized with the cardiac cycle; defibrillation is not synchronized.**
10. Antitachycardia pacing is used to **slow the heart rate—to abort a tachycardia. The pacemaker fires out a series of rapid electrical impulses to interrupt the tachycardia's circuit, thereby stopping that rhythm.** Pacing for bradycardia involves sending out an electrical impulse to increase the heart rate.

Critical Thinking Exercises

1. a. Atrial Fibrillation—**cardiovert.**
   b. V-tach with pulse—**cardiovert.**
   c. V-fib—**defibrillate.**
   d. V-tach without pulse—**defibrillate.**
   e. SVT—**cardiovert.**

2. a. The rhythm **is atrial flutter with two flutter waves to each QRS.** Heart rate is 150.
   b. **The pacemaker is doing nothing** that we can see. We have to assume it is sensing the patient's own rhythm and knows it doesn't need to fire.
   c. Since the patient has a temporary pacemaker in place and therefore has the pulse generator at the bedside in easy reach, **we can use the pacemaker to overdrive this rhythm and slow the heart rate.**
   d. The rhythm is **atrial fibrillation; heart rate mean is 40; range is 19 to 71.**
   e. **The pacemaker is doing nothing.** It's set at a rate of 60 so it shouldn't let the heart rate drop below that.

   f. There is indeed a pacer malfunction—it's **failure to fire.**
   g. **The battery may need to be changed or the pacer wire or cable may need to be changed.**
   h. With the first rhythm, the **heart rate is very rapid, causing decreased time for the ventricles to fill with blood.** Less blood goes in, so less blood is pumped out to the body. With the second rhythm, the **heart rate is very slow. Unless the heart is able to compensate for the decreased heart rate by increasing the amount of blood pumped out with each beat, cardiac output will fall.** Both rhythms can therefore result in Mr. Johnson's low blood pressure and feeling of faintness.

3. a. The symptoms are caused by his use of nitroglycerine and sildenafil together. Sildenafil must not be used with nitrate medications as they can cause a dangerous drop in blood pressure. With a low blood pressure, the heart does not receive adequate blood flow—it can become ischemic and can infarct.
   b. Teach Mr. Lohtrip about the proper use of his medications.

CHAPTER SEVENTEEN
Stress Test Assessment Practice

1. **Continue.** The EKG shows sinus tachycardia, which is expected. There are no ST segment changes that warrant stopping the test.
2. **Terminate.** The heart rate before the test was 70 and now varies from about 33 to 58. Note the P wave shapes vary also. The heart rate during a stress test should increase, not decrease. This decreased heart rate could signal decreased cardiac reserve.
3. **Terminate.** This is third-degree AV block, an ominous development during a stress test. The heart rate should speed up during the test.
4. **Terminate.** There is marked ST segment elevation in Leads II, III, and aVF and V_5 to V_6. This is an indication of an MI in progress. Note the reciprocal ST depression in I, aVL, and V_2 to V_4.
5. **Continue.** Sinus tachycardia is expected during a stress test. As long as the patient is tolerating the rhythm, the test may continue.
6. **False positive.** The stress test is positive for CAD—note the >1.5 mm ST segment depression in I, aVL, and V_5 to V_6. But the angiogram is negative, and that's the gold standard for diagnosing CAD. The stress test result is therefore a false positive.
7. **False negative.** The stress test is negative—no ST depression—but the angiogram is positive.

8. **False positive.** The stress test is positive—striking ST depression in V_1 to V_6—but the angiogram is negative.

9. **True positive.** Both stress test and angiogram are positive. Note the ST depression in V_1 to V_6.

10. **True negative.** Both stress test and angiogram are negative.

Practice Quiz

1. The type of monitor worn for 24 hours to uncover any arrhythmias or ST segment changes that might be causing the patient's symptoms is the **Holter monitor.**

2. Indications for stress testing are the following (choose any three): **to determine the presence or absence of CAD, for post-CABG and post-PTCA evaluation, for diagnosis and treatment of exercise-induced arrhythmias, as follow-up to cardiac rehab, and to evaluate individuals with a family history of heart disease.**

3. Bayes's theorem says that **the validity of a test result depends not only on the test accuracy, but also on the probability that the patient in question would have the disease.**

4. ST segment elevation of 5 mm is **indicative of a positive stress test.** ST elevation that high indicates an infarction beginning.

5. **True.** Patients on beta-blockers and nitrates might be advised to avoid taking these medications for a period of time before the stress test.

6. Target heart rate is **220 minus the patient's age.**

7. Event monitoring differs from Holter monitoring in that **event monitoring can be worn or used over a prolonged period,** whereas Holter monitoring is typically used for only 24 hours. Also, Holter monitoring involves continuous recording of the rhythm, whereas **event monitoring records only abnormalities or rhythms it's programmed to record or that are present when activated by the patient.**

8. The most commonly used protocol for treadmill stress testing is the **Bruce protocol.**

9. The protocol used most often for post-MI patients just before or following hospital discharge is the **Naughton protocol.**

10. A MET is a **metabolic equivalent, a measurement of oxygen consumption, with which 1 MET is the resting oxygen consumption of a seated adult.**

Critical Thinking Exercises

1. Of only slight concern on this EKG is the sinus tachycardia that is present at rest. Mr. Cameron is overweight and a smoker and is probably nervous about the test, so it is not surprising that his heart rate is a little elevated.

2. Mr. Cameron is overweight and a smoker, so his getting short of breath early on is not of too much concern.

3. The test should continue as these changes are normal and expected.

4. The rhythm is a bradycardia with bigeminal PVCs, then ventricular fibrillation.

5. The appropriate course of action is to get Mr. Cameron off the treadmill and to defibrillate him immediately.

6. What you should have done differently was to pay more attention to Mr. Cameron's alarming change in blood pressure and his symptoms—cool, clammy skin, dizziness, pallor, fatigue. He was in distress and the test should have been terminated.

CHAPTER EIGHTEEN
Scenario A: Mr. Johnson

1. Of concern is the **ST segment elevation in Lead II** on this strip. The sinus bradycardia is not a concern, especially since Mr. Johnson had been asleep, but the ST elevation is worrisome.

2. **Mr. Johnson is having an inferior wall MI,** as evidenced by the ST elevation in Leads II, III, and aVF and by the reciprocal ST depression in the anterior leads.

3. **Nitroglycerin dilates coronary arteries and thus increases the flow to the tissues.**

4. **The oxygen will improve tissue concentration of oxygen and can help prevent arrhythmias and decrease the heart's workload.**

5. Thrombolytic medications **dissolve blood clots.**

6. The danger of giving thrombolytics to someone who had recent surgery is that **severe bleeding may occur at the surgical site.**

7. The rhythm is **ventricular tachycardia.** Heart rate is about 300.

8. **Potassium deficit (hypokalemia)** can cause V-tach.

9. **Hypoxia** is another blood abnormality that can cause V-tach.

10. **Amiodarone or lidocaine** could be used to abolish the V-tach.

11. **Morphine** is another medication that can be used to treat chest pain.

12. **The MI is extending into the lateral wall now,** as evidenced by the new ST elevation in Leads V_5 to V_6.

13. This rhythm is **2:1 AV block.** There are two P waves to every QRS on this strip.

14. This rhythm can **cause the cardiac output to drop.**

15. The nurse should now **give atropine** to speed up the heart rate until a transcutaneous pacemaker can be utilized.
16. The block could be at the **AV node or the bundle branches.**
17. If the block were at the bundle branches, **atropine may have no effect on the heart rate.** Atropine speeds up the rate of the sinus node and increases AV conduction, causing the impulses to come more rapidly. The impulses blast through the AV node only to arrive at the still-blocked bundle branches (atropine has no effect on the bundle branches). Epinephrine and/or pacing would be indicated for a block at the bundle branches.
18. This rhythm is **sinus rhythm.**
19. **Mr. Johnson should have no symptoms** from this rhythm. He should in fact feel much better now that his heart rate is more normal.
20. The two coronary arteries blocked were probably the **right coronary artery, which supplies the inferior wall of the left ventricle, and the circumflex, which supplies the lateral wall.**

Scenario B: Ms. Capitano

1. The rhythm is **SVT.** The heart rate is about 150, the rhythm is regular, and P waves are not discernible.
2. The likely cause of this rhythm in this case is **excessive caffeine intake.**
3. **The heart rate slowed dramatically to a junctional bradycardia.** This is not unusual after adenosine administration. In fact, sometimes the heart completely stops for a few seconds before the sinus node kicks back in.
4. **The tachycardia is dropping her cardiac output to dangerously low levels.**

Scenario C: Mr. Farley

1. The rhythm is **slow atrial fibrillation.** Note the wavy, undulating baseline and the absence of P waves.
2. **In atrial fibrillation, there is no atrial kick at all,** thus causing a drop in cardiac output of about 15% to 30%.
3. **Digitalis toxicity can cause almost any arrhythmia, such as junctional tachycardia, atrial tachycardia, sinus arrests, sinus blocks, all degrees of AV blocks, and slow junctional and ventricular rhythms.**
4. The rhythm is **asystole.**
5. **Atropine and epinephrine** would be appropriate to give, as they both work to speed up the heart rate. Vasopressin could be given in place of the first or second dose of epinephrine. Epinephrine and

vasopressin can help restore pumping function in cardiac arrest.
6. A pacemaker would **prevent Mr. Farley's heart rate from going too slow.**
7. Loss of capture is evidenced by the **pacemaker spikes not followed by a QRS complex.**
8. Capture might be restored by **repositioning Mr. Farley in bed or by increasing the voltage sent out by the pacemaker.**
9. A pacemaker provides the possibility of **overdriving the tachycardia.** The pacemaker rate is dialed up to a rate exceeding the patient's heart rate. The pacemaker then assumes control of (usurps) the underlying rhythm. The pacemaker can then be slowly turned down, allowing the sinus node to assume control.
10. **Amiodarone decreases the irritability of the ventricle and makes it less responsive to ventricular impulses.**
11. Mr. Farley should be instructed to **follow his physician's prescription, not to add or subtract doses on his own. If he does not feel well, he should contact his physician or go to the hospital ER.**

Scenario D: Mr. Lew

1. This EKG reveals that **Mr. Lew has suffered an extensive anterior MI,** as evidenced by the ST elevation in I, aVL, and all the precordial leads, along with reciprocal ST depression in the inferior leads.
2. This rhythm is **accelerated idioventricular rhythm.**
3. It usually requires **no treatment.** AIVR is usually well-tolerated.
4. **It was believed in the past that the occurrence of AIVR following use of thrombolytics was a sign of reperfusion of the myocardium,** but recent research has shown that not to be the case.
5. Mr. Lew has now **extended his MI into the inferior wall,** as evidenced by the new ST elevation in II, III, and aVF. This is a catastrophic development.
6. **The right coronary artery is also blocked.**
7. The ST depression in the first EKG was **a reciprocal change.**
8. The rhythm is **ventricular fibrillation.**
9. The rhythm is **agonal rhythm (dying heart).**

Scenario E: Mrs. Epstein

1. The rhythm is **third-degree AV block.** Note that the P-P intervals are regular and the R-R intervals are also regular, but at a different rate. The PR intervals vary.
2. **Her pacemaker is doing nothing.** There are no pacemaker spikes anywhere.

3. The likely cause of this is a **dead pacemaker battery.**
4. The rhythm is **dual-chamber pacing.** Note the pacemaker spikes preceding the P waves and QRS complexes.
5. **The pacemaker is functioning properly.**

Scenario F: Mr. Calico

1. The rhythm is **asystole.** There is a flat line—no P waves, QRS complexes, or T waves.
2. **He would have no pulse, no breathing, no movement. His skin would be cool and ashen or cyanotic in color.**
3. Treatment would include **immediate CPR and administration of intravenous atropine and epinephrine or vasopressin.**
4. The rhythm is **SVT,** heart rate 150. This is a typical reaction to atropine and/or epinephrine—the heart rate speeds up dramatically.
5. There is an **anteroseptal MI.** Note the ST elevation in V_1 to V_4, with reciprocal ST depression in II, III, and aVF.
6. **The ST segment has returned to normal,** indicating the MI has been aborted.
7. **The problem was the nurse tried to cardiovert V-fib.** Cardioversion requires that the electrical shock to the heart be synchronized with the QRS complex. In V-fib there are no QRS complexes with which to synchronize, so the shock is never delivered. The nurse must change the machine setting to **defibrillate** (take it off synchronous mode) and try again.

Scenario G: Mrs. Taylor

1. **Hyperkalemia is elevated blood potassium level.** It can cause tall, pointy T waves and eventually wide QRS complexes. The EKG shows very wide QRS complexes.
2. The rhythm is **idioventricular rhythm,** rate about 28. Note the slow heart rate and the wide QRS complexes.
3. **The QRS complex has narrowed.**

Scenario H: Mr. Foster

1. The rhythm is **atrial fibrillation, heart rate 94 to 167, mean rate 120.**
2. The physician did not want to cardiovert Mr. Foster because **she didn't know how long he'd been in**

atrial fibrillation. Cardioversion could send blood clots out of his atria into the coronary arteries, his brain arteries, or his pulmonary artery, causing MI, stroke, or pulmonary embolus.
3. It's a **STEMI.** There is ST segment elevation.
4. The MI is **extensive anterior.**
5. Cocaine can cause **coronary artery spasm,** which can occlude blood flow to the myocardium in a given area and can cause MIs.

Scenario I: Mr. Frye

1. The rhythm is sinus **rhythm for the first three beats, then changing to PAT.** The fourth beat is a PAC and so are the beats that follow. This "run of PACs" is called PAT.
2. The heart rate starts off **at 100 and then increases to about 187 once in PAT. Mean rate is 170.**
3. The **vagus nerve slows conduction through the AV node and slows the heart rate.**
4. The rhythm is **sinus rhythm with a borderline first-degree AV block. PR interval is 0.20 seconds.**
5. Adenosine can cause **a brief period of asystole.**
6. **No, that is not evident on this strip.**
7. Other treatments could include **beta-blockers, calcium channel blockers, digitalis,** and **electrical cardioversion.**

Scenario J: Mrs. Terry

1. The rhythm is **sinus rhythm with first-degree AV block (PR interval about 0.22 seconds), heart rate 100.**
2. There is **ST segment elevation.**
3. The EKG shows **ST elevation in Leads II, III, and aVF along with reciprocal ST depression in Leads I, aVL, and V_1 to V_5. There's a tiny bit of ST elevation in V_6. Thus there is an inferior MI (II, III, and aVF) with perhaps lateral wall involvement (V_6).**
4. The preferred treatment for this acute MI is **PCI.**
5. The suspected involved coronary artery would be the **left anterior descending** (with maybe a bit starting up in the circumflex, causing that little ST elevation in V_6).

Glossary

Absolute refractory period: The period in which the cardiac cell will not respond to any stimulus, no matter how strong.

Acetylcholine: A hormone released as a result of parasympathetic stimulation.

Action potential: The depolarization and repolarization events that take place at the cell membrane. Also refers to the diagram associated with these polarity events.

Acute: Newly occurring.

AED: A defibrillator meant for use by the lay public.

Age indeterminate: A recent ST elevation MI, but can't be sure of the MI's exact age.

Agonal rhythm: A ventricular rhythm characterized by slow, irregular QRS complexes and absent P waves. Also called *dying heart.*

AICD: An implanted device that shocks the heart out of certain dangerous rhythms.

Algorithm: A flowchart.

Amplitude: The height of the waves and complexes on the EKG.

Angina: Chest pain caused by a decrease in myocardial blood flow.

Anginal equivalent: An individual's version of chest pain. May not involve pain at all—could be shortness of breath, fatigue, or other symptoms.

Angiogram: An invasive procedure in which dye is injected into blood vessels in order to determine their patency (openness).

Antegrade: In a forward direction.

Anterior STEMI: ST elevation MI affecting the anterior wall of the left ventricle.

Anterior wall: The front side of the left ventricle.

Anteroseptal: Pertaining to the anterior and septal walls of the left ventricle.

Anteroseptal STEMI: ST elevation MI affecting the septum and part or all of the anterior wall of the left ventricle.

Antiarrhythmic: Medications used to treat or prevent arrhythmias.

Anticoagulants: Medications used to prevent blood clot formation.

Antihypertensives: Medications used to treat hypertension.

Antitachycardia pacing: A special pacemaker function that interrupts tachycardias and helps convert the rhythm back to sinus rhythm.

Aorta: Largest artery in the body, into which the left ventricle empties.

Aortic stenosis: Narrowed opening to the aortic valve.

Aortic valve: Valve located between the left ventricle and aorta.

Apex: The pointy part of the heart where it rests on the diaphragm.

Arrhythmia: Abnormal heart rhythm.

Arteriole: A small artery that empties into a capillary bed.

Artery: A blood vessel that carries blood away from the heart to the tissues or the lungs.

Artifact: Unwanted jitter or interference on the EKG tracing.

Asystole: No heart beat. Characterized by a flat line on the EKG.

Atrial kick: The phase of diastole in which the atria contract to propel their blood into the ventricles.

Atrial rate: The heart rate of the P waves (or P wave alternatives such as flutter waves).

Atrial tissue: Tissue in the atria.

Atrioventricular block: Also called AV block. A block of impulses moving from atrium to ventricle.

Atrioventricular valves: Also called AV valves. Heart valves located between atrium and ventricle.

Atrium: The upper, thin-walled receiving chambers of the heart.

Augment: Increase.

Automaticity: The ability of cardiac cells to initiate an impulse without outside stimulation.

Automaticity circuit: The "switch" inside cardiac cells that tells the cell to create an impulse.

Autonomic nervous system: The nervous system controlling involuntary biological functions.

AV block (atrioventricular block): A disturbance in conduction in which some or all impulses from the sinus node are either delayed on their trip to the ventricles or do not reach the ventricle at all.

AV dissociation (atrioventricular dissociation): A condition in which the atria and ventricles depolarize and contract independently of each other.

AV junction (atrioventricular junction): Conductive tissue between the AV node and the atria.

AV node (atrioventricular node): The group of specialized cells in the conduction system that slows impulse transmission to allow atrial contraction to occur.

Axillary: Referring to the armpit.

Axis: The mean direction of the heart's current flow.

Axis deviation: An abnormal axis.

Base: The top of the heart; the area from which the great vessels emerge.

Baseline: The line from which the EKG waves and complexes take off. Also called the isoelectric line.

Bayes's theorem: The theorem that states that the predictive value of a test is based not only on the accuracy of the test itself but on the patient's probability of disease, as determined by a risk assessment done prior to the testing.

Beta-blockers: Class of cardiac medications that slows the heart rate, decreases blood pressure, and reduces cardiac workload.

Beta-receptors: Receptors that affect heart rate, contractility, and airway size.

Bigeminy: Every other beat is an abnormal beat.

Bipolar: Having a positive and a negative pole.

Blood pressure: The pressure exerted on the arterial walls by the circulating blood.

Bradyarrhythmia: An arrhythmia with a heart rate less than 60.

Bradycardia: Slow heart rate, usually less than 60.

Bronchodilators: Medications that dilate constricted airway passages in individuals with asthma, bronchitis, or emphysema.

Bundle branch block: A block in conduction through one of the bundle branches.

Bundle branches: Conduction pathways extending from the bundle of His in the lower right atrium to the Purkinje fibers in the ventricles. There is a right and a left bundle branch.

Bundle of His: A confluence of conduction fibers between the AV node and the bundle branches.

Capillary bed: The smallest blood vessels in the body; where nutrient and gas exchange takes place.

Capture: The depolarization of the atrium and/or ventricle as a result of a pacemaker's firing. Determined by the presence of a P wave and/or QRS after the pacemaker spike.

Cardiac arrest: An emergency in which the heart stops beating.

Cardiac cycle: The mechanical events that occur to pump blood. Consists of diastole and systole.

Cardiac output: The amount of blood expelled by the heart each minute. Measured as heart rate times stroke volume.

Cardiogenic shock: Shock induced by heart failure.

Cardioversion: Synchronized electrical shock to the heart to convert an abnormal rhythm to sinus.

Carotid sinus massage: A method of slowing the heart rate by rubbing on the carotid artery in the neck.

Chart speed: EKG machine feature that regulates the speed of the paper printout.

Chordae tendineae: Tendinous cords that attach to the AV valves and prevent them from everting.

Chronotropic incompetence: Inability of the heart rate to increase with stress.

Chronotropic reserve: The ability of the heart rate to increase with exercise.

Circumflex coronary artery: The branch off the left main coronary artery that feeds oxygenated blood to the lateral wall of the left ventricle.

Clockwise: Moving in the direction of clock hands.

Complete compensatory pause: Normally follows PVCs. Measures two R-R cycles from the beat preceding the PVC to the beat following the PVC.

Conduction system: A network of specialized cells whose job is to create and conduct the electrical impulses that control the cardiac cycle.

Conduction system cells: Cardiac cells whose job is to create and conduct electrical signals to trigger a heartbeat.

Conductivity: The ability of a cardiac cell to pass an impulse along to neighboring cells.

Congestive heart failure (CHF):   Fluid buildup in the lungs as a result of the heart's inability to pump adequately.

Contractile cells: Cardiac cells whose job is to contract and cause blood to flow.

Contractility: The ability of a cardiac cell to contract and do work.

Contraindications: Reasons to avoid doing a test or procedure.

Coronary arteries: The arteries that feed oxygenated blood to the myocardium.

Counterclockwise: In a direction opposite the way the clock hands move.

Couplet: A pair of beats.

Coved ST segment: Rounded ST segment elevation typical of an STEMI. Also called convex ST segment elevation.

CPK: Creatine phosphokinase. Chemical released by the heart during an MI.

Critical rate: The rate at which a bundle branch block appears or disappears.

Decreased cardiac output: Inadequate blood flow to meet the body's needs.

Decreased diastolic filling time: Caused by tachycardias. The decreased time between beats for the heart to fill up with blood.

Defibrillation: Asynchronous electrical shock to the heart, used to treat ventricular fibrillation and pulseless V-tach.

Delta wave: A slurred upstroke to the QRS complex, seen in Wolff-Parkinson-White Syndrome.

Depolarization: The wave of electrical current that changes the resting negatively charged cardiac cell to a positively charged one.

Diaphoresis: Sweating, usually a cold sweat. Also referred to as "cold and clammy."

Diastasis: The phase in diastole in which the atrial and ventricular pressures are equalizing.

Diastole: The phase of the cardiac cycle in which the ventricles fill with blood.

Digitalis toxicity: Overabundance of the medication digitalis in the bloodstream.

Dissecting aneurysm: The ballooning out of an artery into the wall of the artery itself.

Dissociation: The lack of relationship between two pacemaker sites in the heart.

Diuretics: Medications given to increase the urine output.

Early repolarization: Phases 1 and 2 of the action potential.

Einthoven's law: The height of the QRS complexes in Lead I + Lead III = Lead II.

Einthoven's triangle: The triangle formed by joining Leads I, II, and III at the ends.

Electrocardiogram: A printout of the electrical signals generated by the heart.

Electrodes: Adhesive patches attached to the skin to receive the electrical signals from the heart.

Electrolytes: Blood chemicals.

Embolus: Blood clot that has broken off and is traveling through a blood vessel.

Endocardium: The innermost layer of the heart.

Epicardium: Outer layer of the heart.

Erectile dysfunction medications: Medications that treat erectile problems in males.

Ergometer: An arm bicycle used in stress testing.

Escape: A safety mechanism in which a lower pacemaker fires at its slower inherent rate when the faster, predominant pacemaker fails.

Escaping: A lower pacemaker taking over when a higher pacemaker fails.

Event monitor: A small device that can be used to determine if sporadic arrhythmias or ischemia is present.

Evolution: The gradual EKG changes that occur in an acute ST elevation MI.

Excitability: The ability of a cardiac cell to depolarize when stimulated.

Extensive anterior STEMI: A large ST elevation MI affecting the anterior and lateral walls of the left ventricle.

Fascicle: A branch.

Fibrillation: The wiggling or twitching of the atrium or ventricle.

Firing: The pacemaker's generation of an electrical impulse.

Fixed-rate pacemaker: An old-fashioned pacemaker that paced at a programmed rate with no regard to the patient's own intrinsic rhythm or beats.

Focus: Location.

Frontal leads: Limb Leads I, II, III, aVR, aVL, and aVF. Leads located on the front of the body.

Fusion beats: A combination of a sinus beat and a PVC. Shape is intermediate between that of the sinus beat and the PVC.

Gain: EKG machine feature that regulates the height of the waves and complexes.

Glaucoma medications: Medications that decrease the eyeball pressure.

Glottis: The flap over the top of the windpipe.

Heart rate: The number of times the heart beats in one minute.

Heart rhythm: A pattern of successive heart beats.

Hemiblock: A block of one of the left bundle branch's fascicles.

Hexiaxial diagram: A diagram of the six frontal leads intersecting at the center; serves as the basis for the axis circle.

Holter monitor: A device used for 24-hour cardiac monitoring to check for arrhythmias or ST segment abnormalities.

Hyperacute changes: Those seen in the earliest stages of a disease or condition.

Hypercalcemia: Elevated blood calcium level.

Hyperkalemia: Elevated blood potassium level.

Hypertension: High blood pressure.

Hypertrophic cardiomyopathy: Heart disease caused by an overgrowth of the interventricular septum.

Hypertrophy: Overgrowth of myocardial tissue.

Hyperventilating: Breathing very rapidly.

Hypocalcemia: Low blood calcium level.

Hypokalemia: Low blood potassium level.

Hypotension: Low blood pressure.

Hypoxia: Low blood oxygen level.

Indeterminate axis: An axis that is between −90 and +−180 degrees.

Indications: Reasons to perform a test or procedure.

Indicative changes: EKG changes that indicate the presence of an MI.

Infarction: Death of tissue. A myocardial infarction (MI) is a heart attack.

Inferior STEMI: ST elevation MI involving the inferior wall of the left ventricle.

Inferior vena cava (IVC): Large vein that returns deoxygenated blood to the right atrium from the lower chest, abdomen, and legs.

Inferior wall: The bottom wall of the left ventricle.

Inherent: Preset.

Injury: Damage to tissue.

Inotropic incompetence: The inability of the blood pressure to increase with exercise.

Inotropic reserve: The ability of the blood pressure to increase with exercise.

Interatrial septum: The muscular band of tissue separating the right and left atria.

Interatrial tracts: The pathways that carry the electrical impulse from the sinus node through the atrial tissue.

Intercostal spaces: Spaces between the ribs.

Internodal tracts: Pathways that carry electrical impulses from the sinus node to the AV node.

Intervals: Measurements of time between EKG waves and complexes.

Interventricular septum: The muscular band of tissue separating right and left ventricles.

Intrinsic: The patient's own. Intrinsic beats are the patient's own beats.

Ions: Electrically charged particles.

Irritability: Also called usurpation. The cardiac cell fires in prematurely, taking control away from the predominant pacemaker.

Ischemia: Oxygen deprivation in the tissues.

Isoelectric line: The flat line between the EKG waves and complexes. Also called the baseline.

Isovolumetric: Maintaining the same volume.

Isovolumetric contraction: The first phase of systole. The ventricles are contracting but no blood flow is occurring because all the valves are still closed.

Isovolumetric relaxation: The final phase of systole. The semilunar valves slam shut and blood flow from the ventricles stops.

J point: The point where the QRS complex and ST segment join together.

Kent bundle: The accessory pathway in WPW.

Lateral wall: The left side wall of the left ventricle.

Lateral wall STEMI: ST elevation MI affecting the lateral wall of the left ventricle.

Lead: An electrocardiographic picture of the heart.

Leakage current: Small amount of electrical current that escapes from an implanted device such as a pacemaker.

Left anterior descending coronary artery: A branch of the left main coronary artery. It feeds oxygenated blood to the anterior wall of the left ventricle.

Left anterior hemiblock: Block of the left anterior fascicle of the left bundle branch.

Left axis deviation: An axis between 0 and −90 degrees.

Left bundle branch: Conduction fibers that carry the cardiac impulses down the left side of the septum to the left ventricle.

Left common bundle branch: The part of the left bundle branch before it divides into its fascicles.

Left main coronary artery: The coronary artery that branches off into the circumflex and left anterior descending coronary arteries.

Left posterior hemiblock: Block of the left posterior fascicle of the left bundle branch.

Macroshock: A large electrical shock caused by improper or faulty grounding of electrical equipment.

Mean rate: The average heart rate.

Mediastinum: The cavity between the lungs, in which the heart is located.

MET: Metabolic equivalent, a measurement of oxygen consumption.

Microshock: A small electrical shock made possible by a conduit, such as a pacemaker, directly in the heart.

Mitral: Valve that separates the left atrium and left ventricle.

Multifocal: Coming from more than one location.

Myocardial infarction: Heart attack.

Myocardium: The muscular layer of the heart.

Necroses: Dies.

Neuropathy: Condition that causes a decrease in sensation, especially pain, in susceptible individuals.

Nitrates: Medications used to dilate coronary arteries and improve coronary blood flow.

Nonconducted PAC: A premature P wave not followed by a QRS complex.

Norepinephrine: The chemical released by the adrenal gland when stimulated by the sympathetic nervous system.

Normal axis: Axis between 0 and +90 degrees.

NSTEMI: Non-ST elevation MI.

Occlusion: Blockage.

Oxygen: An element inhaled from the atmosphere that is necessary for body function.

Pacemaker: The intrinsic or artificial focus that propagates or initiates the cardiac impulse.

Pacing interval: The programmed interval between paced beats.

Papillary muscle: The muscle to which the chordae tendineae are attached at the bottom.

Parasympathetic nervous system: The division of the autonomic nervous system that slows the heart rate, lowers blood pressure, stimulates digestion, and constricts pupils—all signs of the "rest-and-digest" response.

Paroxysmal: Occurring suddenly and stopping just as suddenly.

PCI: Percutaneous coronary intervention. A balloon procedure to open a blocked coronary artery.

Perfusion: The supplying of blood and nutrients to tissues.

Pericardial fluid: Small amount of fluid found between the layers of the pericardial sac.

Pericarditis: An inflammation of the pericardium.

Pericardium: The sac that encloses the heart.

Plateau phase: The phase of the action potential in which the waveform levels off (flattens out). Phase 2 is the plateau phase.

Platelet aggregation: Clumping of platelets to form clots to stop bleeding.

Platelets: Cells responsible for blood clotting.

Polarized: Possessing an electrical charge.

Polymorphic: Possessing multiple shapes.

Postangioplasty evaluation: Evaluation of the patient's condition following a procedure to open up blocked coronary arteries.

Posterior MI: MI affecting the posterior wall of the left ventricle.

Posterior wall: The back wall of the left ventricle.

P-P interval: The distance (interval) between consecutive P waves.

Precordial: Pertaining to the chest.

Pre-excitation: Depolarizing tissue earlier than normal.

PR interval: Measurement of time it takes the cardiac impulse to travel from atrium to ventricle.

Protodiastole: The phase of systole in which the blood flow out of the ventricles slows because of equalizing pressures between the ventricles and the aorta and pulmonary artery.

PR segment: Flat line between the P wave and the QRS complex.

Pulmonary artery: Large artery that takes deoxygenated blood from the right ventricle to the lungs. It is the ONLY artery that carries deoxygenated blood.

Pulmonary embolus: Blood clot in the lung.

Pulmonary veins: Four veins that return oxygenated blood from the lungs to the left atrium. They are the ONLY veins that carry oxygenated blood.

Pulmonic valve: Valve located between the right ventricle and the pulmonary artery.

Purkinje fibers: Fibers at the terminal ends of the bundle branches. Responsible for transmitting the impulses into the ventricular myocardium.

P wave: The EKG wave reflecting atrial depolarization.

QRS complex: The EKG complex representing ventricular depolarization.

QRS interval: The spiked wave on the EKG. Represents ventricular depolarization.

QS wave: A QRS complex with only a downward wave—no upward wave(s).

QT interval: Measures ventricular depolarization and repolarization time.

Quadrigeminy: Every fourth beat is abnormal.

Q wave: A downward wave preceding an R wave in the QRS complex. If a Q wave is present, it is ALWAYS the first wave of the QRS complex.

R′: Pronounced "R prime." Is the second R wave in a QRS complex.

Rapid-filling phase: The first phase of diastole in which the ventricles rapidly fill with blood from the atria.

Rapid repolarization: Phase 3 of the action potential.

Rate-related bundle branch blocks: Bundle branch blocks that appear only at certain heart rates.

Reciprocal changes: EKG changes (ST depression) seen in the area electrically opposite the infarcted area.

Refractory: Resistant to.

Regularity: Spacing of the P waves or QRS complexes.

Relative refractory period: The period in which only a strong stimulus will cause depolarization of the cardiac cell.

Reperfusion arrhythmia: A rhythm, usually AIVR, that was thought to result from the return of blood and oxygen supply to tissues that have been deprived for a period of time.

Repolarization: The wave of electrical current that returns the cardiac cell to its resting, electrically negative state.

Resuscitation: Restoring respirations and/or pulse by way of artificial respiration and cardiac compressions.

Retrograde: In a backward direction.

Rhythm strip: A printout of one or two leads at a time, done on special rolls of paper.

Right axis deviation: An axis between +90 to +−180 degrees.

Right bundle branch: Conduction fibers that carry the cardiac impulses down the right side of the septum to the right ventricle.

Right coronary artery (RCA): The coronary artery that feeds oxygenated blood to the right ventricle and the inferior wall of the left ventricle.

R-on-T phenomenon: The PVC that falls on the T wave of the preceding beat. Predisposes to rapid arrhythmias.

R-R interval: The distance (interval) between consecutive QRS complexes. Usually measured at the peaks of the R waves.

R wave: An upward wave in the QRS complex.

Scooping ST segment: Rounded ST segment seen with digitalis effect.

Segment: The flat line between EKG waves and complexes.

Semilunar valves: Half-moon-shaped. Refers to the aortic and pulmonic valves.

Sensing: The ability of an artificial pacemaker to "see" the intrinsic rhythm in order to determine whether the pacemaker needs to fire.

Sensitivity: The ability of a test to pick out the people who are truly diseased.

Septum: The fibrous tissue that separates the heart into right and left sides.

Sinus node: The normal pacemaker of the heart.

Sleep apnea: Temporary, often repetitive cessation of breathing during sleep.

Sodium-potassium pump: The active transport system that returns the cardiac cell to its resting electrically negative state following depolarization.

Somatic: Referring to the body.

Specificity: The ability of a test to exclude those who are not diseased.

Stenosis: Narrowed opening.

Stenotic: Pertaining to stenosis.

Stent: A wire mesh inserted into a coronary artery to hold it open following PCI.

Sternum: Breastbone.

Stress test: A test done to determine the presence of coronary artery disease. Can be done using exercise or medications to stress the heart.

ST segment: The flat line between the QRS complex and the T wave.

Subendocardial: Referring to the myocardial layer just beneath the endocardium.

Submaximal test: A stress test that is concluded when 70% of the target heart rate is reached.

Superior vena cava (SVC): Large vein that returns deoxygenated blood to the right atrium from the head, neck, upper chest, and arms.

Supernormal period: The period in which the cardiac cell is "hyper" and will respond to a very weak stimulus.

Supine: Back-lying.

Supraventricular: Originating in a pacemaker above the ventricle.

S wave: A negative wave that follows an R wave in the QRS complex.

Sympathetic nervous system: The division of the autonomic nervous system that regulates the "fight-or-flight" response, causing the heart rate and blood pressure to rise, digestion to slow, and pupils to dilate.

Syncope: Fainting spell.

Systole: The phase of the cardiac cycle in which the ventricle contracts and expels its blood.

Tachycardia: Fast heart rate, greater than 100.

T_a wave: The rarely-seen wave that follows the P wave and represents repolarization of the atria.

Telemetry: A method of monitoring a patient's rhythm remotely. The patient carries a small transmitter that relays his or her cardiac rhythm to a receiver located at another location.

Thallium-201: A radioactive medication used to enable special x-ray images to be done following a stress test.

Therapeutic hypothermia: Cooling the post-cardiac arrest patient's body temperature down to 90 to 93 degrees Fahrenheit in order to decrease brain damage and improve brain function.

Thoracic: Referring to the chest cavity.

Three-channel recorder: An EKG recorder that prints out 3 leads simultaneously.

Thrombolysis: The act of dissolving a blood clot.

Thrombolytics: Medications used to dissolve the clot causing an MI or a stroke.

Thyrotoxicosis: Also called thyroid storm. A condition in which the thyroid gland so overproduces thyroid hormones that the body's metabolic rate is accelerated to a catastrophic degree. The body temperature, heart rate, and blood pressure rise to extreme levels.

Trachea: Windpipe.

Transcutaneous: By way of the skin.

Transmembrane potential: The electrical charge at the cell membrane.

Transmural: Through the full thickness of the wall at that location.

Transvenous: By way of a vein.

Triaxial diagram: The diagram of Leads I, II, and III joined at the center or of aVR, aVL, and aVF joined at the center.

Tricuspid: Having three cusps.

Tricuspid valve: Valve that separates the right atrium and right ventricle.

Tricyclic antidepressants (TCA): A kind of medication used for the treatment of depression.

Trigeminy: Every third beat is abnormal.

Troponin: A chemical released by the heart during an MI.

Troubleshooting: Determining and correcting the cause of artifact and recording errors.

T wave: The EKG wave that represents ventricular repolarization.

Unifocal: Coming from one location.

Unipolar: A lead consisting of only a positive pole.

Unstable angina: Chest pain that is increasing in intensity and/or frequency.

Usurpation: The act of a lower pacemaker stealing control from the predominant pacemaker; results in a faster heart rate than before. Also called irritability.

U wave: A small wave sometimes seen on the EKG. It follows the T wave and reflects late repolarization.

Vagus nerve: The nerve that is part of the parasympathetic nervous system. Causes the heart rate to slow when stimulated.

Valve: A structure in the heart that prevents backflow of blood.

Vasoconstrict: To make a blood vessel's walls squeeze down, narrowing the vessel's lumen.

Vasodilate: To make the blood vessel's walls relax, thus widening the blood vessel.

Vasodilators: Medications that relax blood vessel walls.

Vector: An arrow depicting the direction of electrical current flow in the heart.

Vein: A blood vessel that transports deoxygenated blood away from the tissues.

Vena cava: The largest vein in the body; returns deoxygenated blood to the heart.

Ventricles: The lower pumping chambers of the heart.

Ventricular dilatation: Stretching of the myocardial fibers from overfilling or inadequate pumping of blood from the ventricles. Results in a weakened pumping efficiency.

Ventricular ejection: The phase of systole in which the semilunar valves pop open and blood pours out of the ventricles.

Venule: A small vein that drains blood away from a capillary bed.

Wolff-Parkinson-White Syndrome: Also called WPW. A syndrome in which there is an accessory conductive pathway between the atrium and the ventricle. Recognized on the EKG by a delta wave and a short PR interval.

Glossary of Abbreviations

AED: Automated external defibrillator.

AICD: Automated internal cardioverter-defibrillator.

AIVR: Accelerated idioventricular rhythm.

ANS: Autonomic nervous system.

Ao: Aorta.

AV: Atrioventricular.

AVB: Atrioventricular block.

BBB: Bundle branch block.

BP: Blood pressure.

CAD: Coronary artery disease.

CHF: Congestive heart failure.

DDD: A type of dual-chamber pacemaker.

EKG: Electrocardiogram.

IVC: Inferior vena cava.

IVR: Idioventricular rhythm.

LAD: Left axis deviation or left anterior descending coronary artery.

LAHB: Left anterior hemiblock.

LBBB: Left bundle branch block.

LPHB: Left posterior hemiblock.

LVH: Left ventricular hypertrophy.

MAT: Multifocal atrial tachycardia.

MI: Myocardial infarction.

MmHg: Millimeters of mercury, a unit of measurement of blood pressure.

MUGA: Multiple gated acquisition studies.

NSTEMI: Non-ST elevation MI.

PA: Pulmonary artery.

PACs: Premature atrial complexes.

PAT: Paroxysmal atrial tachycardia.

PCI: Percutaneous coronary intervention—a balloon procedure to open occluded coronary arteries.

PE: Pulmonary embolus.

PJCs: Premature junctional complexes.

PNS: Parasympathetic nervous system.

P-P interval: The interval between consecutive P waves.

PR interval: Interval of time between the P wave and QRS complex.

PVC: Premature ventricular complex.

P wave: EKG wave representing atrial depolarization.

QRS: The EKG wave representing ventricular depolarization.

QT interval: The interval of time between the beginning of the QRS complex and the end of the T wave.

RAD: Right axis deviation.

RBBB: Right bundle branch block.

RCA: Right coronary artery.

ROSC: Return of spontaneous circulation.

R-R interval: The interval between consecutive QRS complexes.

RVH: Right ventricular hypertrophy.

RVR: Rapid ventricular response.

SA: Sinoatrial.

SNS: Sympathetic nervous system.

S + S: Signs and symptoms.

STEMI: ST elevation MI.

ST segment: Segment joining the QRS complex and T waves.

SVC: Superior vena cava.

SVT: Supraventricular tachycardia.

TEE: Transesophageal echocardiogram.

TH: Therapeutic hypothermia.

T wave: The EKG wave representing ventricular repolarization.

U wave: The EKG wave sometimes seen following the T wave.

VVI: A type of single-chamber pacemaker.

WAP: Wandering atrial pacemaker.

WPW: Wolff-Parkinson-White syndrome.

Index